2013
YEAR BOOK OF
EMERGENCY MEDICINE®

The 2013 Year Book Series

Year Book of Critical Care Medicine®: Drs Dries, Zanotti-Cavazzoni, Latenser, Martinez, Rincon, and Zwank

Year Book of Emergency Medicine®: Drs Hamilton, Bruno, Handly, Minczak, Quintana, and Ramoska

Year Book of Endocrinology®: Drs Schott, Apovian, Clarke, Eugster, Meikle, Oetgen, Ovalle, Schteingart, and Toth

Year Book of Hand and Upper Limb Surgery®: Drs Yao, Adams, Isaacs, Lee, and Rizzo

Year Book of Medicine®: Drs Barker, Garrick, Gersh, Khardori, LeRoith, Panush, Talley, and Thigpen

Year Book of Neonatal and Perinatal Medicine®: Drs Fanaroff, Benitz, Donn, Neu, Papile, and Van Marter

Year Book of Neurology and Neurosurgery®: Drs Klimo, Minagar, Gandhi, House, Kevill, Liu, Mazia, Panagariya, Ragel, Riesenburger, Robottom, Schwendimann, Shafazand, Uhm, and Yang

Year Book of Obstetrics, Gynecology, and Women's Health®: Drs Dungan and Shulman

Year Book of Oncology®: Drs Arceci, Bauer, Chiorean, Gordon, Lawton, Murphy, Thigpen, and Tsao

Year Book of Ophthalmology®: Drs Rapuano, Cohen, Flanders, Hammersmith, Milman, Myers, Nagra, Nelson, Penne, Pyfer, Sergott, Shields, Talekar, and Vander

Year Book of Orthopedics®: Drs Morrey, Huddleston, Rose, Swiontkowski, and Trigg

Year Book of Otolaryngology-Head and Neck Surgery®: Drs Sindwani, Balough, Franco, Gapany, and Mitchell

Year Book of Pathology and Laboratory Medicine®: Drs Raab and Bissell

Year Book of Pediatrics®: Dr Stockman

Year Book of Plastic and Aesthetic Surgery™: Drs Miller, Boehmler, Gosman, Gutowski, Ruberg, Salisbury, and Smith

Year Book of Psychiatry and Applied Mental Health®: Drs Talbott, Ballenger, Buckley, Frances, Krupnick, and Mack

Year Book of Pulmonary Disease®: Drs Barker, Jones, Maurer, Spradley, Tanoue, and Willsie

Year Book of Sports Medicine®: Drs Shephard, Cantu, Feldman, Galea, Jankowski, Janssen, Lebrun, and Nieman

Year Book of Surgery®: Drs Copeland, Behrns, Daly, Eberlein, Fahey, Huber, Klodell, Mozingo, and Pruett

Year Book of Urology®: Drs Andriole and Coplen

Year Book of Vascular Surgery®: Drs Moneta, Gillespie, Starnes, and Watkins

2013

The Year Book of EMERGENCY MEDICINE®

Editor-in-Chief
Richard J. Hamilton, MD
Professor and Chair, Department of Emergency Medicine, Drexel University College of Medicine, Philadelphia, Pennsylvania

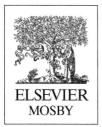

ELSEVIER
MOSBY

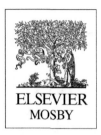

ELSEVIER
MOSBY

Vice President, Continuity: Kimberly Murphy
Editor: Yonah Korngold
Production Supervisor, Electronic Year Books: Donna M. Skelton
Electronic Article Manager: Mike Sheets
Illustrations and Permissions Coordinator: Dawn Vohsen

Composition by TNQ Books and Journals Pvt Ltd, India

Editorial Office:
Elsevier
1600 John F. Kennedy Blvd.
Suite 1800
Philadelphia, PA 19103-2899

International Standard Serial Number: 0271-7964
International Standard Book Number: 978-1-4557-7274-2

Printed and bound by CPI Group (UK) Ltd, Croydon, CR0 4YY

Transferred to digital print 2012

Associate Editors

Eric C. Bruno, MD, FAAEM

Attending Emergency Physician, Middle Tennessee Emergency Physicians, Middle Tennessee Medical Center and Baptist Hospital, Murfreesboro and Nashville, Tennessee

Neal B. Handly, MD, MSc, MS

Associate Professor of Emergency Medicine, Department of Emergency Medicine, Drexel University College of Medicine, Philadelphia, Pennsylvania

Bohdan M. Minczak, MS, MD, PhD

Assistant Professor of Emergency Medicine, EMS Division Head, EMS Fellowship Director, Department of Emergency Medicine, Drexel University College of Medicine, Philadelphia, Pennsylvania

Eileen C. Quintana, MD, MPH

Attending Physician Emergency Medicine, Department of Emergency Medicine, Children's Emergency Department, Lehigh Valley Health Network, Allentown, Pennsylvania

Edward A. Ramoska, MD, MPH

Clinical Associate Professor of Emergency Medicine, Program Director, Emergency Medicine, Department of Emergency Medicine, Drexel University College of Medicine, Philadelphia, Pennsylvania

Table of Contents

JOURNALS REPRESENTED xi

1. Trauma 1
   General Issues 1
   Evaluation 17
   Head and Neck Injury 25
   Thoraco-Abdominal Injury 34
2. Resuscitation 37
   Cardiac Arrest 37
   Shock 41
3. Cardiovascular 45
4. Respiratory Distress 67
   Congestive Heart Failure 67
   Pulmonary Embolism 68
5. Infections and Immunologic Disorders 75
6. Neurology 85
7. Psychiatry 95
8. Gastrointestinal 97
9. Endocrinology 103
10. Pediatric Emergency Medicine 107
    General Issues 107
    Infectious Disease 124
    Neuroscience 132
    Procedures 140
    Pulmonary 159
    Surgery 166
11. Emergency Medical Service Systems 187
    General Issues 187
    Safety and Resource Utilization 194
    Cardiovascular 225
    Treatment and Imaging 229

12. Toxicology 231

13. Emergency Center Activities 267

ARTICLE INDEX 303

AUTHOR INDEX 313

Journals Represented

Journals represented in this YEAR BOOK are listed below.

Academic Emergency Medicine
Air Medical Journal
American Journal of Cardiology
American Journal of Emergency Medicine
American Journal of Medicine
American Journal of Obstetrics and Gynecology
American Journal of Preventive Medicine
American Journal of Public Health
American Journal of Respiratory and Critical Care Medicine
American Journal of Surgery
American Surgeon
Anesthesiology
Annals of Emergency Medicine
Annals of Plastic Surgery
Archives of Disease in Childhood
Archives of Internal Medicine
Archives of Physical Medicine and Rehabilitation
Child's Nervous System
Clinical Pediatrics
Clinical Toxicology
Drugs
Emergency Medicine Journal
Emergency Radiology
European Heart Journal
Gastrointestinal Endoscopy
Injury
Intensive Care Medicine
International Journal of Cardiology
Journal of Cardiothoracic and Vascular Anesthesia
Journal of Emergency Medicine
Journal of General Internal Medicine
Journal of Hypertension
Journal of Nervous and Mental Disease
Journal of Neurological Sciences
Journal of Pediatric Surgery
Journal of Pediatrics
Journal of Pharmacology and Experimental Therapeutics
Journal of the American College of Cardiology
Journal of the American College of Surgeons
Journal of the American Geriatrics Society
Journal of the American Medical Association
Journal of Trauma
Journal of Trauma and Acute Care Surgery
Journal of Urology
Lancet
Medicine and Science in Sports and Exercise
Nephrology Dialysis Transplantation

Neuroradiology
Obstetrics & Gynecology
Orthopedics
Pediatric Emergency Care
Pediatric Infectious Disease Journal
Pediatric Radiology
Pediatrics
Pharmacotherapy
Prehospital Emergency Care
Radiology
Skeletal Radiology
Surgery
Thrombosis Research
Transplantation Proceedings

STANDARD ABBREVIATIONS

The following terms are abbreviated in this edition: acquired immunodeficiency syndrome (AIDS), central nervous system (CNS), cardiopulmonary resuscitation (CPR), cerebrospinal fluid (CSF), computed tomography (CT), deoxyribonucleic acid (DNA), electrocardiography (ECG), emergency department (ED), emergency medical services (EMS), human immunodeficiency virus (HIV), health maintenance organization (HMO), intensive care unit (ICU), intramuscular (IM), intravenous (IV), magnetic resonance (MR) imaging (MRI), ribonucleic acid (RNA), ultrasound (US), and ultraviolet (UV).

NOTE

The YEAR BOOK OF EMERGENCY MEDICINE® is a literature survey service providing abstracts of articles published in the professional literature. Every effort is made to assure the accuracy of the information presented in these pages. Neither the editors nor the publisher of the YEAR BOOK OF EMERGENCY MEDICINE® can be responsible for errors in the original materials. The editors' comments are their own opinions. Mention of specific products within this publication does not constitute endorsement.

To facilitate the use of the YEAR BOOK OF EMERGENCY MEDICINE® as a reference tool, all illustrations and tables included in this publication are now identified as they appear in the original article. This change is meant to help the reader recognize that any illustration or table appearing in the YEAR BOOK OF EMERGENCY MEDICINE® may be only one of many in the original article. For this reason, figure and table numbers will often appear to be out of sequence within the YEAR BOOK OF EMERGENCY MEDICINE®.

1 Trauma

General Issues

Do we glow? Evaluation of trauma team work habits and radiation exposure
Hassan M, Patil A, Channel I et al (West Virginia Univ, Morgantown)
J Trauma Acute Care Surg 73:605-611, 2012

Background.—Health care workers' potential exposure to ionizing radiation has increased. Annual radiation exposure limit for the general public per US Nuclear Regulatory Commission is 100 mrem (1 mSv). The whole-body annual occupational radiation exposure limit is 5,000 mrem (50 mSv). Studies have been done to evaluate patient radiation exposure. To date, there has been no study to evaluate the radiation exposure of trauma team members or evaluate their behaviors and attitudes.

Methods.—Forty primary providers (residents, physician assistants) rotating on the trauma service at an American College of Surgeons Level 1 trauma center participated. Dosimeters were worn by participants, and the radiation doses were measured monthly. A survey detailing the frequency of involvement in radiographic studies, use of protective equipment, and knowledge of education programs was completed monthly.

Results.—The range of radiation measured was 1 mrem to 56 mrem, with an average effective dose of 10 mrem per month. Thirty-two (80%) of 40 reported daily exposure to x-rays and 28 (70%) of 40 to computed tomographic scans. Thirty-four (85%) of 40 reported that they never or seldom wore lead apron in trauma bay as opposed to 1 (3%) of 40 who failed to wear it during fluoroscopy. Twenty (50%) reported that an apron was not available, while 20 (50%) reported that it was too hot or did not fit. Thirty-nine (97%) of 40 reported that they received training in radiation safety.

Conclusion.—Despite inconsistent use of protective equipment by resident staff, the actual radiation exposure remains low. Hospitals should be sure lead aprons and collars are available. Additional education concerning the availability of programs during pregnancy is needed.

Level of Evidence.—Epidemiologic study, level III.

▶ Radiation exposure is a hot topic nowadays. This study from West Virginia University reveals that radiation exposure in trauma team members (as opposed to trauma patients) is low in spite of the fact people do not seem to use protective clothing, such as lead aprons and lead collars. Higher levels of exposure were seen in postgraduate year 2 (PGY2) surgical residents, as opposed to other years. The authors postulated that this was because their PGY2 residents were responsible for care of patients both in the trauma bay and in the intensive care unit (ICU).

The radiation exposure levels reported in this analysis do not put the participants at risk for the deterministic effects of radiation exposure; however, one cannot ignore the stochastic effects of radiation exposure. Stochastic effects are those that occur by chance and consist primarily of cancer and genetic effects. Stochastic effects often show up years after exposure. Increasing dose to an individual increases the probability that cancer or genetic effect will occur. However, at no time is there a threshold dose below which it is certain that an adverse effect cannot occur. Therefore, it is prudent for all of us as practitioners to use available protective clothing in the trauma bay and the ICU. Moreover, as administrators, we should seek out the barriers to the use of protective gear, such as it not being available, being the wrong size, or too hot or too cumbersome to wear, and work to eliminate those impediments to use.

E. A. Ramoska, MD, MPHE

Are All Level I Trauma Centers Created Equal? A Comparison of American College of Surgeons and State-Verified Centers
Smith J, Plurad D, Inaba K, et al (Los Angeles County + USC Med Ctr, CA)
Am Surg 77:1334-1336, 2011

Scant literature investigates potential outcome differences between Level I trauma centers. We compared overall survival and survival after acute respiratory distress syndrome (ARDS) in patients admitted to American College of Surgeons (ACS)-verified *versus* state-verified Level I trauma centers. Using the National Trauma Data Bank Version 7.0, incident codes associated with admission to an ACS-verified facility were extracted and compared with the group admitted to state-verified centers. Overall, there were 382,801 (73.7%) patients admitted to ACS and 136,601 (26.3%) admitted to state centers. There was no adjusted survival advantage after admission to either type (4.9% for ACS *vs* 4.8% for state centers; 1.014 [95% CI, 0.987 to 1.042], $P = 0.311$). However, in the 3,088 cases of ARDS, mortality for admission to the ACS centers was 20.3 per cent (451 of 2,220) *versus* 27.1 per cent (235 of 868) for state centers. Adjusting for injury severity and facility size, admission to an ACS center was associated with a significantly greater survival after ARDS (0.75 [0.654 to 0.860]; $P < 0.001$). Level I verification does not necessarily imply similar outcomes in all subgroups. Federal oversight may become necessary to ensure uniformity of care, maximizing outcomes across all United States trauma systems. Further study is needed.

▶ These authors from Los Angeles County + USC Medical Center raise more questions than they answer with this study. They postulate that not all Level 1 trauma centers are created equal and that although individual state trauma requirements may be similar to American College of Surgeons (ACS) guidelines, the variability that exists in Level I trauma center designation may be associated with differences in patient outcomes. Their analysis of national data show, however, that there is no difference in overall mortality between ACS-verified and state-verified Level I trauma centers.

The authors then pick 1 specific outcome, namely mortality after posttraumatic acute respiratory distress syndrome (ARDS), and find a survival benefit for ACS-verified centers versus state-verified centers. It is unclear why they selected this particular result, other than to say that there are evidence-based treatment guidelines for ARDS that show a survival benefit. Furthermore, their data demonstrate that ACS-verified Level I trauma centers at community hospitals surpass university-based hospitals on this outcome. No such difference is noted in state-verified systems.

What this means is anybody's guess. The overall outcome of mortality shows no disparity between ACS-verified and state-verified centers; however, 1 subgroup shows a survival benefit to ACS-verified centers. This could be just a statistical fluke or it could represent a real finding. Moreover, why should community hospital-based trauma centers outperform university-based ones? I agree with the authors that further study is needed.

E. A. Ramoska, MD, MPHE

Epidemiology of out-of hospital pediatric cardiac arrest due to trauma

De Maio VJ, for the CanAm Pediatric Study Group (WakeMed Health & Hosps, Raleigh, NC; et al)
Prehosp Emerg Care 16:230-236, 2012

Objective.—To determine the epidemiology and survival of pediatric out-of-hospital cardiac arrest (OHCA) secondary to trauma.

Methods.—The CanAm Pediatric Cardiac Arrest Study Group is a collaboration of researchers in the United States and Canada sharing a common goal to improve survival outcomes for pediatric cardiac arrest. This was a prospective, multicenter, observational study. Twelve months of consecutive data were collected from emergency medical services (EMS), fire, and inpatient records from 2000 to 2003 for all OHCAs secondary to trauma in patients aged ≤18 years in 36 urban and suburban communities supporting advanced life support (ALS) programs. Eligible patients were apneic and pulseless and received chest compressions in the field. The primary outcome was survival to discharge. Secondary measures included return of spontaneous circulation (ROSC), survival to hospital admission, and 24-hour survival.

Results.—The study included 123 patients. The median patient age was 7.3 years (interquartile range [IQR] 6.0—17.0). The patient population was 78.1% male and 59.0% African American, 20.5% Hispanic, and 15.7% white. Most cardiac arrests occurred in residential (47.1%) or street/highway (37.2%) locations. Initial recorded rhythms were asystole

(59.3%), pulseless electrical activity (29.1%), and ventricular fibrillation/tachycardia (3.5%). The majority of cardiac arrests were unwitnessed (49.5%), and less than 20% of patients received chest compressions by bystanders. The median (IQR) call-to-arrival interval was 4.9 (3.1–6.5) minutes and the on-scene interval was 12.3 (8.4–18.3) minutes. Blunt and penetrating traumas were the most common mechanisms (34.2% and 25.2%, respectively) and were associated with poor survival to discharge (2.4% and 6.5%, respectively). For all OHCA patients, 19.5% experienced ROSC in the field, 9.8% survived the first 24 hours, and 5.7% survived to discharge. Survivors had triple the rate of bystander cardiopulmonary resuscitation (CPR) than nonsurvivors (42.9% vs. 15.2%). Unlike patients sustaining blunt trauma or strangulation/hanging, most post–cardiac arrest patients who survived the first 24 hours after penetrating trauma or drowning were discharged alive. Drowning (17.1% of cardiac arrests) had the highest survival-to-discharge rate (19.1%).

Conclusions.—The overall survival rate for OHCA in children after trauma was low, but some trauma mechanisms are associated with better survival rates than others. Most OHCA in children is preventable, and education and prevention strategies should focus on those overrepresented populations and high-risk mechanisms to improve mortality.

▶ Pediatric cardiac arrest is an anxiety-provoking event for practically all health care providers from emergency medical services (EMS) to emergency department personnel. This North American epidemiologic study estimated the annual incidence for pediatric traumatic cardiac arrest at 2.3 per 100 000 children. Most of the children were adolescent, male, and African American. Over 36% of arrests occurred in patients from 16 years old to less than 19 years old. The vast majority (over 87%) were in full cardiopulmonary arrest upon EMS arrival and most of those (over 88%) had an initial rhythm of asystole or pulseless electrical activity. Although virtually all of the children received cardiopulmonary resuscitation (CPR), bystanders initiated CPR only about two-fifths of the time.

The median prehospital time from call received to hospital arrival was 27.9 minutes. In almost all cases, EMS initially managed the airway with a bag-valve mask. Endotracheal intubation was attempted in almost 90% of the patients, and it was successful nearly 85% of the time it was attempted.

Only 7 children survived to hospital discharge. Four of the survivors were 10 years of age or younger, 4 were male, and 4 were located at a residence at the time of the traumatic mechanism. Four children had an EMS-witnessed cardiac arrest and 3 were in respiratory arrest on arrival with either sinus or other rhythm on initial recording by EMS. Only 2 of the 7 survivors were successfully intubated. On the whole, these results confirm that survival of out-of-hospital cardiac arrest secondary to trauma in children is low; however, some trauma mechanisms (namely, drowning) may be associated with increased survival.

E. A. Ramoska, MD, MPHE

In a Mature Trauma System, There Is No Difference in Outcome (Survival) Between Level I and Level II Trauma Centers

Rogers FB, Osler T, Lee JC, et al (Lancaster General Health, PA; Univ of Vermont, Burlington)

J Trauma 70:1354-1357, 2011

Background.—The state of Pennsylvania (PA) has one of the oldest, most well-established trauma systems in the country. The requirements for verification for Level I versus Level II trauma centers within PA differ minimally (only in the requirement for patient volume, residency, and research). We hypothesized that there would be no difference in outcome at Level I versus Level II trauma centers.

Methods.—Odds of mortality for 16 Level I and 11 Level II hospitals in PA over a 5-year period (2004 2008) was computed using a random effects logistic regression model. Overall adjusted mortality rates at Level I versus Level II hospitals were compared using the nonparametric Wilcoxon's rank sum test. The crude mortality rates for 140,691 patients over the 5-year period were similar (5.07% Level II vs. 5.48% Level I), but statistically significant (odds ratio mortality at Level I = 1.084, $p = 0.002$ Fisher's exact test).

Results.—Although Level I centers had on average crude mortality rates that were higher than those of Level II centers, median adjusted mortality rates were not different for the two types of centers (Wilcoxon's rank sum test). Performance of Level I versus Level II shows considerable variability among centers (basic random effects model, age, blunt/penetrating, and Injury Severity Score [ISS]). However, Level II centers seem no different from Level I.

Conclusion.— As trauma systems mature, the distinction between Level I and Level II trauma centers blurs. The hierarchal descriptors "Level I" or "Level II" in a mature trauma system is pejorative and implies in those hospitals labeled "Level II" as inferior, and as such should be replaced with nonhierarchal descriptors.

▶ All things being equal (including the patient's age, severity of injury, blunt vs penetrating), do levels I and II trauma differ in terms of survival outcomes? The authors have chosen to compare survival among patients admitted to level I and II centers through review of the Pennsylvania Trauma Outcomes Study (PTOS), a large standardized repository of records of the management of trauma victims.

By selecting to model survival with logistic regression, it is possible to compare similar types of patients (at least among those variables recorded in the PTOS) to determine if there is a difference. This will remove the problem of trying to directly compare survival for, say, a patient with a gunshot wound to the head with a patient from an all-terrain vehicle rollover at low speed. No significant difference in survival was found.

So what does that really mean to the practice of trauma care? The authors' work suggests that although there is no real survival difference for these 2 types of trauma centers regarding clinical performance, there is a stigma applied to the level II center, namely, that the level II center is somehow not as good as a level I center or not worthy of the same level of respect. It would make sense to consider whether there should be alterations in transport rules (which patients should not bypass level II centers). Except for patient outcomes, is there something else the authors are trying to determine? Perhaps bruised egos need mending?

N. B. Handly, MD, MSc, MS

Effect of comorbid illness on the long-term outcome of adults suffering major traumatic injury: a population-based cohort study
Niven DJ, Kirkpatrick AW, Ball CG, et al (Univ of Calgary and Alberta Health Services, Canada)
Am J Surg 204:151-156, 2012

Background.—Few studies have assessed the impact of pre-existing medical comorbidities on long-term survival after major trauma. This study investigated the influence of comorbidities as measured by the Charlson Comorbidity Index (CCI) on the 1-year mortality after major traumatic injury.

Methods.—Adult patients who survived their initial trauma admission in Calgary, Alberta, Canada, between April 1, 2002, and March 31, 2006, defined the study population. Clinical and outcome information was obtained from regional electronic databases.

Results.—The study population consisted of 3,080 patients. The median age was 43.3 years (interquartile range, 26.9—59.3 y), and the median Injury Severity Score was 20 (interquartile range, 16—25). A total of 478 patients (15.5%) had at least one pre-existing comorbidity. The 1-year mortality rate was 2.7% (83 of 3,080). After adjusting for the confounding effects of age, the CCI was independently associated with 1-year mortality with an odds ratio of 1.24 (95% confidence interval, 1.02—1.51; $P = .03$) per point on the CCI. A model that included the CCI and age accurately predicted 1-year mortality (C-statistic, .83; 95% confidence interval, .78—.87; $P < .0001$).

Conclusions.—Comorbid illnesses have an important influence on long-term outcomes after major trauma. Whether this represents an inherent risk for adverse outcome or an opportunity for enhanced medical co-management remains to be defined.

▶ The authors of this study sought to determine if a patient's state of comorbid condition would have any effect on the measure of survival 1 year after a traumatic injury. They note in this report some problems remaining from prior studies that make it difficult up to this point to answer this question well. Some of the problems noted before included not making a focus of those patients who died in the hospital at the time of their index injury or those whose injury severity was low.

They found that it was possible to model 1-year survival using measures of comorbidity beyond what would be possible using demographics and data describing the injuries of the patients.

It should not be so surprising to have found that comorbidity played a significant role in explaining long-term mortality after trauma, but consider a flip to the logic. Would it be possible to show that trauma contributed to an excess 1-year mortality beyond that which would have been found by examining a patient's comorbid state alone?

N. B. Handly, MD, MSc, MS

Are general surgeons behind the curve when it comes to disaster preparedness training? A survey of general surgery and emergency medicine trainees in the United States by the Eastern Association for the Surgery for Trauma Committee on Disaster Preparedness
Dennis AJ, Brandt M-M, Steinberg J, et al (JSH Cook County Trauma Unit, Chicago, IL; St Joseph Mercy Hosp, Ann Arbor, MI; et al)
J Trauma Acute Care Surg 73:612-617, 2012

Purpose.—We think that general surgeons are underprepared to respond to mass casualty disasters. Preparedness education is required in emergency medicine (EM) residencies, yet such requirements are not mandated for general surgery (GS) training programs. We hypothesize that EM residents receive more training, consider themselves better prepared, and are more comfortable responding to disaster events than are GS residents.

Methods.—From February to May 2009, the Eastern Association for the Surgery of Trauma—Committee on Disaster Preparedness conducted a Web-based survey cataloging training and preparedness levels in both GS and EM residents. Approximately 3000 surveys were sent. Chi-squared, logistic regression, and basic statistical analyses were performed with SAS.

Results.—Eight hundred and forty-eight responses were obtained, GS residents represented 60.6% of respondents with 39% EM residents, and four residents did not respond with their specialty (0.4%). We found significant disparities in formal training, perceived preparedness, and comfort levels between resident groups. Experience in real-life disaster response had a significant positive effect on comfort level in all injury categories in both groups (odds ratio, 1.3–4.3, $p < 0.005$).

Conclusion.—This survey confirms that EM residents have more disaster-related training than GS residents. The data suggest that for both groups, comfort and confidence in treating victims were not associated with training but seemed related to previous real-life disaster experience. Given wide variations in the relationship between training and comfort levels and the constraints imposed by the 80-hour workweek, it is critical that we identify and implement the most effective means of training for all residents.

▶ Success in preparation for mass casualty depends on knowing what to do differently when the time comes. Both emergency physicians (EPs) and surgeons need to know that not every resource is available to them and that not every patient can have the full unlimited attention of a physician during the initial course of the event. Additionally, the command and communication structure also changes because teams in the field need feedback from hospitals to plan further site evacuations.

Both types of physicians need to make judgments about which patients are stable enough to leave the acute areas of attention. In the emergency department (ED), the EPs must be able to move low-acuity patients to other care areas (perhaps to hallway and waiting room chairs), provide for space to triage patients that may come by personal transport and by ambulance systems, and coordinate with other hospital services to move patients out of the ED as fast as possible. The surgeon needs to know how to move patients out of low and intensive care unit levels of care to make room for the increased number of patients who might be arriving either directly from the ED or from the operating room.

Patients come from mass casualty events acutely injured and whose care is disrupted by the event.

Surgeons do have a skill set for moving patients through the operating rooms quickly—the skills of damage control surgery. However, in a mass casualty event, surgeons need to shift to a practice to maintain flow that is different because there may not be enough resources to take care of every patient as would occur in other circumstances. It is not easy to shift from normal to mass casualty attitude, so the more experience any practitioner has in this shift, the better will be the performance.

N. B. Handly, MD, MSc, MS

Chronic consequences of acute injuries: Worse survival after discharge
Shafi S, Renfro LA, Barnes S, et al (Baylor Health Care System, Dallas, TX)
J Trauma Acute Care Surg 73:699-703, 2012

Background.—The Trauma Quality Improvement Program uses inhospital mortality to measure quality of care, which assumes patients who survive injury are not likely to suffer higher mortality after discharge. We hypothesized that survival rates in trauma patients who survive to discharge remain stable afterward.

Methods.—Patients treated at an urban Level I trauma center (2006−2008) were linked with the Social Security Administration Death Master File. Survival rates were measured at 30, 90, and 180 days and 1 and 2 years from injury among two groups of trauma patients who survived to discharge: major trauma (Abbreviated Injury Scale score ≥ 3 injuries, n = 2,238) and minor trauma (Abbreviated Injury Scale score ≤ 2 injuries, n = 1,171). Control groups matched to each trauma group by age and sex were simulated from the US general population using annual survival probabilities from census data. Kaplan-Meier and log-rank analyses conditional upon survival to each time point were used to determine changes in risk of mortality after discharge. Cox proportional hazards models with left truncation at the time of discharge were used to determine independent predictors of mortality after discharge.

Results.—The survival rate in trauma patients with major injuries was 92% at 30 days posttrauma and declined to 84% by 3 years ($p > 0.05$ compared with general population). Minor trauma patients experienced a survival rate similar to the general population. Age and injury severity were the only independent predictors of long-term mortality given survival to discharge. Log-rank tests conditional on survival to each time point showed that mortality risk in patients with major injuries remained significantly higher than the general population for up to 6 months after injury.

Conclusion.—The survival rate of trauma patients with major injuries remains significantly lower than survival for minor trauma patients and the general population for several months postdischarge. Surveillance for early identification and treatment of complications may be needed for trauma patients with major injuries.

Level of Evidence.—Prognostic study, level III.

▶ The results of this study stimulate a review of the concepts of prevention—primary, secondary, and tertiary.

Primary prevention in the setting of traumatic injuries would include those interventions that prevent the injury, especially by minimizing risk. Some examples might be educating a population about the relationship between alcohol use and injury (especially driving) or providing warnings written on ladders to not stand on the top step.

Secondary prevention in the setting of traumatic injuries would include those interventions that minimize the extent of injury after it has occurred. Probably the most important intervention has been the development of trauma centers and trauma protocols (eg, advanced trauma life support).

Tertiary prevention in the setting of traumatic injuries would include those interventions that minimize further decay of or inability to regain a quality of life after the hospital-based trauma care has ended.

The authors, by describing the increase in mortality rate after release from the hospital, bring a focus on tertiary prevention. All-cause mortality was chosen and not that of traumatic death. However, it is still worth considering that caring for patients after discharge will be a worthy investment in our patients. It might even be that the interventions we provide to our patients after the injury may even be helpful as a primary preventive tool.

N. B. Handly, MD, MSc, MS

A decade of experience with a selective policy for direct to operating room trauma resuscitations

Martin M, Izenberg S, Cole F, et al (Legacy Emanuel Med Ctr, Portland, OR)
Am J Surg 204:187-192, 2012

Background.—The standard paradigm for acutely injured patients involves evaluation in an emergency department (ED). Our center has employed a policy for bypassing the ED and proceeding directly to the operating room (OR) based on prehospital criteria.

Methods.—This is a retrospective analysis of all trauma patients admitted "direct to OR" (DOR) over 10 years. Demographics, injury patterns, prehospital, and in-hospital data were analyzed.

Results.—There were 1,407 patients admitted as DOR resuscitations. Almost half (47%) had a penetrating mechanism, and 54% had chest or abdominal injury. The mean Injury Severity Score was 19, with altered mentation (Glasgow coma score [GCS] < 9) in 20% and hypotension in 16%. Most patients (68%) required surgical intervention, and 33% required emergency surgery operations (abdominal [70%] followed by thoracic [22%] and vascular [4%]). The median time to intervention was 13 minutes. Mortality was significantly lower than predicted (5% vs 10%). Independent predictors of emergent surgical intervention were a penetrating truncal injury (odds ratio = 9.9), GCS < 9 (odds ratio = 1.9), and hypotension (odds ratio = 1.8).

Discussion.—Our DOR protocol identified a severely injured cohort at high risk for requiring surgery with improved observed survival. High-yield triage criteria for DOR admission include a penetrating truncal injury, hypotension, and a severely altered mental status.

▶ First and foremost, the goal of trauma care is patient care. Should we measure cost of care, survival, and disability, and is it possible to know how well the care is delivered?

The authors present a description of the direct to operating room (DOR) system used at their hospital for 10 years. They offer a look at the types of patients treated, a comparison of mortality data to that predicted by TRISS (Trauma and Injury Severity Score), and analyze the practice variables to identify which patients ultimately end up in the DOR system.

The article stimulates several thoughts. The authors present the fact that DOR patient mortality is much better than would be predicted by TRISS, but they do not compare this value with that seen in the non-DOR patients. Since the DOR system is administered by humans, errors will happen and patients will be inappropriately assigned to care. It is likely that there were patients in the DOR group who actually did not meet criteria discovered in the statistical model and that there were patients in the non-DOR group who would have met the criteria for DOR. Thus, it might be possible to match patients from the non-DOR and DOR groups who were similar using variables that predict assignment to DOR to compare mortality, and this would be a telling result.

Is there any reason to suspect that a TRISS-based mortality prediction needs to be modified? Perhaps trauma center systems have improved and it is time to reset the bar for expected mortality.

If the DOR system were in place in every level I hospital, how would this affect the training of emergency physicians and surgeons who would later practice in non-level I environments? Picture a seriously injured patient brought in by medics to a non-DOR system (a patient who would normally be admitted as DOR when the resources were available)—how would the system at this hospital respond?

N. B. Handly, MD, MSc, MS

Screening for traumatic stress among survivors of urban trauma
Reese C, Pederson T, Avila S, et al (John H. Stroger, Jr Hosp of Cook County, Chicago, IL; Univ of Chicago, IL)
J Trauma Acute Care Surg 73:462-468, 2012

Objective.—This study piloted the use of the Primary Care PTSD (PC-PTSD) screening tool in an outpatient setting to determine its utility for broader use and to gather data on traumatic stress symptoms among direct (patients) and indirect (families) survivors of traumatic injuries.

Methods.—Using the PC-PTSD plus one question exploring openness to seeking help, participants were screened for PTSD in the outpatient clinic of an urban Level 1 trauma center. The survey was distributed during a 23-week period from April to September 2011. The screen was self-administered, a sample of convenience, and participation was voluntary and anonymous.

Results.—With a response rate of 66%, 307 surveys were completed. Forty-two percent of participants had a positive screen. Patients greater than 30 and 90 days from injury had 1.5 and 1.7 times more positive screens than those less than 30 days. Patients with gunshot wounds were 13 times as likely as those with falls and twice as likely as those in a motor vehicle crash to have a positive screen. Sixty percent of patients with a positive screen noted it would be helpful to talk to someone.

Conclusion.—The PC-PTSD was an easy to administer screening tool. Patients reported PTSD symptoms at higher rates than previous studies. Patients with gunshot wounds and those injured greater than 30 days from the time of the screen were more likely to report PTSD symptoms. Although males represented 82% of positive screens, there was no statistical difference in PTSD symptoms between male and female participants because of the small number of females represented. Families also reported significant levels of PTSD. Both patients and families may benefit from additional screening and intervention in the early posttrauma period.

▶ The authors report the results of a study that applies an abbreviated posttraumatic stress disorder (PTSD) assessment tool to their patients returning to outpatient clinics for continued care. Four questions are used in the primary care PTSD survey tool (the basis of this study) to elicit the aspects of definition of PTSD as noted in the Diagnostic and Statistical Manual version IV (DSM IV): reexperiencing, avoidance, hyperarousal, and numbing. Prior work with this primary care PTSD survey suggested that the presence of 3 positive answers was highly sensitive and specific for the PTSD diagnosis.

There are limitations to this study that would prevent using the results alone to establish interventions for the patients. An important one is that there is no way to know if the stress suffered by the subjects of this study was related to the recent injuries for which the victim was attending the outpatient clinic. It may be that many of the subjects manifesting these stress attitudes are in fact responding to traumatic events that have occurred prior.

There are a great number of consequences for PTSD sufferers, their families, and society in general, so finding ways to manage this additional problem that seems to follow the "injury" is very important. Because it is not possible to establish the diagnosis of PTSD at the time of injury according to the definitions in DSM IV, it would be valuable to identify those trauma victims who are most likely to become sufferers of PTSD-like illness. The authors suggest that the type of injury might play a role in predicting later effects. At the same time, it is also noted that a notable fraction of subjects of the study had survey results that suggested that they were not suffering from PTSD. Knowing which patients would be more resistant to PTSD and those that are most sensitive, trauma staff could better identify who needs the most help.

N. B. Handly, MD, MSc, MS

Neighborhood Social Inequalities in Road Traffic Injuries: The Influence of Traffic Volume and Road Design

Morency P, Gauvin L, Plante C, et al (Direction de Santé Publique de Montréal, Québec, Canada; Centre de Recherche du Centre Hospitalier de l'Université de Montréal, Québec, Canada; et al)
Am J Public Health 102:1112-1119, 2012

Objectives.—We examined the extent to which differential traffic volume and road geometry can explain social inequalities in pedestrian, cyclist, and motor vehicle occupant injuries across wealthy and poor urban areas.

Methods.—We performed a multilevel observational study of all road users injured over 5 years (n = 19 568) at intersections (n = 17 498) in a large urban area (Island of Montreal, Canada). We considered intersection-level (traffic estimates, major roads, number of legs) and area-level (population density, commuting travel modes, household income) characteristics in multilevel Poisson regressions that nested intersections in 506 census tracts.

Results.—There were significantly more injured pedestrians, cyclists, and motor vehicle occupants at intersections in the poorest than in the richest areas. Controlling for traffic volume, intersection geometry, and pedestrian and cyclist volumes greatly attenuated the event rate ratios between intersections in the poorest and richest areas for injured pedestrians (-70%), cyclists (-44%), and motor vehicle occupants (-44%).

Conclusions.—Roadway environment can explain a substantial portion of the excess rate of road traffic injuries in the poorest urban areas.

▶ Imagine that you could build a model that predicts risk of roadway traffic injuries. Why would you want to do this? Well, this could help plan for prehospital ambulance distribution, design better roadways, and even become aware of the journey that you will take each day on the way to work.

The authors chose to model the risks at traffic intersections for pedestrians, cyclists, and motor vehicle occupants. Several logical and plausible factors such as roadway size, number of vehicles, and pedestrians crossing at the intersection have been considered previously. In this study, the sources of data allowed the authors to examine a large community without selecting for intersections of low or high acuity or selecting intersections in a small set of neighborhoods. In the Montreal, Quebec, metropolitan area nearly every intersection has been characterized in terms of whether the roads are major or minor and if the junction is 4-way or a "T" shape, injury, and death data associated with that intersection are well documented, and surveys of traffic flows have been completed. Other surveys available contain local information such as the number of people likely to be along or on the roadway at an intersection based on the amount of car ownership and the number using public transport.

In this study, an additional factor, local socioeconomic status (SES) at the level of the census tract that contains each intersection was used to test if this economic variable is a significant and independent factor predicting the risk of injury. The authors used a Poisson model (valuable for infrequent events independent events) and initially found that a variable that described local SES (arranged in quintiles for this region) was a significant factor for predicting injury at intersections.

But, be warned about making an interpretation that low SES independently predicts the likelihood of an injury at an intersection just because it is a statistically significant factor in the model. The authors show how to test if this conclusion is correct by developing multivariate models with SES and intersection type or size of roadways. When these factors already known to affect risk of injury are included in the model, the size of the effect of socioeconomic status is reduced notably. Although the effect of SES did not become nonsignificant, it became apparent that the connection from SES to injury risk was because high-risk intersections were more prevalent in low SES neighborhoods. So when SES was considered as a single factor, it was significant, not because "poverty makes injuries occur" but because locales with low SES are more likely to have the intersections with more foot and cycle traffic, increased car density, larger roads at the intersections, and the shape of intersections that are known to be more dangerous (4 way).

When you talk to your prehospital crews next time, see if you can recognize these patterns of intersection injuries.

N. B. Handly, MD, MSc, MS

Association Between Helicopter vs Ground Emergency Medical Services and Survival for Adults With Major Trauma

Galvagno SM Jr, Haut ER, Zafar SN, et al (Univ of Maryland Med Ctr, Baltimore; Johns Hopkins Univ School of Medicine, Baltimore, MD; Aga Khan Univ, Karachi, Pakistan; et al)
JAMA 307:1602-1610, 2012

Context.—Helicopter emergency medical services and their possible effect on outcomes for traumatically injured patients remain a subject of debate. Because helicopter services are a limited and expensive resource, a methodologically rigorous investigation of its effectiveness compared with ground emergency medical services is warranted.

Objective.—To assess the association between the use of helicopter vs ground services and survival among adults with serious traumatic injuries.

Design, Setting, and Participants.—Retrospective cohort study involving 223 475 patients older than 15 years, having an injury severity score higher than 15, and sustaining blunt or penetrating trauma that required transport to US level I or II trauma centers and whose data were recorded in the 2007-2009 versions of the American College of Surgeons National Trauma Data Bank.

Interventions.—Transport by helicopter or ground emergency services to level I or level II trauma centers.

Main Outcome Measures.—Survival to hospital discharge and discharge disposition.

Results.—A total of 61 909 patients were transported by helicopter and 161 566 patients were transported by ground. Overall, 7813 patients (12.6%) transported by helicopter died compared with 17 775 patients (11%) transported by ground services. Before propensity score matching, patients transported by helicopter to level I and level II trauma centers had higher Injury Severity Scores. In the propensity score—matched multivariable regression model, for patients transported to level I trauma centers, helicopter transport was associated with an improved odds of survival compared with ground transport (odds ratio [OR], 1.16; 95% CI, 1.14-1.17; $P < .001$; absolute risk reduction [ARR], 1.5%). For patients transported to level II trauma centers, helicopter transport was associated with an improved odds of survival (OR, 1.15; 95% CI, 1.13-1.17; $P < .001$; ARR, 1.4%). A greater proportion (18.2%) of those transported to level I trauma centers by helicopter were discharged to rehabilitation compared with 12.7% transported by ground services ($P < .001$), and 9.3% transported by helicopter were discharged to intermediate facilities compared with 6.5% by ground services ($P < .001$). Fewer patients transported by helicopter left level II trauma centers against medical advice (0.5% vs 1.0%, $P < .001$).

Conclusion.—Among patients with major trauma admitted to level I or level II trauma centers, transport by helicopter compared with ground services was associated with improved survival to hospital discharge after controlling for multiple known confounders.

▶ This manuscript illustrates the kind of work necessary to demonstrate the effect of helicopter versus ground transport on survival for major trauma victims.

The data used for the study are extracted from the National Trauma Data Bank (NTDB) that, although carefully collected, still are from a retrospective source. It is not possible to know that adequate confounding variables have been collected. Another problem with the use of these data is that there is no single policy in use by all the contributing trauma centers for helicopters being used for transport. Thus part of this study must attend to the problems of what is collected and why transport has occurred in this way.

The latter problem is managed via a propensity method—essentially, an attempt is made to determine if there are specific factors that are associated with a patient traveling by helicopter or ground. Picture yourself on the ground as the paramedic encountering an injured patient. A very severely injured patient, who in your estimation would need the most rapid transport to a trauma center, might benefit from helicopter transport. Meanwhile, that same day you have a patient who seems less severely injured and could survive the longer journey by ground. A comparison made between these 2 patients might be inappropriate just because of their differences in apparent clinical state. A better comparison would be between individuals who both would have been transported by helicopter or by ground, all things otherwise being equal but that some factor made it so that both could not—perhaps, that there was only room on the helicopter for one of 2 equally severely injured patients as judged by the paramedic team.

An absolute reduction in risk of death before discharge from the hospital has been found by the authors. Unfortunately, there were not adequate data to include distance or time from scene to hospital in their model. If it were available, it might be possible to have also derived some indicators for which patients would be better served by helicopter transport. Even with this information, it will remain tricky to come up with indications for flight because the information about the patients at the scene will always be limited other than those easily observed or collected (eg, vital signs, type of injury whether penetrating vs blunt, mechanism of injury).

N. B. Handly, MD, MSc, MS

A web-based model to support patient-to-hospital allocation in mass casualty incidents

Amram O, Schuurman N, Hedley N, et al (Simon Fraser Univ, British Columbia, Canada; et al)
J Trauma Acute Care Surg 72:1323-1328, 2012

Background.—In a mass casualty situation, evacuation of severely injured patients to the appropriate health care facility is of critical importance. The prehospital stage of a mass casualty incident (MCI) is typically chaotic, characterized by dynamic changes and severe time constraints. As a result, those involved in the prehospital evacuation process must be able to make crucial decisions in real time. This article presents a model intended to assist in the management of MCIs. The Mass Casualty Patient Allocation Model has been designed to facilitate effective evacuation by providing key information about nearby hospitals, including driving times and real-time bed capacity. These data will enable paramedics to make informed decisions in support of timely and appropriate patient allocation during MCIs. The model also enables simulation exercises for disaster preparedness and first response training.

Methods.—Road network and hospital location data were used to precalculate road travel times from all locations in Metro Vancouver to all Level I to III trauma hospitals. Hospital capacity data were obtained from hospitals and were updated by tracking patient evacuation from the MCI locations. In combination, these data were used to construct a sophisticated web-based simulation model for use by emergency response personnel.

Results.—The model provides information critical to the decision-making process within a matter of seconds. This includes driving times to the nearest hospitals, the trauma service level of each hospital, the location of hospitals in relation to the incident, and up-to-date hospital capacity.

Conclusion.—The dynamic and evolving nature of MCIs requires that decisions regarding prehospital management be made under extreme time pressure. This model provides tools for these decisions to be made in an informed fashion with continuously updated hospital capacity information. In addition, it permits complex MCI simulation for response and preparedness training.

▶ Managing care for patients in mass casualty incidents (MCI) is complicated by the number of injuries, the variation in types of injuries, the task of determining which patients need what services, and how to transport the patients to the right care site.

When MCIs occur in cities, often patients who have the lowest degree of injury fall outside these incident management problems because they can transport themselves to the nearest hospital. This begins to consume capacity and may distort the hospital's and incident commander's perspective of the numbers and types of injuries that are a result of the catastrophe. Unfortunately, the tool used in this study does not manage the self-transported, lower acuity patients. It would remain the task of the hospital's triage processes to reserve space for the more severely injured until an adequate description of the event can be communicated to all hospitals.

The authors' system depends on effective communication between hospitals and the incident command team. This could occur with relatively low bandwidth systems since only a few numbers are communicated at each transport decision and during updates at fixed times. The authors discuss the possible problems with power loss; generators at hospitals and batteries in laptops or on-site generators should solve this. Meanwhile, it would probably be easier not to run the computer software on some remote server, and only the data should be copied to a remote site for backup, real-time oversight, and later analysis.

The success of the authors' model can be seen in that the 2 major hospitals reach capacity at about the same time. Thus, neither hospital is confronted with such a large number of severely injured patients that processes become overwhelmed and the quality of care is reduced. We do not have extensive practice with MCIs and we are fortunate not to have many real experiences either. This tool could be integrated with MCI drills and both real-time and later analysis could be helpful in improving MCI response.

N. B. Handly, MD, MSc, MS

Evaluation

Factors Associated With the Interfacility Transfer of the Pediatric Trauma Patient: Implications for Prehospital Triage

Ross DW, Rewers A, Homan MB, et al (American Med Response, Inc, Colorado Springs, CO; Univ of Colorado Denver; et al)
Pediatr Emerg Care 28:905-910, 2012

Objective.—The goal of this study was to identify prehospital factors associated with increased likelihood of interfacility transfer of pediatric trauma patients. Such factors might serve as a basis for improvements in future field pediatric trauma triage guidelines.

Methods.—This was a retrospective cohort study of children aged 12 years or younger with blunt, penetrating, or thermal injuries who were transported by ground emergency medical services from the scene to the emergency department of a Level I, II, or III trauma center within the Denver metropolitan area from January 1, 2000, to December 31, 2008. Characteristics predicting subsequent interfacility transfer to a pediatric trauma center (PTC) were assessed.

Results.—A total of 1673 patients were included in the analysis. Variables hypothesized to be most commonly associated with interfacility transfer were age, sex, mechanism of injury, body region of injury, and Glasgow Coma Scale score. The cohort included 1079 males and 593 females. Logistic regression analysis yielded the following as significant predictors of transfer: younger age (odds ratio [OR], 1.19; 95% confidence interval [CI], 1.15−1.25), lower Glasgow Coma Scale score (OR, 1.08; 95% CI, 1.01−1.16), the presence of burns (OR, 37.52; 95% CI, 7.3−191.7), non-accidental trauma (OR, 6.09; 95% CI, 2.44−15.25), falls (OR, 1.62; 95% CI, 1.06−2.48), other motor vehicle-related incidents (OR, 2.37; 95% CI, 1.08−5.19), abdominal injury (OR, 5.39; 95% CI, 2.31−12.55), head/neck injury (OR, 7.89; 95% CI, 4.21−14.77), limb injury (OR, 5.31; 95% CI, 2.78−10.16), and multiple injuries (OR, 13.01; 95% CI, 5.0−33.8).

Conclusions.—Factors highly associated with transfer of an injured child from a non-PTC to a PTC included younger age, burns, non-accidental trauma, head/neck injury, and multiple injuries in younger children. Further investigation is warranted to determine whether these factors may have applicability in future improvements in field pediatric trauma patient triage guidelines.

▶ It would be ideal if there were criteria that emergency medical services (EMS) could use that would lead to no undertriage of pediatric trauma patients (ie, transport of severely injured children to a non−pediatric trauma center [PTC] rather than a PTC) nor overtriage (transport of minimally injured children to a PTC). Current pediatric trauma triage guidelines tend to be complicated and, therefore, cumbersome for EMS providers to use real-time in the field. This retrospective study over a 9-year period from Denver, Colorado, is an analysis of children younger than 12 years who were transported by ground ambulance to a non-PTC and subsequently transferred to a PTC. Therefore, it examines when adult trauma center staff were uncomfortable providing care for pediatric patients. Injured children had the greatest odds of being transferred if they were younger or if they had burns or nonaccidental trauma, head/neck injuries, or multiple trauma. By identifying a short list of factors and traumatic conditions that result in transfer to a PTC, it might be possible to develop simple, practical field criteria for use by EMS.

E. A. Ramoska, MD, MPHE

Analysis of radiation exposure in trauma patients at a level I trauma center
Sharma OP, Oswanski MF, Sidhu R, et al (Toledo Hosp, OH; Fairview Hosp, Cleveland, OH; et al)
J Emerg Med 41:640-648, 2011

Background.—Trauma patients are exposed to potentially high levels of low-dose radiation during radiologic studies.

Objectives.—To assess the cumulative effective dose (CED) of radiation exposure (RE) in 177 successive patients admitted to a trauma service from January 1 through February 28, 2006.

Results.—Patients received a total of 1505 radiographs and 400 computed tomography (CT) scans in the study period. The CED was 14.56 mSv (0.97 mSv radiographs, 13.59 mSv CT scans) per patient total length of stay (LOS). CED averaged 8.66 mSv in the first hour and 11.76 mSv in the first 24 h after arrival. The most commonly performed CT scan was brain (n = 147), followed by abdomen and pelvis (n = 80), and cervical spine (n = 69). CT scans of the brain and cervical spine were the most commonly performed combined imaging tests (35%). Twelve percent of patients received no radiographs, and 15% received no CT scans. Six or more CT scans were done in 6% of patients. RE increased with longer LOS (> 6 days vs. 3—5 days vs. 1 day, $p < 0.05$). "Pan-scans" (a combination of CTs of the brain, cervical spine, chest, abdomen, and pelvis) were done in 13% (n = 23) of patients. There was a higher total RE from CT scans (25.09 mSv ± 19.48 mSv vs. 4.93 mSv ± 14.20 mSv) in patients with injury severity score (ISS) > 9 vs. ≤ 9 ($p < 0.0001$). First hour and first 24-h RE rates from radiographs were lower in patients younger than 15 years vs. 15—45 years and older-than-45-year age cohorts ($p < 0.05$).

Conclusions.—In this study, CED was 14.56 mSv per patient. CT scans accounted for 21% of radiologic studies and 93% of CED. There was a higher CED rate in patients with ISS > 9 and longer LOS.

▶ This study from The Toledo Hospital (Ohio) confirms what we all suspect: trauma patients are exposed to large cumulative doses of ionizing radiation. Most of that exposure (93% of it in this study) comes from computed tomography (CT) scans and most of it occurs early in the hospital course. Only 12% of the patients did not receive a CT scan at any time during their hospital stay, although the authors note that most of the patients who received no imaging studies were transferred from other facilities where they had radiologic studies performed. It is important to note that in this study 95% of the victims presented with blunt trauma.

The average annual radiation exposure per person from all environmental sources varies from 2.2 to 3.6 mSv. In this analysis, the average trauma patient received 14.56 mSv during their hospital stay. The US Food and Drug Administration estimates 1 cancer event per 2000 patients receiving a 10-mSv effective dose. With the numbers of diagnostic radiologic studies increasing each year, in both trauma and non-trauma patients, we must all be sensible in our use of this technology. Although the risk to any individual patient is small even for high-dose radiologic procedures, major concerns arise when CT scans are used indiscriminately without a proven clinical basis. Alternative modalities without radiation exposure should be considered whenever possible.

E. A. Ramoska, MD, MPHE

A Multisite Assessment of the American College of Surgeons Committee on Trauma Field Triage Decision Scheme for Identifying Seriously Injured Children and Adults
Newgard CD, the WESTRN investigators (Oregon Health & Science Univ, Portland; et al)
J Am Coll Surg 213:709-721, 2011

Background.—The American College of Surgeons Committee on Trauma (ACSCOT) has developed and updated field trauma triage protocols for decades, yet the ability to identify major trauma patients remains unclear. We estimate the diagnostic value of the Field Triage Decision Scheme for identifying major trauma patients (Injury Severity Score [ISS] ≥ 16) in a large and diverse multisite cohort.

Study Design.—This was a retrospective cohort study of injured children and adults transported by 94 emergency medical services (EMS) agencies to 122 hospitals in 7 regions of the Western US from 2006 through 2008. Patients who met any of the field trauma triage criteria (per EMS personnel) were considered triage positive. Hospital outcomes measures were probabilistically linked to EMS records through trauma registries, state discharge data, and emergency department data. The primary outcome defining a "major trauma patient" was ISS ≥ 16.

Results.—There were 122,345 injured patients evaluated and transported by EMS over the 3-year period, 34.5% of whom met at least 1 triage criterion and 5.8% had ISS ≥ 16. The overall sensitivity and specificity of the criteria for identifying major trauma patients were 85.8% (95% CI 85.0% to 86.6%) and 68.7% (95% CI 68.4% to 68.9%), respectively. Triage sensitivity and specificity, respectively, differed by age: 84.1% and 66.4% (0 to 17 years); 89.5% and 64.3% (18 to 54 years); and 79.9% and 75.4% (≥55 years). Evaluating the diagnostic value of triage by hospital destination (transport to Level I/II trauma centers) did not substantially improve these findings.

Conclusions.—The sensitivity of the Field Triage Decision Scheme for identifying major trauma patients is lower and specificity higher than previously described, particularly among elders.

▶ This study was done by the Western Emergency Services Translational Research Network, a consortium of 7 geographic regions and various emergency medical service agencies and hospitals. It reveals that the 2006 American College of Surgeons Committee on Trauma (ACSCOT) field triage decision scheme is not as sensitive as previous research has suggested, especially in older patients (defined here as over 55 years old). ACSCOT suggests that the target for under-triage in a trauma system should be less than 5% (ie, a sensitivity of greater than 95%), while the goal for overtriage should be less than 50% (ie, a specificity of greater than 50%). This analysis revealed that overall the objective for sensitivity is not being met for any age group, but most especially for older patients. It showed that as many as 1 in 5 older patients were not directed to a trauma center for care. If one looks at a breakdown of the results by region, one finds that only 1 of the 7 sites had a sensitivity greater than 95%, and 2 areas were greater than the target if you look at the 95% confidence intervals. The target for overtriage (specificity) is being exceeded in all age groups and for all regions. These results raise doubts about whether the goals for primary (field) trauma triage are realistic and if it is practical to fully concentrate seriously injured patients in high-resource hospitals (trauma centers) through EMS alone. There may be a role for secondary (hospital-based) triage and prompt transfer of identified patients.

E. A. Ramoska, MD, MPHE

Diagnostic Accuracy of Focused Assessment with Sonography for Trauma (FAST) Examinations Performed by Emergency Medical Technicians
Kim CH, Shin SD, Song KJ, et al (Inje Univ College of Medicine, Seoul, Republic of Korea; Seoul Natl Univ College of Medicine, Republic of Korea; Seoul Natl Univ Boramae Med Ctr, Republic of Korea)
Prehosp Emerg Care 16:400-406, 2012

Objective.—We aimed to assess the diagnostic accuracy of focused assessment with sonography for trauma (FAST) examinations when used by emergency medical technicians (EMTs) to detect the presence of free abdominal fluid.

Methods.—Six level 1 EMTs (similar to intermediate EMTs in the United States) who worked at a tertiary emergency department in Korea underwent an educational program consisting of two one-hour didactic lectures that included the principles of ultrasonography, the anatomy of the abdomen, and two hours of hands-on practice. After this educational session, the EMTs performed FAST examinations on a convenience sample of patients from July 1 to October 5, 2009. These patients also received an abdominal computed tomography (CT) scan regardless of their chief complaints. The

CT findings served as the definitive standard and were interpreted routinely and independently by emergency radiologists who were blinded to the study protocol. In addition, the EMTs were blinded to the CT findings. A positive CT finding was defined as the presence of free fluid, as interpreted by the radiologist. The sensitivity, specificity, predictive values, and their 95% confidence intervals (CIs) were calculated. Informed consent was obtained from all participating patients.

Results.—Among the 1,060 eligible patients with abdominal CT scans, 403 patients were asked to participate in the study, and 240 patients agreed. Of these 240 patients, 80 (33.3%) had results showing the presence of free fluid. Fourteen patients had a significant amount of peritoneal cavity fluid, 15 had a moderate amount of peritoneal cavity fluid, and 51 had a minimal amount of peritoneal cavity fluid. Compared with the CT findings, the diagnostic performance of the FAST examination had a sensitivity of 61.3% (95% CI, 50.3%—71.2%), specificity of 96.3% (95% CI, 92.1%—98.3%), positive predictive value of 89.1% (95% CI, 77.0%—95.4%), and negative predictive value of 83.2% (95% CI, 76.9%—88.2%). For a significant or moderate amount of peritoneal cavity fluid, the sensitivity was considerably higher (86.2%).

Conclusion.—EMTs in Korea showed a high diagnostic performance that was comparable to that of surgeons and physicians when detecting peritoneal cavity free fluid in a Korean emergency department setting. The validity of FAST examinations in prehospital care situations should be investigated further.

▶ When I read the title of this study, I had hoped that it might answer a useful question, "Can emergency medical technicians (EMTs) use focused assessment with sonography for trauma (FAST) scans for prehospital triage of trauma patients?" Alas, it does not. This is preliminary work looking to see whether hospital-based EMTs from Seoul, South Korea, can perform a FAST scan and find intraperitoneal fluid. This study has several limitations. Most importantly, these were not trauma patients (40% had neoplasms and the remainder various other conditions), and the FAST scans were not done in the field but in the emergency department. Moreover, there is some methodologic confusion, as the authors state that there are 14 EMTs participating in the study, while later they say that the FAST examinations were performed by 6 EMTs. So it is unclear how many EMTs actually took part in this study.

Using FAST scans in the prehospital setting on trauma patients is essentially using it as a screening test. You would prefer a high sensitivity so that you do not miss any patients with pathology—in this case, intraperitoneal fluid. In this regard, I disagree with the authors' conclusion that the EMTs showed a high diagnostic performance comparable to that of surgeons and physicians. The sensitivity for the 6 EMTs was only 61%. According to the discussion in the article, emergency medicine residents have a sensitivity of 75%; trauma surgeons, 81%; and prehospital physicians, 93%. I do not find these numbers comparable. In any case, this is an interesting area for research. If EMTs or paramedics could adequately screen trauma patients using sonography in the field, it might help reduce the undertriage of patients to trauma centers.

E. A. Ramoska, MD, MPHE

Repeat imaging in trauma transfers: A retrospective analysis of computed tomography scans repeated upon arrival to a Level I trauma center
Emick DM, Carey TS, Charles AG, et al (Univ of North Carolina at Chapel Hill; et al)
J Trauma Acute Care Surg 72:1255-1262, 2012

Background.—The repetition of computed tomography (CT) imaging in caring for injured patients transferred between institutions is common, but it is not well studied. Our objective is to quantify and describe the characteristics associated with repeating chest and abdominal CT images for patients transferred to trauma centers and to determine whether repeat imaging leads to delays in definitive care or disparate outcomes.

Methods.—This is a retrospective review of adult, blunt trauma patients transferred to two Level I trauma centers between January 2004 and May 2008 who underwent CT imaging of the chest, abdomen, or both.

Results.—60% of patients had at least one study repeated upon arrival to the trauma center. Variables associated with repeat imaging include Injury Severity Scores between 24 and 33 versus <15 (odds radio [OR], 1.6; 95% confidence interval [CI], 1.05−2.4), transfer to University of North Carolina (OR, 1.5; 95% CI, 1.01−2.2), transport by helicopter (OR, 1.6; 95% CI, 1.2−2.2), transfer in any year before 2008 (OR, 2.4; 95% CI, 1.6−3.6 for 2007; OR, 3.4; 95% CI, 2.2−5.3 for 2006; OR, 3.0; 95% CI, 1.8−5.0 for 2005; OR, 2.8; 95% CI, 1.7−4.7 for 2004), and triage alert level higher than the least severe level III (OR, 1.6; 95% CI, 1.01−2.7 for level II; OR, 2.2; 95% CI, 1.2−4.1 for level I). In adjusted models, there was no evidence that repeat imaging neither shortened the total time to definitive care nor altered patient outcomes.

Conclusions.—Injured patients often undergo imaging that gets repeated, adding cost and radiation exposure while not significantly altering outcomes. The current policy push to digitize medical records must include provisions for the interoperability and use of imaging software.

Level of Evidence.—III, therapeutic study.

▶ The landscape of medical practice is changing. In an effort to increase the quality of health care delivery and improve efficiency in the utilization of resources, many medical centers have developed into regionalized medical specialty centers. Currently, there are various level trauma centers, chest pain centers, stroke centers, orthopedic centers, eye hospitals, and burn centers operating in many communities. There are also hospitals for neuroscience, spinal injuries, and let's not forget the children's hospitals. However, general community hospitals are still prevalent, and they are attempting to compete in this potpourri of specialty hospitals.

When a patient is injured, emergency medical services (EMS) personnel are summoned. After initial evaluation and stabilization of the patient, EMS personnel have to decide which medical center to take the patient to. At times, the patient is taken to a center not capable of managing all of the patient's injuries. Subsequently, after the patient is evaluated and it is determined that there are injuries that require additional treatment, such as internal traumatic injuries or brain injury, the decision is made to transfer the patient to a specialty center. To complete the transfer, a physician specialist at the receiving hospital must be notified about the patient's condition. The physician must accept the patient, ensure that there is a bed and appropriate resources available, and make sure that a proper transport is arranged. In addition, the records from the initial treating hospital must be copied and sent with the patient and the receiving doctor and nurse must be aware of what was done at the initial facility and what the results of the tests were. After arriving at the receiving facility, another evaluation of the patient is done and treatment proceeds. The records are reviewed and if the situation warrants it more tests are ordered. Few if any of these tests are repeated, unless there is a grossly abnormal value, an unexpected trend, or a new development in the patient's condition such as a significant change in the patient's mental status.

However, when it comes to imaging studies (ie, x-rays, computed tomography scans, or magnetic resonance imaging studies), many of these are repeated at the receiving facility. This exposes the patient to more radiation, causes as increase in contrast dye load for the patient that could adversely affect the kidneys, and increases costs as well as losses in revenue for the hospital. Furthermore, repeating these studies can extend time to disposition of the patient as these studies are repeated.

This study attempted to quantify whether the reimaging of patients had any benefit to the overall care of the patient or if they could possibly be withheld. There appear to be several factors that influence the decision to repeat the studies. Many of the imaging studies are brought as digital data on a disk. When an attempt is made to read the disk at the second facility, often there are software incompatibilities that render the data unreadable. Sometimes, the only data sent are "wet readings" by the radiologist at the sending facility. Many times, the radiologist at the specialized facility may be uncomfortable relying on the reading of the other radiologist, or the treating team may not want to make decisions regarding treatment based on findings from an unfamiliar colleague.

Furthermore, some of the images may be deemed suboptimal, and physicians at the specialty center may request different, specialized views of the patient's injury.

To prevent some of these images from being repeated unnecessarily, because of technical or administrative issues, a possible solution would be to have sending and receiving centers provide reciprocal feedback to each other and develop communication protocols to modify and prevent unnecessary repetition of studies. In addition, if imaging equipment, protocols and data storage were to be standardized so that data from all pertinent facilities could be shared and meaningfully accessed, this would solve many of these problems, reduce unnecessary exposure of patients to radiation, and decrease the rising costs of doing these studies. (By the way, when a study is repeated, payment for these repeat studies is often denied as they are deemed "not allowed.")

This study should be brought to the attention of specialty center leaders so that these issues can be explored and ultimately mitigated.

B. M. Minczak, MS, MD, PhD

A prehospital shock index for trauma correlates with measures of hospital resource use and mortality
McNab A, Burns B, Bhullar I, et al (Univ of Florida College of Medicine–Jacksonville)
Surgery 152:473-476, 2012

Background.—The assessment and treatment of trauma patients begins in the prehospital environment. Studies have validated the shock index as a correlate for mortality and the identification of shock in trauma patients. We investigated the use of the first shock index obtained in the prehospital environment and the first shock index obtained upon arrival in the trauma center as correlates for other outcomes to evaluate its usefulness as a triage tool.

Methods.—This is a retrospective review of data from a level I trauma center. Prehospital and trauma center shock indices for 16,269 patients were evaluated as correlates for duration of hospital stay, duration of stay in the intensive care unit, the number of ventilator days, blood product use, and destination of transfer from the trauma center.

Results.—Pearson correlation coefficients revealed that the relationship of prehospital and trauma center shock indices were correlates for duration of hospital stay, duration of stay in the intensive care unit, the number of ventilator days, and blood product use. A chi-square analysis found that shock indices ≥ 0.9 indicate a higher likelihood of disposition to the intensive care unit, operating room, or death.

Conclusion.—A prehospital shock index for trauma correlates with measures of hospital resource use and mortality. A prospective study is needed to determine the use of this measure as a triage tool.

▶ Although improvements in trauma care continue to develop within the hospital, it is also important to enhance the performance of prehospital care for trauma victims. The Centers for Disease Control and Prevention has taken the position that prehospital care is of significance when considering improvements in patient care of trauma victims.

An aspect of prehospital care important to care is making sure that patients are transported to the most appropriate site; in the setting of severe trauma, the patient should be transported to a trauma center possibly bypassing nontrauma centers.

The authors give a bit more power to the prehospital crew to help decide the final destination of the patient by using the shock index. (This is the ratio of heart rate to systolic blood pressure.) They were able to show that patients with higher levels of shock index assessed in the field received more intensive care in a hospital (more days of admission, more intensive care days, more blood products given, and higher mortality).

It is not clear from this study, however, whether the shock index could be used to decide between transport to different types of hospitals. It is only assumed that specialized trauma care would be of greater importance for those patients needing the greater levels of care.

The shock index is a simple value to calculate, and information can be obtained easily. Field decision making would be greatly enhanced with a tool like this.

N. B. Handly, MD, MSc, MS

Head and Neck Injury

A prehospital shock index for trauma correlates with measures of hospital resource use and mortality
McNab A, Burns B, Bhullar I, et al (Univ of Florida College of Medicine—Jacksonville)
Surgery 152:473-476, 2012

Background.—The assessment and treatment of trauma patients begins in the prehospital environment. Studies have validated the shock index as a correlate for mortality and the identification of shock in trauma patients. We investigated the use of the first shock index obtained in the prehospital environment and the first shock index obtained upon arrival in the trauma center as correlates for other outcomes to evaluate its usefulness as a triage tool.

Methods.—This is a retrospective review of data from a level I trauma center. Prehospital and trauma center shock indices for 16,269 patients were evaluated as correlates for duration of hospital stay, duration of stay in the intensive care unit, the number of ventilator days, blood product use, and destination of transfer from the trauma center.

Results.—Pearson correlation coefficients revealed that the relationship of prehospital and trauma center shock indices were correlates for duration of hospital stay, duration of stay in the intensive care unit, the number of ventilator days, and blood product use. A chi-square analysis found that shock indices ≥ 0.9 indicate a higher likelihood of disposition to the intensive care unit, operating room, or death.

Conclusion.—A prehospital shock index for trauma correlates with measures of hospital resource use and mortality. A prospective study is needed to determine the use of this measure as a triage tool.

▶ The shock index (SI) is the ratio of heart rate to systolic blood pressure. Previous investigations have shown that an SI greater than 0.9 is associated with higher mortality rates. This retrospective review from the University of Florida—Jacksonville examines the utility of the SI as an indicator of resource use in trauma patients. The authors found that SI values of greater than or equal to 0.9 were associated with greater lengths of stay, both general hospital stay and intensive care unit (ICU) stay, and with greater resource use, namely ventilator days and blood product transfusions. They also confirmed higher mortality rates if the SI was above 0.9. There was essentially no difference between the prehospital SI and the SI first reported at the trauma center. Whether incorporating the shock index into the available trauma triage tools, such as the Centers for Disease Control and Prevention's "Guidelines for Field Triage of Injured Patients," the American College of Surgeons trauma triage criteria, or the Loma Linda triage guidelines, would alter the sensitivity and specificity of those tools and increase accuracy is unknown at present and awaits further study. Another consideration that may mitigate against its use is the ability of paramedics to calculate the SI, real time in the chaotic prehospital environment, and to integrate it into their decision-making.

E. A. Ramoska, MD, MPHE

Changing Characteristics of Facial Fractures Treated at a Regional, Level 1 Trauma Center, From 2005 to 2010: An Assessment of Patient Demographics, Referral Patterns, Etiology of Injury, Anatomic Location, and Clinical Outcomes
Roden KS, Tong W, Surrusco M, et al (The Univ of North Carolina at Chapel Hill, NC)
Ann Plast Surg 68:461-466, 2012

Introduction.—Despite improvements in automotive safety, motor vehicle collision (MVC)-related facial fractures remain common and represent preventable injuries. This study examines the changing characteristics of facial fractures treated at a regional, level I trauma center, from 2005 to 2010.

Methods.—We identified all patients with facial fractures admitted to our hospital, from 2005 to 2010, by querying the North Carolina Trauma Registry, using International Classification of Diseases, Ninth Revision codes. Prospectively collected data, sorted by year, were descriptively analyzed for demographics, referral patterns, etiology, anatomic location, and clinical outcomes.

Results.—Number of patients with facial fractures increased from 201 per year to 263 per year (total n = 1508). Although transport distances remained constant at ~85 miles, standard deviation increased from 37 to 68 miles. Transport time increased from 87 to 119 minutes. Referrals came from 28 surrounding counties in 2005 and 43 counties in 2010. Regarding etiology, MVCs decreased from 40% to 27%, all-terrain vehicle crashes decreased from 6% to 2%, falls increased from 8% to 19%, and bicycle accidents increased from 3% to 6%. Regarding anatomic location, frontal sinus fractures increased from 8% to 37%, zygomaticomaxillary fractures increased from 9% to 18%, nasoethmoid fractures decreased from 12% to 6%, orbital floor fractures decreased from 6% to 3%, and mandible fractures decreased from 28% to 18%. Single-site fractures increased from 75% to 90%. Length of intensive care unit and hospital stay remained stable at 3 and 7 days, respectively.

Conclusions.—Despite a decrease in MVC-related facial fractures, the overall increase in facial fractures referred to our trauma center is due to a growing number of patient transfers from rural hospitals, where a paucity of qualified surgeons may exist.

▶ When I first read the title for this article, from the University of North Carolina, I thought it might provide useful information regarding the shifting demographics of facial trauma. And it does to some extent. According to their data both frontal sinus fractures and zygomaticomaxillary fractures increased during the six years of the study. While other types of fractures, notably nasoethmoid, orbital floor, and mandible fractures, showed a reduced incidence. Moreover, the etiology of these fractures has also changed. Falls, motorcycle collisions, and bicycle accidents have all increased, whereas motor vehicle collisions as a cause of facial trauma have decreased.

The major limitation of these data is that the University of North Carolina opened a transfer center to facilitate referrals from outlying hospitals about one-third of the way through the study period. This means that the population base and demographics were altered; therefore, it is unclear whether the changing characteristics the authors describe are due to an actual evolution of injury patterns or just an expanded and different catchment area. Another conclusion of this study is that an outreach program and the development of a transfer center may increase referrals to a trauma center from rural hospitals, thereby increasing their census.

E. A. Ramoska, MD, MPHE

Immediate and Delayed Traumatic Intracranial Hemorrhage in Patients With Head Trauma and Preinjury Warfarin or Clopidogrel Use

Nishijima DK, for the Clinical Research in Emergency Services and Treatment (CREST) Network (UC Davis School of Medicine, Sacramento; et al)
Ann Emerg Med 59:460-468.e7. 2012

Study Objective.—Patients receiving warfarin or clopidogrel are considered at increased risk for traumatic intracranial hemorrhage after blunt head trauma. The prevalence of immediate traumatic intracranial hemorrhage and the cumulative incidence of delayed traumatic intracranial hemorrhage in these patients, however, are unknown. The objective of this study is to address these gaps in knowledge.

Methods.—A prospective, observational study at 2 trauma centers and 4 community hospitals enrolled emergency department (ED) patients with blunt head trauma and preinjury warfarin or clopidogrel use from April 2009 through January 2011. Patients were followed for 2 weeks. The prevalence of immediate traumatic intracranial hemorrhage and the cumulative incidence of delayed traumatic intracranial hemorrhage were calculated from patients who received initial cranial computed tomography (CT) in the ED. Delayed traumatic intracranial hemorrhage was defined as traumatic intracranial hemorrhage within 2 weeks after an initially normal CT scan result and in the absence of repeated head trauma.

Results.—A total of 1,064 patients were enrolled (768 warfarin patients [72.2%] and 296 clopidogrel patients [27.8%]). There were 364 patients

(34.2%) from Level I or II trauma centers and 700 patients (65.8%) from community hospitals. One thousand patients received a cranial CT scan in the ED. Both warfarin and clopidogrel groups had similar demographic and clinical characteristics, although concomitant aspirin use was more prevalent among patients receiving clopidogrel. The prevalence of immediate traumatic intracranial hemorrhage was higher in patients receiving clopidogrel (33/276, 12.0%; 95% confidence interval [CI] 8.4% to 16.4%) than patients receiving warfarin (37/724, 5.1%; 95% CI 3.6% to 7.0%), relative risk 2.31 (95% CI 1.48 to 3.63). Delayed traumatic intracranial hemorrhage was identified in 4 of 687 (0.6%; 95% CI 0.2% to 1.5%) patients receiving warfarin and 0 of 243 (0%; 95% CI 0% to 1.5%) patients receiving clopidogrel.

Conclusion.—Although there may be unmeasured confounders that limit intergroup comparison, patients receiving clopidogrel have a significantly higher prevalence of immediate traumatic intracranial hemorrhage compared with patients receiving warfarin. Delayed traumatic intracranial hemorrhage is rare and occurred only in patients receiving warfarin. Discharging patients receiving anticoagulant or antiplatelet medications from the ED after a normal cranial CT scan result is reasonable, but appropriate instructions are required because delayed traumatic intracranial hemorrhage may occur.

▶ There have been a number of discussions with trauma surgeons at my institution about when a patient should be considered at risk for intracranial bleeding (ICB) if there is a history of "blood thinners." If the patient is using Coumadin, then the patient is going to get a computed tomographic (CT) study of the head and if the patient has therapeutic levels of Coumadin, the patient is going to be admitted, at least for observation overnight. But then what about aspirin or clopidogrel? With newer anticoagulation/antiplatelet drugs being used more and more, we should have some sense of how these may also affect the risk of ICB.

The authors report here an observational study on the risks of intracranial bleeding among patients admitted to emergency departments (EDs) after traumatic injury. They did not study patterns of ICBs after blunt trauma for patients taking aspirin, but they did monitor ICBs for those taking Coumadin or clopidogrel (patients with joint use of Coumadin and clopidogrel were excluded from the study).

I am disappointed that the authors were not consistent about their definitions of ICB. Several times they indicated that immediate and delayed ICB was established by a head CT result. Yet, they included patients in their study who never had a head CT performed at the beginning of the study as well as concluded that no delayed ICB occurred on the basis of telephone interviews. The authors have to be clear: is the measure of ICB based on CT, clinical findings, or both?

Nevertheless, the patterns of ICBs discovered are interesting. Delayed ICBs are rare but not impossible. Patients taking clopidogrel have a higher immediate risk of ICB than those patients taking Coumadin. Those patients taking Coumadin have a small but higher likelihood of ICB than those taking clopidogrel. More patients need to be followed to establish clear magnitudes of risk.

What about other "blood thinners"? Should we ignore the possibility of Arixtra or Pradaxa causing increased risk of ICBs?

N. B. Handly, MD, MSc, MS

Evaluating Age in the Field Triage of Injured Persons
Nakamura Y, the WESTRN Investigators (Oregon Health and Science Univ, Portland; et al)
Ann Emerg Med 60:335-345, 2012

Study Objective.—We evaluate trauma undertriage by age group, the association between age and serious injury after accounting for other field triage criteria and confounders, and the potential effect of a mandatory age triage criterion for field triage.

Method.—This was a retrospective cohort study of injured children and adults transported by 48 emergency medical services (EMS) agencies to 105 hospitals in 6 regions of the western United States from 2006 through 2008. We used probabilistic linkage to match EMS records to hospital records, including trauma registries, state discharge databases, and emergency department databases. The primary outcome measure was serious injury, as measured by an Injury Severity Score greater than or equal to 16. We assessed undertriage (Injury Severity Score ≥ 16 and triage-negative or transport to a nontrauma center) by age decile and used multivariable logistic regression models to estimate the association (linear and nonlinear) between age and Injury Severity Score greater than or equal to 16, adjusted for important confounders. We also evaluated the potential influence of age on triage efficiency and trauma center volume.

Results.—Injured patients (260,027) were evaluated and transported by EMS during the 3-year study period. Undertriage increased for patients older than 60 years, reaching approximately 60% for those older than 90 years. There was a strong nonlinear association between age and Injury Severity Score greater than or equal to 16. For patients not meeting other triage criteria, the probability of serious injury was most notable after 60 years. A mandatory age triage criterion would have decreased undertriage at the expense of overtriage, with 1 patient with Injury Severity Score greater than or equal to 16 identified for every 60 to 65 additional patients transported to major trauma centers.

Conclusion.—Trauma undertriage increases in patients older than 60 years. Although the probability of serious injury increases among triage-negative patients with increasing age, the use of a mandatory age triage criterion appears inefficient for improving field triage.

▶ Trauma undertriage should be on our minds because any system that does not transport patients to the proper level of care (at best, to a trauma center) may lead to poorer outcomes for that patient.

The authors report a technically complicated study that evaluates the role of age in trauma triage. Age is important because at extremes of age there are fewer metabolic reserves to deal with the stress of injury; at the elder end, there are likely to be comorbid conditions that would also put the patient at risk of poor outcome after injuries.

The study is complicated, but not without several good reasons. This is a retrospective study, so concerns about selection bias and missing variables that might describe the patients should be considered. The use of data from a large number of patients seen by multiple prehospital and hospital caregivers should help deal with the former consideration; however, there is no way to be sure that there are other factors that were not collected about these patients. Another challenge in a study is the problem of missing values—that is, when data are expected but not added to the record. The authors used methods of imputation to fill in those missing values and compared the results of analyses with and without the imputed values.

Perhaps the most obscure technique used is that of fractional polynomial multivariate logistic regression to model the nonlinear relationships of variables with the predicted variable. In this study, severe injury was the predicted variable (dependent variable) and age was the primary independent variable. In the setting of significant association of severe injury (Injury Severity Score $\geq$16) with age would suggest that age might have a value in deciding to transport patients to a trauma center. However, it was found that the number to treat to reduce one undertriaged because of age would be between 60 to 65 patients. This is a problem of cost-benefit: do we see more patients who do not have serious injury (with costs of time and money) just to be certain that we do not miss any patients with significant injury (with costs including loss of life, quality of life, productivity)? The final judgment is likely to be based on more than money.

N. B. Handly, MD, MSc, MS

Management of Minor Head Injury in Patients Receiving Oral Anticoagulant Therapy: A Prospective Study of a 24-Hour Observation Protocol

Menditto VG, Lucci M, Polonara S, et al (Ospedali Riuniti di Ancona, Italy; Università Politecnica delle Marche, Ancona, Italy)
Ann Emerg Med 59:451-455, 2012

Study Objective.—Patients receiving warfarin who experience minor head injury are at risk of intracranial hemorrhage, and optimal management after a single head computed tomography (CT) scan is unclear. We evaluate a protocol of 24-hour observation followed by a second head CT scan.

Methods.—In this prospective case series, we enrolled consecutive patients receiving warfarin and showing no intracranial lesions on a first CT scan after minor head injury treated at a Level II trauma center. We implemented a structured clinical pathway, including 24-hour observation and a CT scan performed before discharge. We then evaluated the frequency of death, admission, neurosurgery, and delayed intracranial hemorrhage.

Results.—We enrolled and observed 97 consecutive patients. Ten refused the second CT scan and were well during 30-day follow-up. Repeated CT scanning in the remaining 87 patients revealed a new hemorrhage lesion in 5 (6%), with 3 subsequently hospitalized and 1 receiving craniotomy.

Two patients discharged after completing the study protocol with 2 negative CT scan results were admitted 2 and 8 days later with symptomatic subdural hematomas; neither received surgery. Two of the 5 patients with delayed bleeding at 24 hours had an initial international normalized ratio greater than 3.0, as did both patients with delayed bleeding beyond 24 hours. The relative risk of delayed hemorrhage with an initial international normalized ratio greater than 3.0 was 14 (95% confidence interval 4 to 49).

Conclusion.—For patients receiving warfarin who experience minor head injury and have a negative initial head CT scan result, a protocol of 24-hour observation followed by a second CT scan will identify most occurrences of delayed bleeding. An initial international normalized ratio greater than 3 suggests higher risk.

▶ Patients taking the oral anticoagulant warfarin routinely present to the emergency department after minor head injuries. The authors of this study used a protocol to evaluate the risk of intracranial hemorrhage in this clinical setting. Citing the European Federation of Neurological Societies' recommendation that all patients receiving anticoagulation with a minor head injury warrant initial computed tomography (CT) of the head, followed by 24-hour observation and a second CT prior to discharge. With a negative initial CT, the authors (and the journal's "Editor's Capsule Summary") recommend that patients should be observed for 24 hours and receive a second CT prior to discharge. This approach would have identified additional intracranial hemorrhages (6%). However, 2% of the studied patients were found to have delayed presentations of their intracranial hemorrhages, despite 2 negative CTs and a 24-hour observational period. Understandably, emergency physicians should apply the guidelines to patients with poor social conditions and who lack adequate follow-up, but generalized application of the guidelines would result in numerous negative CTs, unnecessary admissions, and increased health care spending.

E. C. Bruno, MD

Immediate and Delayed Traumatic Intracranial Hemorrhage in Patients With Head Trauma and Preinjury Warfarin or Clopidogrel Use
Nishijima DK, for the Clinical Research in Emergency Services and Treatment (CREST) Network (UC Davis School of Medicine, Sacramento; et al)
Ann Emerg Med 59:460-468.e7, 2012

Study Objective.—Patients receiving warfarin or clopidogrel are considered at increased risk for traumatic intracranial hemorrhage after blunt head trauma. The prevalence of immediate traumatic intracranial hemorrhage and the cumulative incidence of delayed traumatic intracranial hemorrhage in these patients, however, are unknown. The objective of this study is to address these gaps in knowledge.

Methods.—A prospective, observational study at 2 trauma centers and 4 community hospitals enrolled emergency department (ED) patients with blunt head trauma and preinjury warfarin or clopidogrel use from April

2009 through January 2011. Patients were followed for 2 weeks. The prevalence of immediate traumatic intracranial hemorrhage and the cumulative incidence of delayed traumatic intracranial hemorrhage were calculated from patients who received initial cranial computed tomography (CT) in the ED. Delayed traumatic intracranial hemorrhage was defined as traumatic intracranial hemorrhage within 2 weeks after an initially normal CT scan result and in the absence of repeated head trauma.

Results.—A total of 1,064 patients were enrolled (768 warfarin patients [72.2%] and 296 clopidogrel patients [27.8%]). There were 364 patients (34.2%) from Level I or II trauma centers and 700 patients (65.8%) from community hospitals. One thousand patients received a cranial CT scan in the ED. Both warfarin and clopidogrel groups had similar demographic and clinical characteristics, although concomitant aspirin use was more prevalent among patients receiving clopidogrel. The prevalence of immediate traumatic intracranial hemorrhage was higher in patients receiving clopidogrel (33/276, 12.0%; 95% confidence interval [CI] 8.4% to 16.4%) than patients receiving warfarin (37/724, 5.1%; 95% CI 3.6% to 7.0%), relative risk 2.31 (95% CI 1.48 to 3.63). Delayed traumatic intracranial hemorrhage was identified in 4 of 687 (0.6%; 95% CI 0.2% to 1.5%) patients receiving warfarin and 0 of 243 (0%; 95% CI 0% to 1.5%) patients receiving clopidogrel.

Conclusion.—Although there may be unmeasured confounders that limit intergroup comparison, patients receiving clopidogrel have a significantly higher prevalence of immediate traumatic intracranial hemorrhage compared with patients receiving warfarin. Delayed traumatic intracranial hemorrhage is rare and occurred only in patients receiving warfarin. Discharging patients receiving anticoagulant or antiplatelet medications from the ED after a normal cranial CT scan result is reasonable, but appropriate instructions are required because delayed traumatic intracranial hemorrhage may occur.

▶ The decision to order a computed tomography scan of the head (CT head) in the presence of trauma is based on multiple factors. An injury about the clavicles in conjunction with anticoagulant use will generally prompt diagnostic imaging. When an intracranial injury is identified, the disposition of that patient generally includes the involvement of a neurosurgeon. However, the patient may have a negative initial CT head, only to develop a bleed later. In this prospective observational study, the authors assessed the likelihood of an initial injury as well as a delayed one, in the presence of two specific anticoagulants: warfarin and clopidogrel. They were able to demonstrate that patients were more likely to develop an intracranial hemorrhage when taking clopidogrel, whereas those taking warfarin were more likely to present with a delayed bleed. Although the results recognize risk factors for each anticoagulant, the data also reveal something about emergency physicians' practice patterns. About 30% of the enrolled patients received a CT head despite no evidence of trauma about the clavicles. This demonstrates a strong clinical suspicion of the potential for a bleed by the physician.

E. C. Bruno, MD

Subdural Hematomas and Emergency Management in Infancy and Childhood: A Single Institution's Experience

Tehli O, Kazanci B, Türkoğlu E, et al (Marasal Fevzi Çakmak Military Hosp, Erzurum, Turkey; Yozgat Government Hosp, Turkey; et al)
Pediatr Emerg Care 27:834-836, 2011

Objective.—We aimed to identify the incidence, clinical features, management, and outcome of subdural hematomas (SHs) in infancy and childhood.

Methods.—Twenty-one children younger than 11 years with SH were analyzed. Clinical features and possible child abuse were considered in each case.

Results.—Eight children experienced minor injuries due to hitting of solid items on their head. Five of these children also had coagulation disorders. Three of the children suffered from child abuse, only one of the children had head trauma due to car accident. Nine of the patients experienced SH due to fall down. Nine patients have acute SH, 7 had subacute SH, 4 had chronic SH, and 1 had acute and subacute SH together. Clinical presentation varied greatly. Most of them presented with vomiting and seizure. The outcome patterns were different among the patients. Deep coma on admission was associated with an unfavorable outcome.

Conclusions.—Subdural hematoma is common in infancy and childhood and carries a poor prognosis. Most of the cases are due to head trauma, coagulation disorders, and child abuse. We believe that clinical investigation of such children should be carried out in a multidisciplinary approach with the collaboration of pediatricians, social workers, and neurosurgeons.

▶ Pediatric patients presenting for evaluation of a closed head injury is a routine scenario. The principal concerns for all interested parties are identification of serious injury while minimizing exposure to harmful radiation. The authors of this Turkish project identified 21 patients with computed tomography—confirmed subdural hematomas (SDH) and retrospectively present clinical parameters that predict significant injuries. Intuitively, child abuse, head injury, and underlying coagulopathy were identified risk factors. While child abuse may represent a risk factor, suspicion and verification of nonaccidental trauma remain challenges for emergency physicians and subsequently limit the utility of this endpoint. Unfortunately, the small sample size is inadequate and curbs the applicability of the information. The authors, in their objective section, aimed to identify the incidence of SDH in pediatric patients, but they present no population references, that is, number of patients presenting with head injuries that had no SDH. They failed in this goal.

E. C. Bruno, MD

Thoraco-Abdominal Injury

Risk factors that predict mortality in patients with blunt chest wall trauma: A systematic review and meta-analysis

Battle CE, Hutchings H, Evans PA (Univ of Wales Swansea, Morriston, Swansea, UK)
Injury 43:8-17, 2012

Background.—The risk factors for mortality following blunt chest wall trauma have neither been well established or summarised.

Objective.—To summarise the risk factors for mortality in blunt chest wall trauma patients based on available evidence in the literature.

Data Sources.—A systematic review of English and non-English articles using MEDLINE, EMBASE and the Cochrane Library from their introduction until May 2010. Additional studies were identified by hand-searching bibliographies and contacting relevant clinical experts. Grey literature was sought by searching abstracts from all Emergency Medicine conferences. Broad search terms and inclusion criteria were used to reduce the number of missed studies.

Study Selection.—A two step study selection process was used. All published and unpublished observational studies were included if they investigated estimates of association between a risk factor and mortality for blunt chest wall trauma patients.

Data Extraction.—A two step data extraction process using pre-defined data fields, including study quality indicators.

Study Appraisal and Synthesis.—Each study was appraised using a previously designed quality assessment tool and the STROBE checklist. Where sufficient data were available, odds ratios with 95% confidence intervals were calculated using Mantel—Haenszel method for the risk factors investigated. The I^2 statistic was calculated for combined studies in order to assess heterogeneity.

Results.—Age, number of rib fractures, presence of pre-existing disease and pneumonia were found to be related to mortality in 29 identified studies. Combined odds ratio of 1.98 (1.86—2.11, 95% CI), 2.02 (1.89—2.15, 95% CI), 2.43 (1.03—5.72, 95% CI) and 5.24 (3.51—7.82) for mortality were calculated for blunt chest wall trauma patients aged 65 years or more, with three or more rib fractures, pre-existing conditions and pneumonia respectively.

Conclusions.—The risk factors for mortality in patients sustaining blunt chest wall trauma were a patient age of 65 years or more, three or more rib fractures and the presence of pre-existing disease especially cardiopulmonary disease. The development of pneumonia post injury was also a significant risk factor for mortality. As a result of the variable quality in the studies, the results of the selected studies should be interpreted with caution.

▶ Citing a paucity of standard guidelines for the management of blunt thoracic trauma, the authors performed a meta-analysis of the pertinent literature to identify which clinical parameters prognosticated negative outcomes. Patients requiring emergent/urgent surgical intervention or mechanical ventilation were excluded. After sorting through more than 4000 references, the authors whittled down to 29 suitable articles and were able to identify 3 separate risk factors that predict mortality in blunt chest trauma—age greater than 65, 3 or more rib fractures, and the presence of a preexisting condition. Although the cutoff of age 65 years was used, this age is not a rigid indicator, because included studies used younger benchmarks. The treating clinician should be aware that advancing age forecasts a worse outcome. The criterion of 3 fractures demonstrated a statistically significant increase in mortality, though some discrepancy was present. The authors referenced 4 studies in which the number of fractures was inconsequential. The presence of a preexisting condition also predicted detrimental events. The included studies specifically identified congestive heart failure, but the authors extrapolated this link to all cardiopulmonary disorders. The authors suggest that patients lacking these findings are suitable for discharge, but the emergency physician must be vigilant for other reasons for admission or transfer, including anticoagulation, pain medication requirements, or concomitant injuries.

E. C. Bruno, MD

Patients With Rib Fractures Do Not Develop Delayed Pneumonia: A Prospective, Multicenter Cohort Study of Minor Thoracic Injury
Chauny JM, Émond M, Plourde M, et al (Hôpital du Sacré-Coeur de Montréal, Quebec, Canada; Hôpital de l'Enfant-Jésus, Quebec, Canada; Hôpital Saint-François d'Assise, Quebec, Canada; et al)
Ann Emerg Med 2012 [Epub ahead of print]

Study Objective.—Patients admitted to emergency departments (EDs) for minor thoracic injuries are possibly at risk of delayed pneumonia. We aimed to evaluate the incidence of delayed pneumonia post–minor thoracic injury and the associated risk factors.

Methods.—A prospective, multicenter cohort study was conducted in 4 Canadian EDs, from November 2006 to November 2010. All consecutive patients aged 16 years and older with minor thoracic injury who were discharged from the ED were screened for eligibility. Uniform clinical and radiologic evaluations were performed on the initial ED visit and were repeated at weeks 1 and 2. Relative risk analyses quantified incidence with comparison by age, sex, smoking status, alcohol intoxication, pulmonary comorbidity, ability to cough atelectasis, pain level, and number of rib fractures.

Results.—Of the 1,057 participants recruited, 347 (32.8%) had at least 1 rib fracture, 87 (8.2%) had asthma, and 36 (3.4%) had chronic obstructive pulmonary disease. Only 6 patients (0.6%; 95% confidence interval 0.24% to 1.17%) developed pneumonia during the follow-up period. The relative risk for patients with preexistent pulmonary disease and radiologically proven rib fractures was 8.6 ($P = .045$; 95% confidence interval 1.05 to 70.9). Sex, smoking habit, initial atelectasis, ability to cough, and alcohol intoxication were not significantly associated with delayed pneumonia.

Conclusion.—This prospective cohort study of nonhospitalized patients with minor thoracic injuries revealed a low incidence of delayed pneumonia. Nonetheless, our results support tailored follow-up for asthmatic or chronic obstructive pulmonary disease patients with rib fracture.

▶ Emergency physicians have several concerns once a patient with thoracic trauma is diagnosed with 1 or more rib fractures. A principal worry is the development of posttraumatic pneumonia. The authors of this prospective, multicenter project looked to determine this incidence of pneumonia in patients with thoracic trauma as well as identify potential risk factors. Patients with significant injuries, such as a hemothorax or a pneumothorax were excluded, leaving only those with minor trauma to be followed. At the 2-week follow-up evaluation, 0.6% of the patients had developed delayed pneumonia, and none had pneumonia at the 4- or 12-week interviews. The researchers did root out that the combination of pre-existing pulmonary disease and rib fracture portends a marked increased risk of posttraumatic pneumonia. They also suggest that patients not felt to be low risk by the treating physician were not included in the sample population. Patients viewed as high risk by mechanism, physical examination, or underlying comorbidities are candidates for admission.

E. C. Bruno, MD

2 Resuscitation

Cardiac Arrest

Implication of cardiac marker elevation in patients who resuscitated from out-of-hospital cardiac arrest
Oh SH, Kim YM, Kim HJ, et al (Catholic Univ of Korea, Seoul, South Korea)
Am J Emerg Med 30:464-471, 2012

Objectives.—It is often difficult to diagnose acute myocardial infarction (AMI) in patients who resuscitated after out-of-hospital cardiac arrest (OHCA) and had a delayed elevation in cardiac marker. This study explored whether elevations in cardiac marker were due to coronary artery occlusion or resulted from other causes.

Methods.—The study included 19 non–ST-segment elevation patients who resuscitated after OHCA and underwent delayed coronary angiography. We checked patients' serial creatine kinase–myocardial band (CK-MB) and troponin I (cTnI) levels on arrival and 6, 12, 24, 48, 72, and 96 hours postarrest. Based on the association of elevated cTnI and the results of their delayed angiographies, the patients were retrospectively divided into 2 groups: an AMI group (n = 5) and a non-AMI group (n = 14). We then analyzed the serial cardiac marker measurements in each group.

Results.—Peak marker levels were significantly higher in the AMI group than in the non-AMI group (CK-MB, 177.0 ± 112.7 vs 66.4 ± 85.2 ng/mL; $P = .033$ and cTnI, 40.4 ± 14.5 vs 10.6 ± 13.5 ng/mL; $P = .005$). After adjusting for covariates, the peak and 6-, 12-, and 24-hour cTnI and 6-hour CK-MB were significantly different between the 2 groups ($P = .005$, $P = .004$, $P = .005$, $P = .020$, and $P = .007$). In the non-AMI group, 3 patients had cTnI values that were within the reference range at all of the evaluated times. Most patients had only low cTnI elevations that rapidly fell back to normal.

Conclusion.—The resuscitation of patients who experience sudden OHCA but do not have an AMI may lead to elevations of cardiac markers. However, these elevations are low and normalize early.

▶ I am not sure how to interpret this study from the Catholic University of Korea (Seoul, South Korea). Certainly, their conclusion that patients who are resuscitated after out-of-hospital cardiac arrest (OHCA) but do not have an acute myocardial infarction (AMI) may have elevated cardiac markers is correct. Nonetheless, this analysis does not prove it.

37

The authors note that the peak level of creatine troponin I (cTnI) was significantly higher in the AMI group than in the non-AMI group. However, there is considerable overlap in the values, and it does not appear that there is a distinct cutoff for AMI versus non-AMI. Furthermore, they state that the time course of cardiac marker elevation is different in AMI patients when compared with non-AMI patients. Again, a comparison of their graphs reveals substantial overlap in the changes of cTnI over time. To me, this is analogous to using a white blood count (WBC) to diagnose appendicitis. We all know that the WBC is elevated in patients with appendicitis as compared with patients without appendicitis; however, the overlap is sizable and this single test is not definitive.

This investigation has some major limitations that should be mentioned. First, it is based on a total of only 19 OHCA patients. This is an extremely small sample size. Second, the gold standard used to diagnose a patient with an AMI is unclear. The diagnosis was based on a delayed coronary angiography of at least 5 to 30 days postarrest, and it appears that they used the very same cardiac markers in determining whether the patient had an AMI. Until further studies are conducted, I would not rely exclusively on serial cardiac marker measurement to differentiate patients who experience OHCA because of coronary artery occlusion from those who arrest because of other causes.

E. A. Ramoska, MD, MPHE

Time to first compression using Medical Priority Dispatch System compression-first dispatcher-assisted cardiopulmonary resuscitation protocols
Van Vleet LM, Hubble MW (Wake County EMS, Raleigh, NC; Western Carolina Univ, Cullowhee)
Prehosp Emerg Care 16:242-250, 2012

Introduction.—Without bystander cardiopulmonary resuscitation (CPR), cardiac arrest survival decreases 7%—10% for every minute of delay until defibrillation. Dispatcher-assisted CPR (D-CPR) has been shown to increase the rates of bystander CPR and cardiac arrest survival. Other reports suggest that the most critical component of bystander CPR is chest compressions with minimal interruption. Beginning with version 11.2 of the Medical Priority Dispatch System (MPDS) protocols, instructions for mouth-to-mouth ventilation (MTMV) and pulse check were removed and a compression-first pathway was introduced to facilitate rapid delivery of compressions. Additionally, unconscious choking and third-trimester pregnancy decision-making criteria were added in versions 11.3 and 12.0, respectively. However, the effects of these changes on time to first compression (TTFC) have not been evaluated.

Objective.—We sought to quantify the TTFC of MPDS versions 11.2, 11.3, and 12.0 for all calls identified as cardiac arrest on call intake that did not require MTMV instruction.

Methods.—Audio recordings of all D-CPR events for October 2005 through May 2010 were analyzed for TTFC. Differences in TTFC across versions were compared using the Kruskal-Wallis test.

Results.—A total of 778 cases received D-CPR. Of these, 259 were excluded because they met criteria for MTMV (pediatric patients, allergic reaction, etc.), were missing data, or were not initially identified as cardiac arrest. Of the remaining 519 calls, the mean TTFC was 240 seconds, with no significant variation across the MPDS versions ($p = 0.08$).

Conclusions.—Following the removal of instructions for pulse check and MTMV, as well as other minor changes in the MPDS protocols, we found the overall TTFC to be 240 seconds with little variation across the three versions evaluated. This represents an improvement in TTFC compared with reports of an earlier version of MPDS that included pulse checks and MTMV instructions (315 seconds). However, the MPDS TTFC does not compare favorably with reports of older, non-MPDS protocols that included pulse checks and MTMV. Efforts should continue to focus on improving this key, and modifiable, determinant of cardiac arrest survival.

▶ Over the past few decades, resuscitation of out of hospital cardiac arrest (OHCA) has been scrutinized by many studies. From analysis of the data, many modifications have been made to the sequence of steps designed to restore normal mechanical activity of the heart and to restore spontaneous circulation of blood. Of all the proposed changes, times to first effective chest compression and early defibrillation are proving to be most effective in improving survival rates for patients.

Many progressive communities have taken the initiative and provided access to cardiopulmonary resuscitation (CPR) training programs and implemented public access defibrillation (PAD) programs in an effort to improve the potential for survivability from OHCA. However, when a patient collapses and becomes unresponsive, many bystanders fail to initiate CPR, let alone apply an automatic external defibrillator (AED). In many instances, bystanders wait for the arrival of emergency medical personnel before any substantial resuscitation begins.

Currently, when a 911 call is placed by a bystander, the dispatchers are trained to assess the nature of the call and send the appropriate response team. In addition, the dispatchers provide verbal directions to the caller, instructing them how to perform compressions on a patient who is in cardiac arrest. This is described as dispatcher-assisted CPR. Because the sequence of steps of CPR has been modified, initiation of chest compressions has taken priority. Directions that are provided to the caller have been simplified; this has demonstrated that more bystanders are initiating chest compressions on unresponsive, pulseless, apneic patients. However, although several steps (ie, the pulse check and ventilations) have been put further down the timeline in the sequence, there are still delays in initiation of chest compressions. Now that more victims are receiving chest compressions, a more in-depth look needs to be taken as to why it can take up to 4 minutes from collapse to "hands-only" CPR. Remember that for each minute of "down time," the potential for a successful resuscitation decreases by 7% to

10%. Let's revisit those dispatcher-assisted CPR versions and see where some time can be trimmed off to decrease time to first compression even more.

B. M. Minczak, MS, MD, PhD

Mild hypothermia treatment in patients resuscitated from non-shockable cardiac arrest

Storm C, Nee J, Roser M, et al (Charité Universitätsmedizin Berlin, Germany; German Heart Centre Berlin, Germany)

Emerg Med J 29:100-103, 2012

Objective.—Therapeutic hypothermia has proved effective in improving outcome in patients after cardiac arrest due to ventricular fibrillation (VF). The benefit in patients with non-VF cardiac arrest is still not defined.

Methods.—This prospective observational study was conducted in a university hospital setting with historical controls. Between 2002 and 2010 387 consecutive patients have been admitted to the intensive care unit (ICU) after cardiac arrest (control n = 186; hypothermia n = 201). Of those, in 175 patients the initial rhythm was identified as non-shockable (asystole, pulseless electrical activity) rhythm (control n = 88; hypothermia n = 87). Neurological outcome was assessed at ICU discharge according to the Pittsburgh cerebral performance category (CPC). A follow-up was completed for all patients after 90 days, a Kaplan–Meier analysis and Cox regression was performed.

Results.—Hypothermia treatment was not associated with significantly improved neurological outcome in patients resuscitated from non-VF cardiac arrest (CPC 1–2: hypothermia 27.59% vs control 18.20%, $p = 0.175$). 90-Day Kaplan–Meier analysis revealed no significant benefit for the hypothermia group (log rank test $p = 0.82$), and Cox regression showed no statistically significant improvement.

Conclusions.—In this cohort patients undergoing hypothermia treatment after non-shockable cardiac arrest do not benefit significantly concerning neurological outcome. Hypothermia treatment needs to be evaluated in a large multicentre trial of cardiac arrest patients found initially to be in non-shockable rhythms to clarify whether cooling may also be beneficial for other rhythms than VF.

▶ Acknowledging that patients resuscitated from nonventricular tachycardia arrhythmias have poor prognosis, the authors of this project looked to determine whether therapeutic hypothermia (TH) affected neurological outcomes in this cohort of cardiac arrest survivors. Using the institution's accepted protocol, patients were divided into the TH and non-TH groups. They were able to demonstrate trends toward improved neurological outcomes as well as shorter ventilator times and intensive care unit stays in the TH group. Though not statistically significant, the favorable trend of improved outcomes with the TH supports broader application of the intervention. The authors also did not see an increase in negative outcomes, suggesting that TH is low risk with potential for high gain. The treating physician must be reminded that the TH is aimed at improving neurological outcomes and will not improve survival. Additionally, the emergency physician should not prognosticate on outcomes while the patient is in the emergency department because this practice is extremely unreliable and may give the patient's family and friends an incorrect impression.

E. C. Bruno, MD

Shock

Lightweight noninvasive trauma monitor for early indication of central hypovolemia and tissue acidosis: A review
Soller BR, Zou F, Ryan KL, et al (Reflectance Med, Inc, Westboro, MA; US Army Inst of Surgical Res, Fort Sam Houston, TX; et al)
J Trauma Acute Care Surg 73:S106-S111, 2012

Background.—Hemorrhage is a major cause of soldier death; it must be quickly identified and appropriately treated. We developed a prototype patient monitor that noninvasively and continuously determines muscle oxygen saturation (S_mO_2), muscle pH (pH_m), and a regional assessment of blood volume (HbT) using near-infrared spectroscopy. Previous demonstration in a model of progressive, central hypovolemia induced by lower body negative pressure (LBNP) showed that S_mO_2 provided an early indication of impending hemodynamic instability in humans. In this review, we expand the number of subjects and provide an overview of the relationship between the muscle and sublingual microcirculation in this model of compensated shock.

Methods.—Healthy human volunteers (n = 30) underwent progressive LBNP in 5 minute intervals. Standard vital signs, along with stroke volume (SV), total peripheral resistance, functional capillary density, S_mO_2, HbT, and pH_m were measured continuously throughout the study.

Results and Discussion.—S_mO_2 and SV significantly decreased during the first level of central hypovolemia (−15 mm Hg LBNP), whereas vital signs were later indicators of impending cardiovascular collapse. S_mO_2 declined with SV and inversely with total peripheral resistance throughout LBNP. HbT was correlated with declining functional capillary density, suggesting vasoconstriction as a cause for decreased S_mO_2 and subsequently decreased pH_m.

Clinical Translation.—The monitor has been miniaturized to a 58-g solid-state sensor that is currently being evaluated on patients with dengue hemorrhagic fever. Early results demonstrate significant decreases in S_mO_2 similar to those observed with progressive reductions in central blood volume. As such, this technology has the potential to (1) provide a monitoring capability for both nontraumatic and traumatic hemorrhage and

(2) help combat medics triage casualties and monitor patients during lengthy transport from combat areas.

▶ The authors studied a near-infrared (nIR) tool for assessing deep tissue perfusion and pH levels with a model of varied central hypovolemia. This hypovolemia was created by applying negative pressure on the lower body of healthy volunteers.

Correlation of the nIR tool to a number of other cardiovascular measures expected to be related to hypovolemia was also part of this study. What is important is that changes to the parameters measured in the deep tissue were more sensitive to lower body negative pressure than classically examined vital signs suggesting then that changes in these deep tissue characteristics would be an earlier warning of hypovolemic shock.

The tool has been packaged for real-world application (only 58 g!) for studying hemorrhagic shock in dengue hemorrhagic fever patients to further validate these measurements. The final challenge will be to determine the optimal therapy for these tissue changes and to show that correcting these values will yield patient-oriented improvements.

N. B. Handly, MD, MSc, MS

Damage Control Immunoregulation: Is There a Role for Low-Volume Hypertonic Saline Resuscitation in Patients Managed with Damage Control Surgery?

Duchesne JC, Simms E, Guidry C (Tulane Univ School of Medicine, New Orleans, LA; et al)
Am Surg 78:962-968, 2012

Hypertonic saline (HTS) is beneficial in the treatment of head-injured patients as a result of its potent cytoprotective effects on various cell lines. We hypothesize that low-volume resuscitation with 3 per cent HTS, when used after damage control surgery (DCS), improves outcomes compared with standard resuscitation with isotonic crystalloid solution (ICS). This is a 4-year retrospective review from two Level I trauma centers. Patients included had 10 units or more of packed red blood cells during initial DCS. On arrival to the trauma intensive care unit (TICU), patients were resuscitated with low-volume 3 per cent HTS or with conventional ICS. A cohort analysis was performed comparing resuscitation strategies. Univariate analysis of continuous data was done with Student t test followed by multivariate analysis. Of 188 patients included, 76 were in the low-volume HTS group and 112 in the ICS group. Demographics were similar between the groups. Over the next 48 hours after DCS in HTS *versus* ISC groups, intravenous fluids were given: 1920 ± 455 mL *versus* 8400 ± 1200 mL ($P < 0.0001$); urine output was 4320 ± 480 mL *versus* 1940 ± 480 mL ($P < 0.0001$); mean TICU length of stay was 10 ± 8 *versus* 16 ± 15 days ($P < 0.01$); prevalence of acute respiratory distress syndrome was 4.0 *versus* 13.4 per cent ($P = 0.02$); sepsis was 6.6 *versus* 15.2 per cent ($P = 0.06$); multisystem organ failure was: 2.6 *versus* 16.1 per cent ($P < 0.01$); and 30-day mortality was 5.3 *versus* 15.2 per cent ($P = 0.03$). There was no difference for prevalence of renal failure at 5.3 *versus* 3.6 per cent ($P = 0.58$). Low-volume resuscitation with HTS administered after DCS on arrival to the TICU may have a protective effect on the polytrauma patient. We believe that this study demonstrates a role for low-volume resuscitation with HTS to improve outcomes in patients undergoing DCS.

▶ There is a body of work developed around the role of hypertonic saline resuscitation in the setting of trauma care.

In this study, the authors compare outcomes among those patients treated with hypertonic saline and those treated with isotonic saline. There appear to be significant benefits to using hypertonic saline, which the authors attribute to a modulation of inflammatory processes perhaps by the decrease in total volume administered. Parts of the rationale are clear: increased volume infused will lead to extensive extravascular edema and can also modify behavior of vascular endothelia and immunomodulator release.

This study included patients who underwent damage control surgery accompanied by at least 10 units of packed red cells. Clearly these were severely injured individuals. Is it possible that the immunomodulatory effects of hypertonic saline can be used to manage other injured patients? How about patients suffering from vascular injury and shock in other forms (eg, sepsis, influenza)?

N. B. Handly, MD, MSc, MS

3 Cardiovascular

A new site for venous access: superficial veins of portal collateral circulation
Turc J, Gergelé L, Attof R, et al (Desgenettes Military Hosp, Lyon, France; Univ of Lyon, Saint Etienne, France; Univ of Lyon, Pierre Bénite, France; et al)
Am J Emerg Med 30:258.e1-258.e2, 2012

In case of failure of peripheral vascular access, classical alternatives are central venous or intraosseous access. We report a new site of vascular access necessitating no specific material. A 53-year-old patient with cirrhosis-induced coagulopathy, portal hypertension, and collateral abdominal porto-systemic circulation required parenteral antibiotherapy. After failure of peripheral vein catheterization, he was addressed to our resuscitation room for central venous access. To avoid the risks associated with this invasive procedure, we chose an alternative approach. After skin preparation, a 20-gauge peripheral venous catheter was inserted in a dilated subcutaneous vein of abdominal wall. To our knowledge, it is the first human report of insertion of a catheter in a superficial vein of abdominal wall. It could be an alternative approach for vascular access after failure of peripheral veni-puncture in patients with portal hypertension (Fig 1).

▶ Securing venous access is one of the first steps in the resuscitation of any patient. The inability to insert an intravenous (IV) catheter can be a source of consternation for the emergency department staff in a patient with poor veins or a coagulopathy. Alternatives to peripheral IV access include placing a central venous catheter or obtaining intraosseous access. These authors from Lyon, France, describe a cirrhotic patient in whom they placed a 20-gauge IV catheter in a superficial vein of the abdominal wall. They were able to use the line for 2 days. They injected several boluses of crystalloids under pressure and infused 4 doses of antibiotics with no extravasation or discomfort.

Cirrhosis and portal hypertension lead to a collateral portosystemic circulation, which becomes visible when it causes dilatation of the superficial veins of the abdominal wall. The blood flow in these veins is upward above the umbilicus and downward below. This can be verified clinically by applying pressure on the vein and watching it refill. The bioavailability of drugs was not assessed in this patient. The authors postulate that a first-pass metabolism is unlikely to occur because the flow is strictly portosystemic. This technique for IV access, while not reported previously, may represent another tool in the armamentarium of emergency physicians.

E. A. Ramoska, MD, MPHE

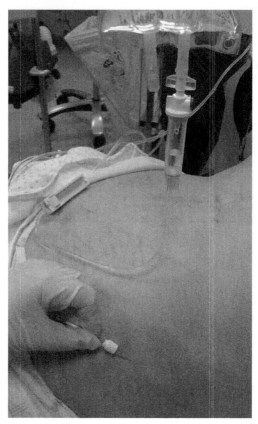

FIGURE 1.—The catheter is inserted in a superficial vein of the abdominal wall. (Reprinted from the American Journal of Emergency Medicine, Turc J, Gergelé L, Attof R, et al, A new site for venous access: superficial veins of portal collateral circulation. *Am J Emerg Med*. 2012;30:258.e1-258.e2. Copyright 2012, with permission from Elsevier.)

Gender Differences in Calls to 9-1-1 During an Acute Coronary Syndrome
Newman JD, Davidson KW, Ye S, et al (Columbia Univ Med Ctr, NY; et al)
Am J Cardiol 111:58-62, 2013

Calling 911 during acute coronary syndromes (ACS) decreases time to treatment and may improve prognosis. Women may have more atypical ACS symptoms compared to men, but few data are available on differences in gender and ACS symptoms in calling 911. In this study, patient interviews and structured chart reviews were conducted to determine gender differences in calling 911. Calls to 911 were assessed by self-report and validated by medical chart review. Of the 476 patients studied, 292 (61%) were diagnosed with unstable angina and 184 (39%) with myocardial infarctions (MIs). Overall, only 23% of patients called 911. Similar percentages of women

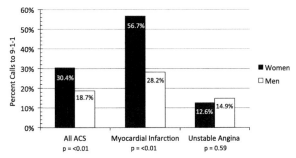

FIGURE 1.—Women versus men on calls to 911. The p values are reported for the difference between women and men on calls to 911. (Reprinted from Newman JD, Davidson KW, Ye S, et al. Gender differences in calls to 9-1-1 during an acute coronary syndrome. *Am J Cardiol.* 2013;111:58-62, Copyright 2013, with permission from Elsevier.)

and men with unstable angina called 911 (15% and 13%, respectively, $p = 0.59$). In contrast, women with MIs were significantly more likely to call 911 than men (57% vs 28%, $p < 0.001$). After adjustment for sociodemographic factors, health insurance status, history of MI, the left ventricular ejection fraction, Global Registry of Acute Coronary Events (GRACE) score, and ACS symptoms, women were 1.79 times more likely to call 911 during an MI than men (prevalence ratio 1.79, 95% confidence interval 1.22 to 2.64, $p < 0.01$). In conclusion, the findings of the present study suggest that initiatives to increase calls to 911 are needed for women and men (Fig 1).

▶ This study from Columbia University Medical Center in New York demonstrates that fewer than 1 in 4 patients with acute coronary syndromes called 911 to get to the emergency department. Furthermore, women appear to use the 911 system more often than men; although all of their increased use is due to myocardial infarction rather than unstable angina (Fig 1). This finding of a sex difference in a health-seeking behavior is certainly consistent with other research, which shows that men seek help and use health services less frequently than women do. Although this is a relatively small, urban, single-site study, its results are in concert with other investigations that reveal women who are having myocardial infarctions call 911 more frequently than men do. In any case, public health initiatives are needed to get more people with symptoms of ACS to use the 911 system.

E. A. Ramoska, MD, MPHE

Intraosseous Versus Intravenous Vascular Access During Out-of-Hospital Cardiac Arrest: A Randomized Controlled Trial

Reades R, Studnek JR, Vandeventer S, et al (Methodist Hosp System, Dallas, TX; Carolinas Med Ctr and the Ctr for Prehospital Medicine, Charlotte, NC; Baylor Univ Med Ctr, Dallas, TX)
Ann Emerg Med 58:509-516, 2011

Study Objective.—Intraosseous needle insertion during out-of-hospital cardiac arrest is rapidly replacing peripheral intravenous routes in the out-of-hospital setting. However, there are few data directly comparing the effectiveness of intraosseous needle insertions with peripheral intravenous insertions during out-of-hospital cardiac arrest. The objective of this study is to determine whether there is a difference in the frequency of first-attempt success between humeral intraosseous, tibial intraosseous, and peripheral intravenous insertions during out-of-hospital cardiac arrest.

Methods.—This was a randomized trial of adult patients experiencing a nontraumatic out-of-hospital cardiac arrest in which resuscitation efforts were initiated. Patients were randomized to one of 3 routes of vascular access: tibial intraosseous, humeral intraosseous, or peripheral intravenous. Paramedics received intensive training and exposure to all 3 methods before study initiation. The primary outcome was first-attempt success, defined as secure needle position in the marrow cavity or a peripheral vein, with normal fluid flow. Needle dislodgement during resuscitation was coded as a failure to maintain vascular access.

Results.—There were 182 patients enrolled, with 64 (35%) assigned to tibial intraosseous, 51 (28%) humeral intraosseous, and 67 (37%) peripheral intravenous access. Demographic characteristics were similar among patients in the 3 study arms. There were 130 (71%) patients who experienced initial vascular access success, with 17 (9%) needles becoming dislodged, for an overall frequency of first-attempt success of 113 (62%). Individuals randomized to tibial intraosseous access were more likely to experience a successful first attempt at vascular access (91%; 95% confidence interval [CI] 83% to 98%) compared with either humeral intraosseous access (51%; 95% CI 37% to 65%) or peripheral intravenous access (43%; 95% CI 31% to 55%) groups. Time to initial success was significantly shorter for individuals assigned to the tibial intraosseous access group (4.6 minutes; interquartile range 3.6 to 6.2 minutes) compared with those assigned to the humeral intraosseous access group (7.0 minutes; interquartile range 3.9 to 10.0 minutes), and neither time was significantly different from that of the peripheral intravenous access group (5.8 minutes; interquartile range 4.1 to 8.0 minutes).

Conclusion.—Tibial intraosseous access was found to have the highest first-attempt success for vascular access and the most rapid time to vascular access during out-of-hospital cardiac arrest compared with peripheral intravenous and humeral intraosseous access.

▶ This randomized trial of intraosseous (IO) access versus peripheral intravenous (PIV) access in nontraumatic out-of-hospital cardiac arrest comes from the Mecklenburg County emergency medical services (EMS) and Carolinas Medical Center (North Carolina). It is a follow-up to a previous observational study comparing tibial IO access and humeral IO access.[1] The current study reveals both a greater initial success rate and a greater overall success rate with tibial IO access as compared with either humeral IO or PIV access. The humeral IO route had a longer time to placement and a larger displacement rate than either the tibial IO lines or the peripheral intravenous (PIV) lines. Moreover, the medics felt either comfortable or very comfortable in placing either the tibial IO or the PIV lines in virtually all cases (98% and 96%, respectfully) whereas they felt that way in less than half (48%) of the humeral IO attempts. Taken together, all of this suggests that tibial IO access might be the preferred method of vascular access during out-of-hospital cardiac arrest.

There are, however, several limitations to keep in mind before you generalize these results to your emergency medical service. First, this study was conducted by a single EMS agency, and the specifics of their situation may not be comparable to others. Second, they did not have a mechanism to report complications or morbidity and mortality. The tibial IO line may be faster and easier, but it may not make a difference in the overall outcome. Third, the average patient weight of the humeral IO group (103.9 kg) was greater than either the PIV group (97.7 kg) or the tibial IO group (91.5 kg). This piece of information, coupled with the fact that there were 13 protocol violations that favored the tibial IO route, suggests that confounding variables may have biased the results.

There are certainly good reasons to think that the tibial IO route may be superior to other forms of IO access. The proximal tibia has a larger surface area, less subcutaneous tissue, and is easier to identify than the humeral head. In addition, the stability of a proximal humeral IO line may be tenuous during cardiac arrest because it is centered near the upper torso, where resuscitation efforts are occurring.

The tibial IO line seems to have many positive aspects associated with its use. Whether it is the optimal vascular access route for out-of-hospital cardiac arrest is still unclear, although this study adds more evidence to the discussion.

E. A. Ramoska, MD, MPHE

Reference

1. Reades R, Studnek JR, Garrett JS, Vandeventer S, Blackwell T. Comparison of first attempt success between tibial and humeral intraosseous insertions during out-of-hospital cardiac arrest. *Prehosp Emerg Care*. 2011;15:278-281.

Prehospital care of left ventricular assist device patients by emergency medical services

Schweiger M, Vierecke J, Stiegler P, et al (Med Univ of Graz, Austria; German Heart Inst, Berlin, Germany)
Prehosp Emerg Care 16:560-563, 2012

Left ventricular assist devices (LVADs) are frequently implanted as permanent (bridge to destination BTD) or temporary (bridge to transplantation BTT) cardiac support. When LVAD patients are discharged to home, they are very likely to require emergency medical services (EMS), but there is very little literature on out-of-hospital emergency care for patients with LVADs. We present two typical cases of LVAD patients for whom EMS was called. In the first case, the patient was in an ambulance two hours distant from our university hospital when a pulsatile system malfunctioned. In the second case, EMS was called to an unconscious LVAD patient.

Emergency reference cards, training programs for emergency medical staff, and a 24-hour emergency hotline for the local VAD team are advisable.

▶ Advances in medicine, computer science, and biomedical engineering have led to the development of smaller, more efficient, sophisticated medical equipment that can be implanted into a patient and function by providing life-supporting actions, such as maintaining circulation. One such device is the left ventricular assist device (LVAD). As these devices become more available and are more frequently used, patients outside the hospital will be calling emergency medical services (EMS) when these devices malfunction. Having the knowledge and training to intervene in an emergency when a particular device malfunctions will become a prerequisite for responding to these emergencies. Failure to comply with attaining this information can lead to the demise of the patient.

This publication provides 2 case reports to put this problem into perspective. The authors also list some suggestions as to what can be done to facilitate dealing with emergencies related to this type of special equipment.

Some of the actions that need to be taken in the future to help the patient when these pieces of equipment malfunction are:

- To provide education for the families and EMS personnel on how the equipment works, what it specifically does, and how to assess if the equipment is functioning appropriately.
- What has to be done when the equipment malfunctions in order to prevent an immediate threat to the patients' well-being?
- Teach paramedics and family what can go wrong and how to deal with it.
- Provide reference material in the form of easy to understand cards, pictures, and illustrations that can guide a rescuer in what to do during an emergent event.
- Provide a 24-hour contact number to the appropriate support personnel who are familiar with the equipment and who can provide useful guidance to the individual providing the rescue actions for the patient.

The bottom line is that there is a need to provide education for the families, EMS personnel, and emergency department physicians and nurses regarding what has to be done when an emergent malfunction occurs with one of these devices.

B. M. Minczak, MS, MD, PhD

Potential utility of near-infrared spectroscopy in out-of-hospital cardiac arrest: an illustrative case series
Frisch A, Suffoletto BP, Frank R, et al (Univ of Pittsburgh, PA)
Prehosp Emerg Care 16:564-570, 2012

Objective.—We evaluated the measurement of tissue oxygen content (StO_2) by continuous near-infrared spectroscopy (NIRS) during and following cardiopulmonary rescuscitation (CPR) and compared the changes in StO_2 and end-tidal carbon dioxide ($ETCO_2$) as a measure of return of spontaneous circulation (ROSC) or rearrest.

Methods.—This was a case series of five patients who experienced out-of-hospital cardiac arrest. Patients included those who had already experienced ROSC, who were being transported to the hospital, or who were likely to have a reasonable amount of time remaining in the resuscitation efforts. Patients were continuously monitored from the scene using continuous $ETCO_2$ monitoring and a NIRS StO_2 monitor until they reached the hospital. The $ETCO_2$ and StO_2 values were continuously recorded and analyzed for comparison of the time points when patients were clinically identified to have ROSC or rearrest.

Results.—Four of five patients had StO_2 and $EtCO_2$ recorded during an episode of CPR and all were monitored during the postarrest period. Three patients experienced rearrest en route to the hospital. Downward trends were noted in StO_2 prior to each rearrest, and rapid increases were noted after ROSC. The StO_2 data showed less variance than the $ETCO_2$ data in the periarrest period.

Conclusions.—This preliminary study in humans demonstrates that StO_2 dynamically changes during periods of hemodynamic instability in postarrest patients. These data suggest that a decline in StO_2 level may correlate with rearrest and may be useful as a tool to predict rearrest in post–cardiac arrest patients. A rapid increase in StO_2 was also seen upon ROSC and may be a better method of identifying ROSC during CPR than pauses for pulse checks or $ETCO_2$ monitoring.

▶ When cardiac arrest occurs, the electromechanical activity of the heart is compromised, causing the cardiac output to drop to zero. As a result, blood pressure falls precipitously and blood flow through the vasculature is interrupted. This lack of blood flow to the various organ systems causes tissue ischemia with subsequent cellular hypoxia. Carbon dioxide removal from the tissues ceases because of the lack of circulation and delivery of blood containing carbon dioxide to the lungs for removal via pulmonary ventilation is interrupted. Assessment of the patient demonstrates no palpable pulse, apnea, no blood pressure, and an indeterminate pulse oximeter reading. The cardiac monitor might show ventricular fibrillation, pulseless ventricular tachycardia, or possibly asystole. If the patient has an advanced airway in place, there will be no measurable carbon dioxide in the expired gas as a result of the interruption in blood flow through the lungs.

Initiation of prompt cardiopulmonary resuscitation, access to timely defibrillation, and medications (vasopressors) may mitigate this condition by restoring cardiac output (ie, correcting the electromechanical compromise of the heart) and restoring blood pressure with subsequent return of spontaneous circulation (ROSC).

When ROSC occurs, pulmonary and systemic blood flow resume, oxygen levels in the tissues increase, carbon dioxide levels in the tissues slowly return to normal, and blood flow to the lungs returns to baseline, thus removing the carbon dioxide produced by normal organ function. The pulse returns, blood pressure can be measured, oxygen saturation levels of the hemoglobin, as determined by the pulse oximeter, rise and the end-tidal carbon dioxide levels in the expired respiratory gases ($ETCO_2$) rise. Thus, the aforementioned parameters can be used to determine the efficacy of the cardiac resuscitation of a patient in cardiac arrest. However, many of these patients rearrest and do not fare well. Immediately after ROSC, there is a period of hemodynamic instability. Monitoring the parameters mentioned previously, especially the $ETCO_2$, which is currently being used to scrutinize the efficacy of the cardiopulmonary resuscitation in progress are not very helpful in predicting if a patient will rearrest. However, a fairly new technique has surfaced that can determine the level of tissue oxygen content via spectroscopy. This technique is described as noninvasive near-infrared spectroscopy (NIRS). This technique does not require placement of an advanced airway, nor is it directly affected by real-time pulmonary ventilation. Simply put, hemodynamic instability causes changes in NIRS values (ie, oxygen content of the tissues [StO_2]). A drop in StO_2 often occurs before loss of pulses. This may be useful in predicting and possibly preventing rearrest.

This study compares the utility of $ETCO_2$ and the use of NIRS. This study was done in the prehospital setting, thus providing an additional avenue for determining the usefulness of NIRS versus $ETCO_2$ in the efficacy of out-of-hospital cardiac arrest resuscitation. The data in this study suggest that this technique has better utility in potentially predicting rearrest in cardiac arrest patients. It is the opinion of this reviewer that this modality will become an important parameter in the future evaluation of cardiac resuscitations.

B. M. Minczak, MS, MD, PhD

Impact of delayed and infrequent administration of vasopressors on return of spontaneous circulation during out-of-hospital cardiac arrest

Cantrell CL Jr, Hubble MW, Richards ME (Western Carolina Univ, Cullowhee, NC; Univ of New Mexico, Albuquerque)
Prehosp Emerg Care 17:15-22, 2013

Introduction.—Epinephrine and vasopressin are the only vasopressors associated with return of spontaneous circulation (ROSC). While current guidelines recommend rapid and frequent vasopressor administration during cardiac arrest, delays in their administration in the out-of-hospital setting remain a concern.

Objective.—This study evaluated delays in vasopressor administration and their effect on field ROSC.

Methods.—This retrospective review included all adult patients who experienced cardiac arrest of medical origin and received field resuscitative efforts among 10 emergency medical services (EMS) systems. Data were abstracted from the EMS medical record and included response time intervals, calculated first-dose and interdosing intervals of vasopressors, and ROSC. Data were analyzed using Mann-Whitney tests, chi-square tests, and t-tests, survival analysis, and logistic regression, with $p \leq 0.05$ indicating significance.

Results.—A total of 660 cardiac arrest patients were enrolled in the study. The mean EMS response time was 8.8 minutes; 52.7% of patients had witnessed cardiac arrests, 46.2% received bystander cardiopulmonary resuscitation (CPR), 23.0% had shockable initial rhythms, and 19.5% experienced field ROSC. In total, 1,913 doses of epinephrine and 111 doses of vasopressin were administered, with mean and 90th-percentile scene arrival—to—first drug intervals of 9.5 and 17 minutes, respectively. The mean and 90th-percentile interdosing intervals were 6.1 and 10 minutes, respectively. Patients experiencing ROSC had shorter scene arrival—to—first drug intervals than those without ROSC (8.1 vs. 9.8 min, $p < 0.01$), but there was no difference in the mean interdosing interval (6.8 vs. 6.0 min, $p = 0.57$). In the logistic regression analysis of ROSC, the adjusted odds ratio for call receipt—to—first drug interval ≤ 10 minutes was 1.91 ($p = 0.04$). Patients receiving advanced airway control prior to vasopressor administration were less likely to have a call receipt—to—first drug interval within 10 minutes (4.0% vs. 17.3%, $p < 0.01$) and were less likely to attain ROSC (15.7% vs. 25.4%, $p < 0.01$).

Conclusion.—The interval between scene arrival and first administration of vasopressors is significantly shorter among patients who experience ROSC compared with those who do not. Airway control procedures delay vasopressor administration and reduce the likelihood of ROSC. Although the interdosing intervals of most patients were not consistent with current recommendations, there was no difference in the mean interdosing times between those who achieved ROSC and those who did not.

▶ The goal of cardiac resuscitation is to reestablish electromechanical activity of the heart and to establish a stable return of spontaneous circulation (ROSC).

After a patient suffers a cardiac arrest, the chance of successful resuscitation decreases significantly without intervention; survivability decreases by a factor of 10% for every minute without circulation. If cardiopulmonary resuscitation (CPR) is initiated by bystanders and there is access to prompt defibrillation (ie, via a public access defibrillation program), the chances of survival improve modestly. However, when the resuscitation proceeds beyond the initial performance of CPR and defibrillation, administration of vasopressors such as epinephrine and/or vasopressin may enhance the possibility for survival.

To date, the current emphasis in the resuscitation sequence is on prompt chest compressions and timely defibrillation. Several studies have analyzed the relationship between ROSC and the administration of vasopressors. The data from these studies suggest that victims of cardiac arrest who receive epinephrine or vasopressin early on during the resuscitation effort have a better chance of achieving ROSC and surviving to hospital admission. This study supports these findings and attempts to describe some of the factors that contribute to delays in the administration. These factors are identified as securing the airway, and establishing intravenous access or intraosseous access.

Crew configuration (ie, 1 or more paramedics present on scene) during the resuscitation also affect time to drug. If there are more medics on scene, multiple tasks can be performed simultaneously thus facilitating earlier administration of the medications.

In addition to the aforementioned issues, this study also attempted to describe how response times may also affect time to vasopressors, time from the 9-1-1 call to scene arrival, and so on. More data need to be collected before definitive conclusions can be drawn.

In reviewing this particular study, it can be concluded that the "time to vasopressors" can be affected by many factors and that for patients to survive out-of-hospital cardiac arrest, timely access to CPR, defibrillation, and vasopressors is important. To this end, current protocols to make this happen need to be revised and the resources required must be made available. These issues should become a priority in social and governmental actions.

Of note, it would be interesting to reassess the types of electrical cardiac rhythms present on arrival of the medics in an effort to determine how the initial cardiac electrophysiology may be affecting time to ROSC.

B. M. Minczak, MS, MD, PhD

Prehospital Point-of-Care Testing for Troponin: Are the Results Reliable?
Venturini JM, Stake CE, Cichon ME (Loyola Univ of Chicago, Maywood, IL)
Prehosp Emerg Care 17:88-91, 2012

Background.—Swift assessment of patients presenting with chest pain results in faster treatment and improved outcomes. Allowing ambulance crews to use point-of-care (POC) devices to measure cardiac troponin I levels during transport of patients to the emergency department (ED) may result in earlier diagnosis of acute myocardial infarction, particularly in those patients without ST-segment elevation. The ability of POC devices to measure cardiac troponin I levels reliably in a moving ambulance has not previously been tested.

Objective.—This study was conducted to determine whether POC devices operated in a moving ambulance reliably duplicate the measurement of cardiac troponin I levels obtained by POC devices in the ED.

Methods.—Blood samples were obtained in the ED and the hospital from patients reporting chest pain or other cardiac complaints. Troponin I assays were then performed in a moving ambulance using two POC devices. The POC devices were placed on flat surfaces in the rear of the ambulance. The ambulance driver was instructed to keep the ambulance moving in traffic while each assay was completed. A variety of routes were taken. Each set of two assays was completed entirely during a single simulated run. The results of the two assays performed in the moving ambulance were then compared with the results of the control assay, which was performed simultaneously in the ED on the same sample.

Results.—Forty-two whole-blood samples underwent troponin I assays in a moving ambulance. Thirteen (30.9%) assays were positive. One (2.4%) was excluded because of cartridge error. Two (4.8%) were excluded because of interfering substance. No significant difference in whole-blood troponin results was found between the assays performed in the moving ambulance and those performed in the ED (intraclass correlation coefficient 0.997; 95% confidence interval 0.994 to 0.998; $p < 0.005$).

Conclusions.—When used in a moving ambulance, the POC device provided results of cardiac troponin I assays that were highly correlated to the results when the device was used in the ED. The feasibility, practicality, and clinical utility of prehospital use of POC devices must still be assessed.

▶ Early detection of injury to the myocardium decreases morbidity and mortality. Under ideal conditions, when an undifferentiated chest pain call goes out as a 911 call to the emergency medical services (EMS), the medics arrive, they evaluate the patient, and those that have 12-lead cardiac monitors obtain an electrocardiogram (ECG) and look for evidence of an ST segment elevation myocardial infarction (STEMI). If the patient is having a STEMI, then the medics notify the destination chest pain center and promptly transport the patient to that destination. If there is no evidence of a STEMI, the urgency of the call decreases. The patient may not even be taken to a chest pain center, but a local facility without catheter laboratory services, with the assumption that this is not an acute myocardial infarction (MI). If the patient is nonetheless taken to a chest pain center, most likely he or she will be placed in an emergency department bed and the workup for chest pain with repeat ECG and so on will be carried out in a routine rather than an expedient manner.

As the cardiac enzymes are drawn and ultimately return for this patient, and it is discovered that the myoglobin and or the CPK are elevated, the notion of doing "a rule out" is entertained and there is a slight elevation in the urgency that returns to the patient's evaluation. If the troponin is found to be elevated, the urgency returns and everyone becomes concerned about the patient "ruling in for an MI."

If the prehospital EMS providers have the capability of assessing troponin in the prehospital setting while the patient is on the ambulance stretcher, another valuable diagnostic parameter may be obtained. Henceforth, even if the ECG is negative, and the troponin I is found to be elevated, the patient will be presented to the emergency department as a patient with chest pain, nondiagnostic ECG, and a positive troponin. (Consider the response of the emergency department when a patient arrives with ECG findings positive for a STEMI and positive troponin I.) This changes the perception and urgency of the patient's emergency department encounter.

This study provides evidence that point of care testing can be done both accurately and precisely in the ambulance before arrival of the patient at the hospital. This procedure should be examined closely by medical directors with the intent of incorporating this test into the prehospital protocols of undifferentiated chest pain.

Just an afterthought, if medics must deal with sophisticated equipment such as left ventricular assist devices, intra-aortic balloon pumps, cardiac pacers, and continuous positive airway pressure devices, why not do field troponin I levels?

B. M. Minczak, MS, MD, PhD

Cardiac arrest survival is rare without prehospital return of spontaneous circulation

Wampler DA, Collett L, Manifold CA, et al (Univ of Texas Health Science Ctr at San Antonio; Univ of Cincinnati, OH)
Prehosp Emerg Care 16:451-455, 2012

Background.—Emergency medical services (EMS) are crucial in the management of out-of-hospital cardiac arrest (OHCA). Despite accepted termination-of-resuscitation criteria, many patients are transported to the hospital without achieving field return of spontaneous circulation (ROSC).

Objective.—We examine field ROSC influence on OHCA survival to hospital discharge in two large urban EMS systems.

Methods.—A retrospective analysis of prospectively collected data was conducted. Data collection is a component of San Antonio Fire Department's comprehensive quality assurance/quality improvement program and Cincinnati Fire Department's participation in the Cardiac Arrest Registry to Enhance Survival (CARES) project. Attempted resuscitations of medical OHCA and cardiac OHCA for San Antonio and Cincinnati, respectively, from 2008 to 2010 were analyzed by city and in aggregate.

Results.—A total of 2,483 resuscitation attempts were evaluated. Age and gender distributions were similar between cities, but ethnic profiles differed. Cincinnati had 17% ($p = 0.002$) more patients with an initial shockable rhythm and was more likely to initiate transport before field ROSC. Overall survival to hospital discharge was 165 of 2,483 (6.6%). More than one-third (894 of 2,483, 36%) achieved field ROSC. Survival with field ROSC was 17.2% (154 of 894) and without field ROSC was 0.69% (11 of 1,589). Of the 11 survivors transported prior to field ROSC, nine received defibrillation by EMS. No asystolic patient survived to hospital discharge without field ROSC.

Conclusion.—Survival to hospital discharge after OHCA is rare without field ROSC. Resuscitation efforts should focus on achieving field ROSC. Transport should be reserved for patients with field ROSC or a shockable rhythm.

▶ Emergency medical services (EMS) today are capable of providing a high level of care to victims of cardiac arrest in the prehospital environment. In addition, many communities now have public access defibrillation (PAD) programs in place as well as programs available to educate the lay public in the techniques of cardiopulmonary resuscitation (CPR). Thus victims of out-of-hospital cardiac arrest (OHCA), given the "right set of circumstances," have a reasonable chance of surviving this medical insult. With prompt recognition of the arrest, immediate initiation of CPR, short time to "first compression" early defibrillation, and a timely EMS response to the OHCA, it is not unreasonable, barring unusual medical circumstances, to expect that the resuscitation effort initiated on the victim of the cardiac arrest has a strong probability of achieving return of spontaneous circulation (ROSC). If ROSC is achieved, the patient needs to be brought to the hospital for further treatment and stabilization in an effort to preserve neurological function. However, if there are delays in recognizing an OHCA, such as an unwitnessed arrest, CPR is delayed or there is no bystander CPR, defibrillation is not performed and/or there is a delay in the summoning and the arrival of EMS, then the possibility of the resuscitation effort achieving ROSC is less likely. (Remember that the possibility of successful resuscitation decreases 7% to 10% for every minute that resuscitation is delayed.)

This study attempted to describe the relationship of achieving ROSC in the prehospital environment and survival of the victim to hospital discharge. The data support the conclusion that failure to achieve ROSC in the prehospital setting correlates to a very low survival rate to hospital discharge from an OHCA. Very few patients who did not achieve ROSC in the field survived to hospital discharge. Those that did survive had a shockable rhythm reported during their resuscitations.

The aforementioned conclusion raises a new question. Should patients who have not achieved ROSC in the field be transported to the hospital. If there were extraneous circumstances that prevented the restoration of a heartbeat and spontaneous, self-sustaining circulation in the field, should the rescuers consider termination of the resuscitation (TOR) because of the potential futility of continuing care? Will transfer to the hospital increase the chances of ROSC and survival to discharge? Is there any reason for the resuscitation to continue during transport to the hospital? Transfer of the patient to a hospital while conducting resuscitation can be fraught with hazards to the EMS personnel and to the public as the ambulance speeds to the hospital with lights and sirens. On arrival at the hospital, what else can be done? Also, the patient will be without ROSC that much longer and probably have an even smaller possibility of survival to discharge.

The aforementioned issues need to be revisited by progressive community leaders, EMS directors, hospital medical leaders, and police departments in an effort to revise protocols on how to deal with the deceased if transport is not initiated and a TOR field pronouncement is completed.

Communities that have CPR/PAD programs and a progressive EMS system need to consider the possibility of TOR protocols and the revision of protocols regarding unnecessary or unwarranted transport of patients without field ROSC to the hospital. Acceptance of TOR will take some time because family and bystanders may have difficulty dealing with the issues of disposition of the deceased (eg, coroner evaluation, calling the undertaker, contacting organ harvesting groups, clergy). Protocols and a position statement on TOR are currently available from EMS organizations. However, realizing the potential consequences that may occur as a result of TOR, community leaders may become more motivated to seek out ways to improve prehospital resuscitation in an effort to increase the possibility of achieving ROSC in the prehospital environment and improving survival from an OHCA.

B. M. Minczak, MS, MD, PhD

Genetics of myocardial infarction: a progress report

Schunkert H, Erdmann J, Samani NJ (Universität zu Lübeck, Germany; Univ of Leicester, UK)
Eur Heart J 31:918-925, 2010

A small region on chromosome 9p21.3, discovered in parallel by three groups in the year 2007, is typical of the new understanding of the genetic basis of myocardial infarction (MI). The finding emerged from the application of novel high-throughput genome-wide approaches, the risk-associated allele is frequent, acts independently of traditional risk factors, and confers a modest yet highly reproducible hazard. Since then, another 10 chromosomal regions have been identified to affect the risk of MI or coronary artery disease (CAD). Although the number of risk alleles is growing rapidly, several conclusions can already be drawn from the findings to date. First, it appears that multiple hitherto unknown molecular mechanisms—initiated by these chromosomal variants—ultimately precipitate CAD. Secondly, essentially all Caucasians carry a variable number of risk alleles such that disease manifestation is affected to some extent by these inherited factors in basically all individuals. This means that a better understanding of underlying functional genomic mechanisms may offer novel opportunities to neutralize a broadly based genetic susceptibility for CAD in a large proportion of the population. In parallel, the newly discovered genes open novel opportunities for disease prediction. In summary, modern MI genetics carries the promise to identify individuals at high risk and to improve prevention and therapy of this important disease.

▶ This is not the latest report on the link between genes and the development of myocardial infarction (MI); however, this is an important review of the state of the art.

A perfect storm of technology and sampling has made it possible to hunt for genetic loci, and these authors cited cases of allelic variants that are associated with risk of disease independent of a family history of MI. Likely, it will turn out that some allelic variation will be related to processes way upstream from hypertension or diabetes, such as changing receptor signaling in cells. No doubt at the same time the study of the mechanisms of how these newly discovered genetic elements can control the risk of MI will both reinforce our current understanding of and suggest new systems for genetic regulation.

Prevention of MI based on genetic analysis is still not ready for primetime, but the connection of genetic analysis and clinical outcome is starting to find its way.

N. B. Handly, MD, MSc, MS

Effect of Long-Term Thoracic Epidural Analgesia on Refractory Angina Pectoris: A 10-Year Experience

Richter A, Cederholm I, Fredrikson M, et al (Linköping Univ Hosp, Sweden; Linköping Univ, Sweden; et al)
J Cardiothorac Vasc Anesth 26:822-828, 2012

Objectives.—In patients with refractory angina, the adjuvant effects of long-term home self-treatment with thoracic epidural analgesia on angina, quality of life, and safety were evaluated.

Design.—A prospective, consecutive study.

Setting.—A university hospital.

Participants and Intervention.—Between January 1998 and August 2007, 152 consecutive patients with refractory angina began treatment with thoracic epidural analgesia by intermittent injections of bupivacaine (139 home treatment and 13 palliative). Data were collected until August 2008; therefore, the follow-up for each patient was between 1 and 9 years.

Measurements and Main Results.—All but 7 of the patients improved symptomatically, and the improvement was maintained throughout the period of treatment (median = 19 months; range, 1 month-8.9 years). After 1 to 2 weeks, the median (interquartile range [IQR]) Canadian Cardiovascular Society angina class decreased from 4.0 (3.0-4.0) to 2.0 (1.0-2.0), the mean ± standard deviation frequency of anginal attacks decreased from 36 ± 19 to 4.4 ± 6.8 a week, the nitroglycerin intake decreased from 27.7 ± 15.7 to 2.7 ± 4.9 a week, and the median (IQR) overall self-rated quality of life assessed by the visual analog scale increased from 25 (20-30) to 70 (50-75) (all $p < 0.001$). About one-third of the patients had a dislodgement of the epidural catheter. Apart from 1 epidural hematoma that appeared in 1 patient with a previously undiagnosed bleeding defect, no other serious catheter-related complications occurred.

Conclusions.—Long-term self-administered home treatment with thoracic epidural analgesia is a safe, widely available adjuvant treatment for patients with severe refractory angina. It produces symptomatic relief of angina and improves quality of life. The technical development of the method to protect the catheter against dislodgement is needed.

▶ Just what is the nature of your patients' medical management when no further invasive approaches are being considered for angina? These are the patients coming to the emergency department (ED) because the pain persists after taking 3 nitroglycerin tablets. They are no longer eligible for coronary artery bypass grafting or percutaneous interventions either because of diffuse vessel disease or significant comorbidities.

If they are taking their medications, there may not be much you can do in the ED besides screen for acute coronary syndromes. But if a patient is suffering from refractory angina and myocardial oxygen demand is well-controlled, there may be very little benefit that can be provided by a hospital visit.

It is not clear how many patients suffer from refractory angina; the number has been estimated to be at least 5% to 15%. What fraction appears in the ED is also not known.

The authors report their results of providing treatment for patients with refractory angina using transcutaneous epidural anesthesia (TEA) to block sympathetic innervation at the thoracic 3-5 levels. Notable is decrease in nitroglycerin use, improvement in function (increased activity without symptoms), and quality of life with the use of TEA. This sounds wonderful, but this treatment modality is not possible without significant patient attention to care: the patients self-administer bupivacaine, maintain sterility, and change bio-filters. So the success of this type of treatment is based on a culture of self-care and personal responsibility that may not be present among a number of patients. Adverse effects appear to be relatively limited among the study sample: 1 epidural hematoma and approximately 1/3 of patients had displaced catheters, but no spinal cord infections.

The study needs prospective validation and a screening tool needs to be developed to find those patients who can take care of themselves. If patients can enjoy better quality of life and seek fewer ED visits, I for one would be happy to support the use of TEA.

N. B. Handly, MD, MSc, MS

Community-based gender perspectives of triage and treatment in suspected myocardial infarction
Ravn-Fischer A, Caidahl K, Hartford M, et al (Sahlgrenska Univ Hosp, Göteborg, Sweden)
Int J Cardiol 156:139-143, 2012

Background.—The gender perspectives of the triage of acute coronary syndromes (ACS) in a community are insufficiently explored.

Methods.—Patients ($n = 3224$) with symptoms of ACS, in whom ECG was sent by the ambulance crew to a coronary care unit (CCU)/cath lab, were investigated in the municipality of Göteborg in 2004–2007. Background, triage priority, investigations and treatment were analysed (p-values age adjusted) in relation to gender. Data were compared with three published studies (1995–2002: Surveys 1–3).

Results.—Women were directly admitted to the CCU significantly less frequently than men (23 versus 35%, $p < 0.0001$). Adjusted for ECG findings, age, symptoms and medical history, odds ratio and 95% confidence limits (for direct admission; men versus women) were 0.61; 0.46–0.82.

Survey 1.—Patients with ACS, aged <80, in CCU at a university hospital ($n = 1744$). Only minor differences between women and men, with regard to investigations and treatment, were found.

Survey 2.—Patients discharged from hospital (dead or alive) with AMI, regardless of type of ward ($n = 1423$). Fewer women than men were admitted to CCU and fewer women underwent coronary angiography (21% versus 40%; $p = 0.02$) and coronary revascularisation (12% versus 27%; $p = 0.004$).

Survey 3.—Patients with symptoms of AMI ($n = 930$) and patients with a confirmed AMI ($n = 130$) from a pre-hospital perspective. Women tended to be given lower priority than men both by the ambulance dispatchers and by the ambulance crew.

Conclusion.—In our practice setting, men are given priority over women in admission to CCU, but no gender differences are seen thereafter.

▶ This analysis is based on a series of retrospective surveys performed over a 12-year period (1995-2007) within the Municipality of Göteborg, Sweden. It reveals that women and men (younger than 80 years of age) who were admitted to the critical care unit (CCU) were treated similarly in terms of echocardiography, exercise testing, coronary angiography, and coronary revascularization (including percutaneous coronary intervention and coronary artery bypass graft [CABG]). Although CABG was performed more frequently in the male group, that may be explained by the fact that more advanced vessel disease was seen in the male group. However, a considerable number of patients suffering from an acute myocardial infarction (AMI) are treated outside of the CCU, and it is in these patients that gender disparities emerge.

Among all patients with acute chest pain, or other symptoms suggestive of AMI, who called for an ambulance, women were given significantly lower priority than men at the dispatch center. Furthermore, women were admitted to the CCU less frequently than men, there was a longer period between arrival at the hospital and admission for women as compared with men, and women underwent exercise testing and coronary angiography less frequently than men. The authors suggest that some of this diagnosis inequality may be because women have more diffuse symptoms than men. In their study, women had more neck and back pain and more dyspnea and nausea than men. On the other hand, women had less diaphoresis and syncope. Although the authors note that this study was not designed to address outcomes, they report that there was a tendency (not statistically significant) toward higher mortality in women.

For more than a decade, researchers have noted gender differences in the diagnosis and treatment of acute coronary syndrome (ACS). This study shows that although men and women were treated the same once they got to the CCU, women were treated less aggressively before that time. All emergency physicians must keep in mind that women have different symptomatology than men. Actually, all health care providers need to understand this concept because even the ambulance dispatchers were guilty of a male bias in sending out ambulances to patients with possible ACS. Remember, women have what appear to be atypical symptoms when compared with men. We all need to be more willing to consider ACS in women and to treat it just as aggressively as we would in a male patient.

E. A. Ramoska, MD, MPHE

A new electrocardiographic criteria for emergent reperfusion therapy

Hennings JR, Fesmire FM (Univ of Tennessee College of Medicine Chattanooga)

Am J Emerg Med 30:994-1000, 2012

The benefit of emergency reperfusion therapy with fibrinolytics or primary percutaneous coronary intervention in patients with ST-segment elevation (STE) acute myocardial infarction (MI) is well known. However, what is not well known are which subgroups of MI patients with ST-segment depression (STD) on the 12-lead electrocardiogram (ECG) may benefit from emergent reperfusion therapy. Current clinical guidelines recommend against administering emergent reperfusion therapy to MI patients with STD on the ECG unless a true posterior MI is suspected. Overlooked subgroups of patients with STD on the initial ECG who may potentially benefit from emergent reperfusion therapy are patients with multilead STD with coexistent STE in lead aVR. This finding has been reported in MI patients with occlusion of the left main artery, occlusion of the proximal left anterior descending artery, and MI in the presence of severe multivessel coronary artery disease. Because these patients have a higher mortality in the setting of MI, we believe that this ECG finding be considered a STEMI equivalent and that patients with this finding receive consideration for emergent reperfusion therapy preferably at a center with both primary percutaneous coronary intervention and coronary artery bypass grafting capability. In this report, we present 3 such patients to heighten the awareness of the emergency physician to this phenomenon.

▶ I have been an aVR "ignorer" except for toxicological events. Sure, I am more suspicious when I see significant ST segment depression, but I do not think I have ever activated a STEMI (ST segment elevation myocardial infarction) alert based on the findings described by these authors.

A few years ago it seems that recognizing posterior MI was added to the cluster of STEMI activations by electrocardiogram (ECG) appearance. It seems that we are not done decoding the information in ECGs that signals when patients need emergent reperfusion therapy. The authors present 3 cases and highlight the literature regarding the value of recognizing the appearance of these ECGs.

Of course 3 cases do not make a proof nor can one calculate sensitivity and specificity of this presentation any time soon. Can you imagine a study that would take every patient with ST elevations in aVR and multiple area ST depressions to the catheterization lab (the gold standard)?

N. B. Handly, MD, MSc, MS

Body Mass Index and Mortality in Acute Myocardial Infarction Patients

Bucholz EM, Rathore SS, Reid KJ, et al (Yale Univ School of Medicine, New Haven, CT; Mid America Heart Inst of St Luke's Hosp, Kansas City, MO; et al)
Am J Med 125:796-803, 2012

Background.—Previous studies have described an "obesity paradox" with heart failure, whereby higher body mass index (BMI) is associated with lower mortality. However, little is known about the impact of obesity on survival after acute myocardial infarction.

Methods.—Data from 2 registries of patients hospitalized in the US with acute myocardial infarction between 2003-2004 (PREMIER) and 2005-2008 (TRIUMPH) were used to examine the association of BMI with mortality. Patients (n = 6359) were categorized into BMI groups (kg/m^2) using baseline measurements. Two sets of analyses were performed using Cox proportional hazards regression with fractional polynomials to model BMI as categorical and continuous variables. To assess the independent association of BMI with mortality, analyses were repeated, adjusting for 7 domains of patient and clinical characteristics.

Results.—Median BMI was 28.6. BMI was inversely associated with crude 1-year mortality (normal, 9.2%; overweight, 6.1%; obese, 4.7%; morbidly obese; 4.6%; $P < .001$), which persisted after multivariable adjustment. When BMI was examined as a continuous variable, the hazards curve declined with increasing BMI and then increased above a BMI of 40. Compared with patients with a BMI of 18.5, patients with higher BMIs had a 20% to 68% lower mortality at 1 year. No interactions between age ($P = .37$), sex ($P = .87$), or diabetes mellitus ($P = .55$) were observed.

Conclusions.—There appears to be an "obesity paradox" among patients after acute myocardial infarction such that higher BMI is associated with lower mortality, an effect that was not modified by patient characteristics and was comparable across age, sex, and diabetes subgroups.

▶ Imagine a world where increasing body mass index (BMI) would mean that you are more likely to survive your heart attack? Wait, you do not need to imagine any such thing as these authors found this exact result when they examined records in previously collected registries of heart attack sufferers. Their result is consistent with another study that compared survival with BMI after congestive heart failure.

Note that their work does not conclude that increasing BMI is associated with less likelihood of a heart attack. But what aspects of the study might have influenced their findings?

This study looked at the survival of those individuals who did have a heart attack and lived long enough in the hospital (1 to 3 days) to consent to the study and complete several surveys. How many patients and with what BMI values did not live to join the study? Perhaps proportionally more of the higher BMI patients who had heart attacks had already died before joining the study.

The authors noted that about 5% of the records reviewed did not have documented BMI values (BMI-less). These patients had significantly higher mortality.

The authors missed a chance to perform several sensitivity analyses within this group of patients. They could have assigned them in proportion to the known BMI distribution to each BMI group categorically or to a continuous distribution. In each assignment, the probability of death would be based randomly on the overall BMI-less death probability. Another sensitivity analysis would be to assign all these BMI-less patients to each BMI category one at a time (with the probability of death as before). This way, the authors might be able to better answer the effect of the BMI-less patients in the overall picture. Essentially they would be able to establish a range of possible values for mortality versus BMI.

If it does bear out that higher BMI provides some all-cause survival benefit after a heart attack, then it would be essential to look at specific causes of death so that we can develop an understanding of how to prevent as many deaths as possible.

N. B. Handly, MD, MSc, MS

Posterior myocardial infarction: are we failing to diagnose this?
Khan JN, Chauhan A, Mozdiak E, et al (Sandwell & West Birmingham Hosps NHS Trust, Birmingham, UK)
Emerg Med J 29:15-18, 2012

Introduction.—Isolated posterior ST-elevation myocardial infarction (STEMI) accounts for up to 7% of STEMIs. The diagnosis is suggested by indirect anterior-lead ECG changes. Confirmation requires presence of ST-elevation in posterior-leads (V7—V9). We investigated the ability of hospital doctors and paramedics to diagnose posterior STEMI (PMI).

Methods.—Doctors in the emergency department and acute medical unit at two teaching hospitals and West Midlands Ambulance Service Paramedics were asked to interpret a 12-lead ECG illustrating ST-depression and dominant R-wave in V1-V2 in the context of cardiac chest pain, and identify PMI as a potential diagnosis. Their ability to identify PMI was compared with their ability to diagnose anterolateral STEMI on a 12-lead ECG. We assessed whether doctors knew that posterior-leads were required to confirm PMI and whether doctors and nurses could position posterior-leads.

Results.—44 of the 117 doctors (38%) identified PMI as a potential diagnosis. PMI was identified by 73% of registrars, 30% of senior house-officers and 18% of house-officers. 50% of doctors who identified potential PMI knew that posterior-leads were required to confirm the diagnosis. 20% of doctors correctly positioned these and 19% knew the diagnostic criteria for PMI (ST-elevation ≥ 1 mm in V7—V9). 13 of the 60 nurses (22%) in the emergency department and acute medical unit correctly positioned posterior-leads. Five of the 50 (10%) paramedics identified PMI as a potential diagnosis. Doctors and paramedics were significantly better at diagnosing anterolateral STEMI than PMI.

Conclusions.—A significant proportion of doctors and paramedics were unable to diagnose PMI. Hence, the majority of PMIs may be being missed.

Routine use of posterior-leads in the standard assessment of patients with chest pain may identify up to an additional 7% of STEMIs, allowing prompt reperfusion therapy, which would reduce morbidity and mortality.

▶ Cardiovascular disease remains the top killer of Americans, and failure to diagnose acute coronary syndrome may result in catastrophic consequences. Identification of the posterior myocardial infarction (PMI) is a particular challenge because of the shortcomings of conventional electrocardiogram (ECG). Representing 7% of all myocardial infarctions (MIs), PMIs may only be seen if the treating physician requests posterior ECG leads. The authors of this project presented emergency physicians (EPs) with an ECG that has findings concerning for a PMI and determined what percentage of EPs were able to identify the PMI and what percentage of EPs requested the important posterior leads. Unfortunately, the authors found that only 38% of the surveyed population recognized the potential for PMI—and only half of those EPs knew to ask for the posterior leads. The authors extrapolate that the majority of PMIs are therefore being missed, increasing morbidity and mortality. It is unclear if these MIs are truly being missed. An experienced physician may establish an irregularity in the tracing and "flip the ECG" to evaluate for a PMI. Additionally, patients with concerning history and risk factors may receive cardiology consultation and undergo cardiac catheterization because of persistent pain.

E. C. Bruno, MD

Electrocardiographic Differentiation of Early Repolarization From Subtle Anterior ST-Segment Elevation Myocardial Infarction

Smith SW, Khalil A, Henry TD, et al (Hennepin County Med Ctr, Minneapolis, MN; Abbott Northwestern Hosp, Minneapolis, MN; Univ of Minnesota School of Medicine, Minneapolis; et al)
Ann Emerg Med 60:45-56, 2012

Study Objective.—Anterior ST-segment elevation myocardial infarction (STEMI) can be difficult to differentiate from early repolarization on the ECG. We hypothesize that, in addition to ST-segment elevation, T-wave amplitude to R-wave amplitude ratio (T-wave amplitude$_{avg}$/R-wave amplitude$_{avg}$), and R-wave amplitude in leads V2 to V4, computerized corrected QT interval (QTc) and upward concavity would help to differentiate the 2. We seek to determine which ECG measurements best distinguish STEMI versus early repolarization.

Methods.—This was a retrospective study of patients with anterior STEMI (2003 to 2009) and early repolarization (2003 to 2005) at 2 urban hospitals, one of which (Minneapolis Heart Institute) receives 500 STEMI patients per year. We compared the ECGs of nonobvious ("subtle") anterior STEMI with emergency department noncardiac chest pain patients with early repolarization. ST-segment elevation at the J point and 60 ms after the J point, T-wave amplitude, R-wave amplitude, QTc, upward concavity, J-wave notching, and T waves in V1 and V6 were measured. Multivariate logistic regression modeling was used to identify ECG measurements independently predictive of STEMI versus early repolarization in a derivation group and was subsequently validated in a separate group.

Results.—Of 355 anterior STEMIs identified, 143 were nonobvious, or subtle, compared with 171 early repolarization ECGs. ST-segment elevation was greater, R-wave amplitude lower, and T-wave amplitude$_{avg}$/R-wave amplitude$_{avg}$ higher in leads V2 to V4 with STEMI versus early repolarization. Computerized QTc was also significantly longer with STEMI versus early repolarization. T-wave amplitude did not differ significantly between the groups, such that the T-wave amplitude$_{avg}$/R-wave amplitude$_{avg}$ difference was entirely due to the difference in R-wave amplitude. An ECG criterion based on 3 measurements (R-wave amplitude in lead V4, ST-segment elevation 60 ms after J-point in lead V3, and QTc) was derived and validated for differentiating STEMI versus early repolarization, such that if the value of the equation ([1.196 × ST-segment elevation 60 ms after the J point in lead V3 in mm]+[0.059 × QTc in ms]−[0.326 × R-wave amplitude in lead V4 in mm]) is greater than 23.4 predicted STEMI and if less than or equal to 23.4, it predicted early repolarization in both groups, with overall sensitivity, specificity, and accuracy of 86% (95% confidence interval [CI] 79, 91), 91% (95% CI 85, 95), and 88% (95% CI 84, 92), respectively, with positive likelihood ratio 9.2 (95% CI 8.5 to 10) and negative likelihood ratio 0.1 (95% CI 0.08 to 0.3). Upward concavity, upright T wave in V1 or T wave, in V1 greater than T wave in V6, and J-wave notching did not provide important information.

Conclusion.—R-wave amplitude is lower, ST-segment elevation greater, and QTc longer for subtle anterior STEMI versus early repolarization. In combination with other clinical data, this derived and validated ECG equation could be an important adjunct in the diagnosis of anterior STEMI.

▶ Emergency physicians (EPs) are routinely presented with patients and their accompanying electrocardiograms (ECGs) and must decide when to activate the cardiac catheterization laboratory (cath lab) based on the findings of an acute ST-segment elevation myocardial infarction (STEMI). At times, this decision can be blatant. However, factors can be less obvious when the ECG has ST-segment elevations in the requisite distribution, but the pattern may be more consistent with J-point elevation. The authors attempted to tease out which patients with the more benign appearing J-point elevation might actually be candidates for the cath lab. After eliminating patients with ECGs that demonstrated the straightforward STEMI and focusing on the less clear cases, they identified 3 separate ECG findings that trended toward STEMI. In STEMI, the ECGs tended to have lower R-wave amplitude, greater ST-segment elevation, and longer QTc intervals. The conclusions are broad based when compared with the results, and the results provide more details. However, these details are not conducive to a rapid emergency department assessment. EPs and the interventional cardiologists must continue to accept a certain false-positive rate in order to meet the requisite door-to-balloon guidelines.

E. C. Bruno, MD

4 Respiratory Distress

Congestive Heart Failure

Feasibility of continuous positive airway pressure by primary care paramedics
Cheskes S, Thomson S, Turner L (Sunnybrook—Osler Centre for Prehospital Medicine, Toronto, Ontario, Canada)
Prehosp Emerg Care 16:535-540, 2012

Introduction.—Continuous positive airway pressure (CPAP) has been used effectively in the prehospital environment for a wide range of respiratory emergencies. The feasibility of CPAP when used by primary care paramedics (PCPs) has not been established.

Objective.—We sought to study the feasibility of prehospital CPAP when used by paramedics trained to the primary care paramedic (PCP) level compared with those trained to the advanced care paramedic (ACP) level. Our hypothesis was that the feasibility of CPAP use by paramedics trained to the PCP level is similar to that of paramedics trained to the ACP level.

Methods.—We conducted an observational study of 302 consecutive cases of CPAP use over one year beginning June 25, 2009. We defined compliant use as 100% adherence to the provincial CPAP medical directive. The criteria for compliance included specifics of patient presentation, vital signs, and appropriate documentation by the paramedic, as well as proper use, titration, and discontinuation of CPAP equipment according to protocol. Data were abstracted from ambulance call reports.

Results.—Using the criteria set out for compliant CPAP use, the highest level of compliance among the ACPs and the PCPs was 98.6% and 98.9%, respectively, for documenting indication for CPAP use. The lowest level of compliance among the ACPs was 84.4% for titration of CPAP during treatment, and the lowest level of compliance among the PCPs was 90% for adherence to criteria for CPAP application according to patients' vital signs. Overall, the criteria for compliant use of CPAP were met for 76.8% (232/302) of the call reports examined. The rate of compliant use of CPAP was 75.9% (161/212) for ACP calls and 78.9% (71/90) for PCP calls. The difference between rates of compliant use for ACP calls versus PCP calls was not statistically significant (χ^2 [1 df] $= 0.31$, $p = 0.66$).

Conclusions.—This study found no significant difference in the compliant use of prehospital CPAP between paramedics trained to the PCP level and those trained to the ACP level. This study suggests that CPAP use by

PCP-level paramedics may be feasible. Further study is required to determine whether compliance translates to safe use of prehospital CPAP by PCP-level paramedics.

▶ When speaking about "airway" management, most listeners think about endotracheal intubation, placement of a laryngeal mask airway (LMA), a King airway, Combitubes, Bougies, and so on. Now, with the advent of continuous positive airway pressure (CPAP) and its debut in the prehospital arena, the combined use of a mask and a pressurized oxygen source that can be regulated has changed both the perception of airway management based on preliminary data analysis. This technique has improved the final treatment outcomes of patients in various forms of respiratory distress.

Endotracheal intubation in both the in-hospital and prehospital venue has its potential risks and benefits; unrecognized esophageal intubations, broken teeth, tracheal injury, aspiration of secretions into the trachea-bronchial tree or cardiac arrest secondary to a failed airway, and/or prolonged apnea from either the disease process or the use of pharmacological agents. The application of CPAP does not require manipulation of the airway, nor does it require the use of paralytics and is less likely to cause problems when compared with endotracheal intubation. Endotracheal intubation may decrease the possibility of aspiration, whereas CPAP does not provide protection from aspiration.

By applying an appropriate face mask and providing pressure to the patients airway, especially at the end of expiration, via, for example, CPAP, the trachea-bronchial tree has lower resistance to inspiration and expiration, alveoli are recruited via the pores of Kohn, the intra-alveolar pressure favors the movement of oxygen into the pulmonary vasculature, and the removal of carbon dioxide from the pulmonary circulation. Training for the use of CPAP is easily accomplished and use of CPAP by advanced care paramedics has had a favorable history.

This study attempts to quantify the use of CPAP by medics with lesser training. The initial data suggest that CPAP has a future with medics with various levels of training. It is not unreasonable to speculate that CPAP may even its way into the treatment protocols of emergency medical technicians in the future, as have automatic external defibrillators.

B. M. Minczak, MS, MD, PhD

Pulmonary Embolism

Ordering CT pulmonary angiography to exclude pulmonary embolism: defense versus evidence in the emergency room
Rohacek M, Buatsi J, Szucs-Farkas Z, et al (Univ Hosp Bern, Freiburgstrasse, Switzerland)
Intensive Care Med 38:1345-1351, 2012

Purpose.—To identify reasons for ordering computed tomography pulmonary angiography (CTPA), to identify the frequency of reasons for CTPA reflecting defensive behavior and evidence-based behavior, and to identify the impact of defensive medicine and of training about diagnosing pulmonary embolism (PE) on positive results of CTPA.

Methods.—Physicians in the emergency department of a tertiary care hospital completed a questionnaire before CTPA after being trained about diagnosing PE and completing questionnaires.

Results.—Nine hundred patients received a CTPA during 3 years. For 328 CTPAs performed during the 1-year study period, 140 (43 %) questionnaires were completed. The most frequent reasons for ordering a CTPA were to confirm/rule out PE (93 %), elevated D-dimers (66 %), fear of missing PE (55 %), and Wells/simplified revised Geneva score (53 %). A positive answer for "fear of missing PE" was inversely associated with positive CTPA (OR 0.36, 95 % CI 0.14-0.92, $p = 0.033$), and "Wells/simplified revised Geneva score" was associated with positive CTPA (OR 3.28, 95 % CI 1.24-8.68, $p = 0.017$). The proportion of positive CTPA was higher if a questionnaire was completed, compared to the 2-year comparison period (26.4 vs. 14.5 %, OR 2.12, 95 % CI 1.36-3.29, $p < 0.001$). The proportion of positive CTPA was non-significantly higher during the study period than during the comparison period (19.2 vs. 14.5 %, OR 1.40, 95 % CI 0.98-2.0, $p = 0.067$).

Conclusion.—Reasons for CTPA reflecting defensive behavior-such as "fear of missing PE"-were frequent, and were associated with a decreased odds of positive CTPA. Defensive behavior might be modifiable by training in using guidelines.

▶ Pulmonary embolism (PE), as a diagnosis, eludes physicians of all specialties. The authors of this survey-based study assessed the reasons why European emergency physicians order computed tomography pulmonary angiography (CTPA) in the quest to find the next PE. Citing a scarcity of data regarding defensive medicine practices, the European-based emergency physicians may be subject to a less litigious society when compared with their American counterparts.

PE pretest probability training may have made the greatest impact in the process, giving focused information on the assessment of and further diagnostic testing in the evaluation of patients with suspected PE. The results demonstrated that "fear of missing PE" was referenced in 55% of the cases, bringing the combination of concern for the patient and medical malpractice to the forefront. However, this specific concern was actually inversely related to a positive CTPA. In contrast, evidence-based medicine tools such as the Wells/Geneva score did correlate with finding PEs.

The data are somewhat limited in that only 43% of the possible 328 CTPAs during the study period had surveys completed.

E. C. Bruno, MD

Evaluation of pulmonary embolism in the emergency department and consistency with a national quality measure: quantifying the opportunity for improvement

Venkatesh AK, Kline JA, Courtney DM, et al (Brigham and Women's Hosp-Massachusetts General Hosp—Harvard Affiliated Emergency Medicine Residency, Boston)

Arch Intern Med 172:1028-1032, 2012

Background.—The National Quality Forum (NQF) has endorsed a performance measure designed to increase imaging efficiency for the evaluation of pulmonary embolism (PE) in the emergency department (ED). To our knowledge, no published data have examined the effect of patient-level predictors on performance.

Methods.—To quantify the prevalence of avoidable imaging in ED patients with suspected PE, we performed a prospective, multicenter observational study of ED patients evaluated for PE from 2004 through 2007 at 11 US EDs. Adult patients tested for PE were enrolled, with data collected in a standardized instrument. The primary outcome was the proportion of imaging that was potentially avoidable according to the NQF measure. Avoidable imaging was defined as imaging in a patient with low pretest probability for PE, who either did not have a D-dimer test ordered or who had a negative D-dimer test result. We performed subanalyses testing alternative pretest probability cutoffs and imaging definitions on measure performance as well as a secondary analysis to identify factors associated with inappropriate imaging. χ^2 Test was used for bivariate analysis of categorical variables and multivariable logistic regression for the secondary analysis.

Results.—We enrolled 5940 patients, of whom 4113 (69%) had low pretest probability of PE. Imaging was performed in 2238 low-risk patients (38%), of whom 811 had no D-dimer testing, and 394 had negative D-dimer test results. Imaging was avoidable, according to the NQF measure, in 1205 patients (32%; 95% CI, 31%-34%). Avoidable imaging owing to not ordering a D-dimer test was associated with age (odds ratio [OR], 1.15 per decade; 95% CI, 1.10-1.21). Avoidable imaging owing to imaging after a negative D-dimer test result was associated with inactive malignant disease (OR, 1.66; 95% CI, 1.11-2.49).

Conclusions.—One-third of imaging performed for suspected PE may be categorized as avoidable. Improving adherence to established diagnostic protocols is likely to result in significantly fewer patients receiving unnecessary irradiation and substantial savings.

▶ The National Quality Forum, a group that advises the federal government's Agency for Healthcare Research and Quality, has endorsed an effort to decrease the number of computed tomography and nuclear medicine imaging studies for suspected pulmonary embolism (PE). Retrospective analysis determined that between 7% and 25% of PE imaging was unnecessary. Further using these recommendations, the authors of this multicenter study prospectively tested these measures, looking to determine the number of unnecessary imaging studies performed. They reported that 38% of the low-risk patients, determined by hemodynamic stability and a low-risk Wells score, underwent imaging, including nearly 400 patients (11%) with negative D-dimer tests. No explanation for the imaging decision was given, though a search for alternative diagnosis may be the justification. Of the patients determined to have an avoidable imaging procedure, 1.3% actually were found to have a PE. These findings call into question the acceptable miss rate and the practice of defensive medicine. When faced with a patient with PE in the differential, an accurately calculated Wells score, derived from the information provided by the patient, and a negative D-dimer should absolve the emergency physician from any further pursuit of PE.

Unfortunately, the primary outcome studied in the project was not the presence of PE, but rather the proportion of imaging that was potentially avoidable based on the endorsed protocol.

E. C. Bruno, MD

Normalization of Vital Signs Does Not Reduce the Probability of Acute Pulmonary Embolism in Symptomatic Emergency Department Patients
Kline JA, Corredor DM, Hogg MM, et al (Carolinas Med Ctr, Charlotte, NC)
Acad Emerg Med 19:11-17, 2012

Objectives.—In a patient with symptoms of pulmonary embolism (PE), the presence of an elevated pulse, respiratory rate, shock index, or decreased pulse oximetry increases pretest probability of PE. The objective of this study was to evaluate if normalization of an initially abnormal vital sign can be used as evidence to lower the suspicion for PE.

Methods.—This was a prospective, noninterventional, single-center study of diagnostic accuracy conducted on adults presenting to an academic emergency department (ED), with at least one predefined symptom or sign of PE and one risk factor for PE. Clinical data, including the first four sets of vital signs, were recorded while the patient was in the ED. All patients underwent computed tomography pulmonary angiography (CTPA) and had 45-day follow-up as criterion standards. Diagnostic accuracy of each vital sign (pulse rate, respiratory rate, shock index, pulse oximetry) at each time was examined by the area under the receiver operating characteristic curve (AUC).

Results.—A total of 192 were enrolled, including 35 (18%) with PE. All patients had vital signs at triage, and 174 (91%), 135 (70%), and 106 (55%) had second to fourth sets of vital signs obtained, respectively. The initial pulse oximetry reading had the highest AUC (0.63, 95% confidence interval [CI] = 0.50 to 0.76) for predicting PE, and no other vital sign at any point had an AUC over 0.60. Among patients with an abnormal pulse rate, respiratory rate, shock index, or pulse oximetry at triage that subsequently normalized, the prevalences of PE were 18, 14, 19, and 33%, respectively.

Conclusions.—Clinicians should not use the observation of normalized vital signs as a reason to forego objective testing for symptomatic patients with a risk factor for PE.

▶ Further evidence of the difficulty in diagnosing a pulmonary embolism (PE) is unnecessary. Despite the volumes of literature presented over the last 15 years or more, the diagnosis is elusive. After a clinical evaluation and potential use of 1 or more scoring systems, the emergency physician (EP) must then decide if a diagnostic test (eg, D-dimer, computed tomography pulmonary angiography) is warranted. The EP may choose to monitor the patient to see if concerning clinical parameters, such as tachycardia, low pulse oximetry, or blood pressure, would improve during an observational period in the emergency department. The authors of this observational, noninterventional study found that normalization of abnormal vital signs was not adequate to rule out PE. The presenting vital signs were fundamental to the evaluation of patients with suspected PEs, and normalization of the abnormal vital signs did not predict a lower risk of having a PE. They also found the hypoxia was the most predictive of disease in this patient population.

E. C. Bruno, MD

Risk factors associated with delayed diagnosis of acute pulmonary embolism
Smith SB, Geske JB, Morgenthaler TI (Mayo Clinic College of Medicine, Rochester, MN)
J Emerg Med 42:1-6, 2012

Background.—Prompt diagnosis and treatment of acute pulmonary embolism (PE) is essential to reduce mortality. Risk factors for PE are well known, but factors associated with delayed diagnosis are less clear.

Objective.—Our objective was to identify clinical factors associated with delayed diagnosis of patients with acute PE presenting to a tertiary-care emergency department (ED).

Methods.—We studied 400 consecutive adults who presented to our ED with acute, symptomatic PE. All patients were diagnosed by computed tomography (CT) angiography. Early diagnosis was defined as CT diagnosis <12 h from ED arrival, and delayed diagnosis as CT diagnosis >12 h. Univariate and multiple logistic regression models were used to identify factors associated with delayed diagnosis. Odds ratios with 95% confidence intervals are reported.

Results.—The median time from arrival to diagnosis was 2.4 h (interquartile range 1.4–7.6), and 73 (18.3%) patients had delayed diagnosis. Patients aged >65 years and those with coronary artery disease or congestive heart failure had longer times from ED arrival to CT diagnosis, whereas patients with recent immobility had shorter times. Patients diagnosed >12 h were older and had higher rates of morbid obesity and coronary artery disease, whereas patients diagnosed <12 h had higher rates of tachycardia. In multiple regression modeling, tachycardia and recent immobility remained associated with early diagnosis, whereas morbid obesity remained associated with delayed diagnosis.

Conclusions.—Older patients with cardiovascular comorbidities had longer times from ED arrival to CT diagnosis. Our data suggest that these patients represent more of a diagnostic challenge than those presenting with traditional risk factors for PE, such as tachycardia and recent immobilization. Physicians should consider these factors to diagnosis acute PE promptly in the ED.

▶ The diagnosis of an acute pulmonary embolism (PE) requires clinical suspicion and appropriate testing. Causes for delays, real or perceived, in diagnosing a PE are multifactorial. The authors of this retrospective review assessed 400 patients with confirmed symptomatic PEs and attempted to identify risk factors that predicted delay in diagnosis. They found that patients with elements of the Wells score for PE trended toward more rapid diagnosis; those patients with potential alternative etiologies for their symptoms, specifically coronary artery disease (CAD), congestive heart failure (CHF), and age greater than 65 were more likely to experience the delay in identification of the offending PE. Delay in diagnosis may not translate to delay in management because patients (CAD and CHF) may receive supplemental oxygen and anticoagulation during the admission, and the diagnosis of PE may reveal itself after other potential etiologies are ruled out. A point of information that warrants discussion is the definition of a delay in diagnosis. The authors report 12 hours from arrival in the emergency department (ED) as a postponement, not 3 hours (ie, an average length of stay in the ED). Treating emergency physicians therefore are not obligated to diagnose every PE in the ED, despite the best efforts of the admitting physicians.

E. C. Bruno, MD

5 Infections and Immunologic Disorders

Lower mortality in sepsis patients admitted through the ED vs direct admission
Powell ES, Khare RK, Courtney DM, et al (Northwestern Univ, Chicago, IL)
Am J Emerg Med 30:432-439, 2012

Purpose.—Early aggressive resuscitation in patients with severe sepsis decreases mortality but requires extensive time and resources. This study analyzes if patients with sepsis admitted through the emergency department (ED) have lower inpatient mortality than do patients admitted directly to the hospital.

Procedures.—We performed a cross-sectional analysis of hospitalizations with a principal diagnosis of sepsis in institutions with an annual minimum of 25 ED and 25 direct admissions for sepsis, using data from the 2008 Nationwide Inpatient Sample. Analyses were controlled for patient and hospital characteristics and examined the likelihood of either early (2-day postadmission) or overall inpatient mortality.

Findings.—Of 98 896 hospitalizations with a principal diagnosis of sepsis, from 290 hospitals, 80 301 were admitted through the ED and 18 595 directly to the hospital. Overall sepsis inpatient mortality was 17.1% for ED admissions and 19.7% for direct admissions ($P < .001$). Overall early sepsis mortality was 6.9%: 6.8% for ED admissions and 7.4% for direct admissions ($P = .005$). Emergency department patients had a greater proportion of comorbid conditions, were more likely to have Medicaid or be uninsured (12.5% vs 8.4%; $P < .001$), and were more likely to be admitted to urban, large bed-size, or teaching hospitals ($P < .001$). The risk-adjusted odds ratio for overall mortality for ED admissions was 0.83 (95% confidence interval, 0.80-0.87) and 0.92 for early mortality (95% confidence interval, 0.86-0.98), as compared with direct admissions to the hospital.

Conclusion.—Admission for sepsis through the ED was associated with lower early and overall inpatient mortality in this large national sample.

▶ Septic patients may have a mortality rate up to 60%. Although controversy surrounds the early goal-directed therapy bundle and associated dedicated time and resources, the discussion has likely resulted in emergency physicians being more aware of and more aggressive in the management of these septic patients. However, patients do not always arrive through the emergency department (ED) waiting room or ambulance bay. Patients may also be admitted directly by their primary physician, but this may raise concern about the timeliness of interventions and resuscitation. The authors of this cross-sectional analysis retrospectively assessed the mortality differences between patients admitted through the ED and those admitted directly. Patients transferred from an outside facility were excluded because they may have received resuscitative measures (eg, intravenous fluids, antibiotics, vasopressors) prior to transportation to the receiving facility. With statistical significance, the authors demonstrated a lower mortality in the ED group, despite having more comorbidities than the compared set. These findings are further evidence that emergency physicians and the ED nurses and staff are uniquely trained and qualified to treat critically ill patients, despite countless complaints and snide remarks regarding the quality of ED care by primary physicians.

E. C. Bruno, MD

Advanced endotracheal tube biofilm stage, not duration of intubation, is related to pneumonia
Wilson A, Gray D, Karakiozis J, et al (West Virginia Univ, Morgantown)
J Trauma Acute Care Surg 72:916-923, 2012

Background.—Biofilms are complex communities of living bacteria surrounded by a protective glycocalyx. Biofilms have been implicated in the development of infections such as dental caries and hardware infections. Biofilms form on endotracheal tubes (ETT) and can impact airway resistance. The lifecycle of a biofilm has four stages. We hypothesize that there is a relationship between the stage of biofilm on the ETT and development of pneumonia.

Methods.—Thirty-two ETT were analyzed for biofilms and staged. Staging was performed by a microbiologist blinded to all patient information. Data included development of pneumonia, duration of intubation, comorbidities, and microbiology. Pneumonia was defined as presence of fever, WBC > 12 K or < 4 K, infiltrate on chest X-ray, and purulent sputum with +lower airway culture (bronchoalveolar lavage or brush). Statistics were performed by a biostatistician; $p < 0.05$ defined significance.

Results.—There were 11 women and 21 men with a mean age of 50 years. Mean intensive care unit days were 13 (standard deviation ± 9.9) and mean length of intubation was 7.4 days (standard deviation ± 5.0). Half (16 of 32) the patients developed pneumonia while intubated. Eight of 10 patients with a stage IV biofilm had pneumonia. There was a relationship between increasing biofilm stage with the incidence of pneumonia ($p < 0.05$). Stage IV biofilms were associated with pneumonia ($p < 0.02$). There was no relationship to duration of intubation, patient age or hospital stay and biofilm stage.

Conclusions.—Advanced biofilm stage (stage IV) is associated with pneumonia. Duration of intubation does not predict biofilm stage.

▶ Intubated patients are at risk for pneumonia because of a loss of protective reflexes and more direct access of pathogens to the deep lung tissues. There is a bundle of procedures expected to prevent pneumonias, and each should reduce the risk of bacterial infiltration. It appears that our respiratory friend, the endotracheal tube (ETT), is a double-edged sword.

Our understanding of bacterial growth has increased by the recognition of free-floating monocellular and attached film polymicrobial aspects. Four stages of film growth are highlighted in the manuscript, each having a functional role for the bacteria. On ETTs, the last stage suggestive of a growth beyond nutritional resources or an increase of toxic wastes is followed by a breakup of the film and may be important to seeding infections elsewhere such as in the lungs. The authors chose to compare characteristics of patients on ventilators including patterns of biofilms on ETTs and the risk of pneumonia.

In a small sample of patients who had been intubated, it was possible to identify the stage of biofilm after the patient was extubated. The most significant correlation of pneumonia was that the ETT demonstrated the last stage of biofilm growth. Duration of intubation, days' stay in the intensive care unit, and other factors such as comorbidities were all unrelated to pneumonia.

If it can be shown that an ETT with late-stage biofilm status is a causal factor for development of ventilatory-associated pneumonia, it will be essential to work with our engineer brothers to find materials that will resist biofilm growth.

N. B. Handly, MD, MSc, MS

Viral Meningitis: Which Patients Can Be Discharged from the Emergency Department?
Mohseni MM, Wilde JA (Med College of Georgia, Augusta)
J Emerg Med 2012 [Epub ahead of print]

Background.—Even in an era when cases of viral meningitis outnumber bacterial meningitis by at least 25:1, most patients with clinical meningitis are hospitalized.

Objective.—We describe the clinical characteristics of an unusual outbreak of viral meningitis that featured markedly elevated cerebrospinal fluid white blood cell counts (CSF WBC). A validated prediction model for viral meningitis was applied to determine which hospital admissions could have been avoided.

Methods.—Data were collected retrospectively from patients presenting to our tertiary care center. Charts were reviewed in patients with CSF pleocytosis (CSF WBC > 7 cells/mm^3) and a clinical diagnosis of meningitis between March 1, 2003 and July 1, 2003. Cases were identified through hospital infection control and by surveying all CSF specimens submitted to the microbiology laboratory during the outbreak.

Results.—There were 78 cases of viral meningitis and 1 case of bacterial meningitis identified. Fifty-eight percent of the viral meningitis cases were confirmed by culture or polymerase chain reaction to be due to Enterovirus. Mean CSF WBC count was 571 cells/mm^3, including 20 patients with a CSF WBC count > 750 cells/mm^3 (25%) and 11 patients with values > 1000 cells/mm^3 (14%). Sixty-four of 78 patients (82%) were hospitalized. Rates of headache, photophobia, nuchal rigidity, vomiting, and administration of intravenous fluids in the Emergency Department were no different between admitted and discharged patients. Only 26/78 (33%) patients with viral meningitis would have been admitted if the prediction model had been used.

Conclusions.—Although not all cases of viral meningitis are necessarily suitable for outpatient management, use of a prediction model for viral meningitis may have helped decrease hospitalization by nearly 60%, even though this outbreak was characterized by unusually high levels of CSF pleocytosis.

▶ When faced with patients with signs and symptoms (headache, nuchal rigidity, and photophobia) concerning for meningitis, emergency physicians must first perform the lumbar puncture and then analyze the results to determine the presence or absence of meningitis. The decision to admit patients for further management not only focuses on the determination of bacterial versus viral meningitis, but also on the need for supportive care (intravenous fluid hydration, antiemetics, and pain control). The authors of this cohort study looked to determine if some patients could be safely managed as outpatients when diagnosed with a viral etiology. Using a previously validated scoring model, the authors retrospectively reviewed the charts of a specific cohort—patients afflicted with meningitis during a spring outbreak of viral meningitis. The scoring system assessed the spinal fluid's gram stain, absolute neutrophil count, and protein as well as the peripheral absolute neutrophil count and the presence of seizure-like activity.

The product is admittedly biased by the predominance of viral meningitis patients in the presence of the epidemic, and limited by the retrospective nature of the study. However, the results do demonstrate that some patients with viral meningitis could be safely managed as an outpatient if the only parameters are the diagnostic test results. The patient's comfort and hydration status must be considered when attempting to disposition them.

E. C. Bruno, MD

The degree of bandemia in septic ED patients does not predict inpatient mortality

Ward MJ, Fertel BS, Bonomo JB, et al (Univ of Cincinnati, OH)
Am J Emerg Med 30:181-183, 2012

Background.—A delay in diagnosis of sepsis and appropriate treatment increases subsequent mortality. An association with the degree of bandemia, or the presence of immature neutrophils in the white blood cell count, has not been explored in septic patients presenting to the emergency department (ED). We hypothesized that the presenting band levels would be higher in septic patients who die in hospital compared with survivors.

Methods.—This study reviewed charts of ED patients presenting with sepsis to a single urban, academic, tertiary care ED with an annual census of 80,000 visits. Patients were included if they had bandemia assessed and were eligible for early goal-directed therapy. Reviewers blinded to the study purpose abstracted data using predetermined definitions. The band level was compared between patients who died and those who survived to discharge using the Mann-Whitney *U* test. Logistic regression was used to estimate the effect of bandemia levels on the odds of death.

Results.—Ninety-six patients meeting inclusion criteria were enrolled; 2 were excluded with incomplete data. Mean age was 59 years, 53% were white, and 51% were male. Thirty-two patients (34%) died during admission. The median band levels in patients who died was 17% (range, 0%-67%); and in patients surviving to discharge, the median band level was 9% (range, 0%-77%) (difference in medians, 8%; CI_{95}, −27.04 to 11.04; $P = .222$).

Conclusions.—The band level on presentation was not found to be associated with inpatient mortality in ED patients with sepsis who are eligible for early goal-directed therapy.

▶ With the anticipated increase in sepsis cases because of the aging population, identification of which patients are in need of more aggressive measures is important. A complete blood count (CBC) with manual differential may be included in the standard order set for the diagnostic workup of patients with findings consistent with sepsis. Bandemia, representing immature white blood cells of greater than 10% is indicative of systemic inflammatory response syndrome and may press the patient into the population that warrants early goal-directed therapy. The authors of this retrospective review attempted to draw a correlation between bandemia and mortality from sepsis. The authors emphatically report that the presence of bandemia did not predict mortality (17% vs 8%). Unfortunately, the study is limited strongly by a small sample size and retrospective chart review design. Considering the prevalence of sepsis, a larger prospective project could be undertaken. Dogma dictates that physician viewing the CBC with 17% bands is going to be even more concerned about the patient's well-being.

E. C. Bruno, MD

Acute meningitis prognosis using cerebrospinal fluid interleukin-6 levels

Vázquez JA, Adducci MdC, Coll C, et al (Hosp Italiano de San Justo, Buenos Aires, Argentina; Univ of Buenos Aires, Argentina; et al)

J Emerg Med 43:322-327, 2012

Background.—Improved diagnostic tests would aid in diagnosing and treating community-acquired meningitis.

Objective.—To analyze the diagnostic value of interleukin-6 (IL-6) in the cerebrospinal fluid (CSF) of patients presenting with symptoms of acute meningitis.

Material and Methods.—In a 6-month prospective, observational, cross-sectional emergency department (ED) study, serum and CSF samples were obtained from all patients with a headache and fever in whom the physician suspected meningitis. Patients were excluded if computed tomography findings contraindicated a lumbar puncture, if they had bleeding disorders, or if their serum indicated bleeding. IL-6 levels were measured and compared in patients with (Group A) and without (Group B) bacterial meningitis.

Results.—Samples were obtained from 53 patients, of whom 40 were ultimately found to have meningitis. These 40 patients averaged 49.6 ± 21.9 years, with number of men 18 (45%), hospitalizations 21 (52%), mortality 3 (.07%), and IL-6 average rating 491 (median: 14.5; range 0000−6000). Findings in the two groups were: Group A (with meningitis): n = 13, average IL-6 level: 1495 (median: 604; 25/75 percentiles: 232.5−2030; 95% confidence interval [CI] 371.7−2618.6; range 64−6000). Group B (with aseptic meningitis): n = 27, average IL-6 level: 7.34 (median: 5; 25/75 percentiles: 0.0/15.1; 95% CI 3.94−10.73; range 0−23.6). Mann-Whitney rank sum test: $p < 0.0001$.

Conclusions.—In patients with acute bacterial meningitis, CSF cytokine concentrations are elevated. Measuring CSF inflammatory cytokine levels in patients with acute meningitis could be a valuable ED diagnostic tool. Using this tool could improve the prognosis of patients with bacterial meningitis by allowing more rapid initiation of antibiotic treatment.

▶ Headache is a common presenting complaint, but when it coincides with fever and neck stiffness, the emergency physician (EP) must consider the more dire diagnosis of meningitis. The current standard to identify the presence of meningitis remains the diagnostic lumbar puncture. This procedure can be technically difficult, especially with the growing obesity epidemic. EPs would likely embrace an alternative diagnostic test that did not involve the more invasive spinal needle. The authors of this study evaluated the effectiveness of the interleukin-6 (IL-6) level to determine the presence of meningitis.

The report should be described as a preliminary effort. The clinical applicability of the use of IL-6 remains limited because of the small collection of patients. The inclusion criteria can only be described as generous, considering a patient with acute appendicitis (fever, nausea/vomiting, and more than 1 systemic inflammatory response syndrome criteria) would be included in the studied cohort. However, the results are promising. No patient diagnosed with bacterial diagnosis had a low IL-6 level, but was also elevated in those patients with aseptic meningitis. The authors also found a correlation between the absolute IL-6 level and mortality. At this point, more robust analysis of the application of IL-6 level in the diagnostic evaluation of acute meningitis is necessary and EPs are not absolved of the need to perform the spinal tap.

E. C. Bruno, MD

Ambulatory Intravenous Antibiotic Therapy for Children With Preseptal Cellulitis
Brugha RE, Abrahamson E (Chelsea and Westminster NHS Trust, London, UK)
Pediatr Emerg Care 28:226-228, 2012

Objective.—This study aimed to compare the use of outpatient ambulatory care versus admission for intravenous antibiotics in the management of preseptal cellulitis.

Methods.—This is a retrospective consecutive cohort study of children younger than 16 years presenting to an Inner London Paediatric Emergency Department with signs and symptoms of preseptal cellulitis.

Results.—A total of 94 cases were identified during a 17-month period. Of them, 30 children were prescribed oral antibiotics. One child did not receive treatment. Of the 63 children prescribed with intravenous antibiotics, 42 were managed on an ambulatory basis and 21 were admitted. There was no significant difference in duration of treatment in days between those on ambulatory management and those admitted (2.79 ± 0.8 vs 2.76 ± 1.9, $P = 0.94$) or in the rate of complications. The net cost saving was \$205,924 (£131,065; €147,578) overall, equal to \$4900 (£3120; €3513) per patient.

Conclusions.—Ambulatory intravenous antibiotics with daily review are a safe and cost-effective alternative to inpatient admission in simple preseptal cellulitis for children in our population who require parenteral antibiotics.

▶ Preseptal, or periorbital, cellulitis is a facial soft tissue infection that is generally managed with oral antibiotics, supportive care, and close follow-up. The emergency physician must be convinced that the presenting condition is the periorbital cellulitis and not the more sinister cousin, orbital cellulitis. Elimination of findings consistent with orbital cellulitis, including ophthalmoplegia, proptosis, and loss of visual acuity, can reassure the treating emergency physician that the condition is preseptal, but intravenous antibiotics may still be warranted in the more concerning cases of periorbital cellulitis.

The authors of this retrospective review assess the feasibility of an outpatient intravenous antibiotics service to manage periorbital cellulitis. Patients fall into 3 groups: oral antibiotics, outpatient intravenous antibiotics, and inpatient intravenous antibiotics. The results reviewed an extremely low complication rate in all 3 divisions, and only one patient in the study was ultimately diagnosed with orbital cellulitis and was treated nonoperatively. Without blinding patients, the results further suggest that clinical impression of the severity of illness should guide management, specifically inpatient versus outpatient. Furthermore, obtaining outpatient intravenous therapy services, especially in the nontertiary care centers, is a challenge, making the option of ambulatory intravenous antibiotic therapy from the emergency department less desirable.

E. C. Bruno, MD

U.S. Emergency Department Visits for Meningitis, 1993–2008

Takhar SS, Ting SA, Camargo CA Jr, et al (Brigham and Women's Hosp, Boston, MA; Massachusetts General Hosp, Boston, MA)
Acad Emerg Med 19:632-639, 2012

Objectives.—Large-scale epidemiologic studies of meningitis in the emergency department (ED) setting are lacking. Using a nationwide sample, the authors determined the frequency of meningitis visits and characterize management.

Methods.—Using National Hospital Ambulatory Medical Care Survey (NHAMCS) data, 1993 through 2008, meningitis diagnoses were studied and national rates were estimated via standard weighting procedures.

Results.—Meningitis was diagnosed at 1,048,000 visits (95% confidence interval [CI] = 893,000 to 1,203,000) during 1993 through 2008. This is 66,000 cases annually, or 62 per 100,000 visits, with no change over time ($p = 0.20$). ED diagnoses were unspecified (60%), viral (31%), bacterial (8%), and fungal (1%) meningitis. Median age was 24 years (interquartile range = 9 to 40 years). While 1.97 times as many adults were diagnosed with meningitis (95% CI = 1.83 to 2.13), meningitis accounted for a similar proportion of visits among children and adults (ratio = 1.33, 95% CI = 0.58 to 2.63). Per population, children were more likely to have a meningitis visit (31 vs. 21 per 100,000; ratio = 1.48, 95% CI = 1.003 to 2.10); children aged younger than 3 years had the highest rate (98 per 100,000, 95% CI = 63 to 133). Spring and summer visits were 1.25 times as numerous as fall and winter (95% CI = 1.15 to 1.36). Third-generation cephalosporins were administered in 42%, analgesics in 19%, and antiemetics in 15% of cases, and 66% were admitted to the hospital (95% CI = 58% to 73%).

Conclusions.—Meningitis is rare, diagnosed at 62 per 100,000 ED visits. Rates have been stable over time. Children are 1.48 times more likely to have a visit for meningitis, although adults make twice as many visits. Absence of consensus guidelines for patients suspected of having viral meningitis but being tested for bacterial meningitis may lead to variability in admission and prescribing decisions.

▶ This study uses a large national database to estimate meningitis rates over a 16-year period. Since they used only emergency department (ED) data and reported just ED diagnoses, it is not surprising that unspecified meningitis was the most common diagnosis, accounting for 60% of diagnoses. Approximately one-third of the patients with a diagnosis of meningitis were discharged from the ED. The data suggest that while you will see more adults with meningitis, children, especially young children, are more likely to be diagnosed with the disease.

This analysis also implies that there is practice variation in the treatment of meningitis in the ED. Various national guidelines recommend that for bacterial meningitis, virtually everyone should receive a third-generation cephalosporin and vancomycin, while those at risk for *Listeria* also should receive ampicillin. Many guidelines will advocate for corticosteroids as well. The authors found that 48% of patients diagnosed with meningitis received at least 1 antibiotic (which means that a majority did not get antibiotics) and that a third-generation cephalosporin was given in 42% while vancomycin was only given in 6%. Corticosteroids were rarely given. Unquestionably, antibiotics and steroids are not indicated in a patient with viral meningitis. However, there is no clear standard of care for what to do with patients suspected of having viral meningitis but who is being tested for bacterial meningitis. A number of studies have shown that delays in administering antibiotics are associated with a poorer prognosis. That being said, it would seem from these data that many clinicians do not give antibiotics in this latter scenario. It is certainly my practice to give an initial dose of antibiotics in most patients in whom I have a moderate to high suspicion for meningitis. Whether this is the best practice has never been addressed by research.

E. A. Ramoska, MD, MPHE

6 Neurology

Cheerio, Laddie! Bidding Farewell to the Glasgow Coma Scale
Green SM (Loma Linda Univ Med Ctr and Children's Hosp, CA)
Ann Emerg Med 58:427-430, 2011

Background.—The Glasgow Coma Scale (GCS) was originally devised to serve in repeated bedside assessments for neurosurgical patients to determine changing states of consciousness and measure coma duration. However, it has become the undisputed universal standard for determining mental status and a fundamental part of emergency medical culture, out-of-hospital care, trauma surgery, and neurosurgery. Although it has the advantages of face validity, wide acceptance, and established statistical associations with adverse neurologic outcomes, it also has powerful limitations. Based on these failings, it should now be considered obsolete for use in acute care medicine because it is confusing, unreliable, and unnecessarily complex.

Problems.—To be accurate and useful, a clinical scale must be reproducible. The GCS is unreliable and has multiple subjective elements and low interrater reliability.

Clinical scales must also be easy to use and remember, but the GCS again fails. It is not consistently remembered, is widely viewed as complicated, and takes more than a few seconds to use. In 2003 it was found that a third of British hospitals were using the original 12-point GCS instead of the current 13-point version and no one had noticed.

The GCS is also limited to gross predictions. Although statistically associated with events such as the presence of brain injury, the need for neurosurgical intervention, and ultimate mortality, the GCS's prognostic value is weak enough that it cannot accurately predict outcomes for individual patients. Its sensitivity and specificity combinations are similar to those of weather forecasters to predict rain.

Summing the three scales is inherently unsound and infers that each gradation of each subscale has a similar magnitude of clinical importance, which is both unlikely and statistically incorrect. The 13 possible GCS values can yield 120 combinations depending on how they are calculated. The summary score is actually less informative than the separate component scores.

Alternatives.—Several investigations have shown essentially equivalent test performance for the individual subscales compared to the total. The 6-point motor component has the best performance and could be used alone. Two 4-point scores (AVPU and ACDU) give comparable results to GCS assessments. The use of 3 of the 6 points in the GCS motor scale essentially define its entire performance and have been used to form the Simplified

Motor Scale or Test Responsiveness: Obeys, Localizes, or Less (TROLL), which has performed as well as the total GCS. It provides the same information, was statistically derived, is simple, has been externally validated, and demonstrates better interrater reliability. The scale is so basic that some say it is no better than clinical judgment alone, and that suggests that health care providers may have been using judgment all along, with the GCS calculation just a ritual.

Conclusions.—Why has the GCS remained in use if it has such drawbacks? The answer may be psychological, with the scale bringing apparent order out of disorder. Its seeming accuracy and precision can be appealing. Based on evidence, simple unstructured clinical judgment may be as accurate. If a tool is needed, it should be easier to learn, use, and retain. The Simplified Motor Scale/TROLL may be the best choice.

▶ A trauma victim arrives or a stroke patient is about to go to the computed tomography scanner. You quickly break out your trusty Glasgow Coma Scale (GCS) calculator from your memory—bingo. Do you remember correctly? Do you get in fights with others in the team about who remembered it correctly?

At my institution, the trauma team insists on a full team activation for any patient with a GCS under 14. How many times is the response dependent on ethanol-fueled belligerence? Wait, what was the patient's best response when testing the GCS? Besides, my patients often get tired of having to answer repetitive questions from residents and then attendings.

Do not even get me started on the use of mean (average) GCS reported in studies. Sure you can calculate it, but it does not mean anything statistically. Why do we put up with this silliness?

Once we used to have to explain our decision to intubate patients based on the values from blood gases. Do we need to calculate the GCS to know if an airway is at risk?

When I think of the GCS, I feel a bit like Steve Martin playing his Saturday Night Live role as Theodoric of York musing about the future of medicine. Could there be a better way to describe patient outcomes and the need for intubation to protect airways? Theodoric would resign himself to blood letting. I want to find that future now and Dr Green leads the way with this editorial.

N. B. Handly, MD, MSc, MS

Does primary stroke center certification change ED diagnosis, utilization, and disposition of patients with acute stroke?
Ballard DW, Reed ME, Huang J, et al (Massachusetts General Hosp, Boston, MA)
Am J Emerg Med 30:1152-1162, 2012

Background and Purpose.—We examined the impact of primary stroke center (PSC) certification on emergency department (ED) use and outcomes within an integrated delivery system in which EDs underwent staggered certification.

Methods.—A retrospective cohort study of 30 461 patients seen in 17 integrated delivery system EDs with a primary diagnosis of transient ischemic attack (TIA), intracranial hemorrhage, or ischemic stroke between 2005 and 2008 was conducted. We compared ED stroke patient visits across hospitals for (1) temporal trends and (2) pre- and post-PSC certification—using logistic and linear regression models to adjust for comorbidities, patient characteristics, and calendar time, to examine major outcomes (ED throughput time, hospital admission, radiographic imaging utilization and throughput, and mortality) across certification stages.

Results.—There were 15 687 precertification ED visits and 11 040 postcertification visits. Primary stroke center certification was associated with significant changes in care processes associated with PSC certification process, including (1) ED throughput for patients with intracranial hemorrhage (55 minutes faster), (2) increased utilization of cranial magnetic resonance imaging for patients with ischemic stroke (odds ratio, 1.88; 95% confidence interval, 1.36-2.60), and (3) decrease in time to radiographic imaging for most modalities, including cranial computed tomography done within 6 hours of ED arrival (TIA: 12 minutes faster, ischemic stroke: 11 minutes faster), magnetic resonance imaging for patients with ischemic stroke (197 minutes faster), and carotid Doppler sonography for TIA patients (138 minutes faster). There were no significant changes in survival.

Conclusions.—Stroke center certification was associated with significant changes in ED admission and radiographic utilization patterns, without measurable improvements in survival.

▶ This is a noteworthy article from the Kaiser Permanente Division of Research. They retrospectively looked at data from 17 hospitals that served over 3.1 million members in their system. They discovered that process-oriented statistics, such as MRI utilization, timing of radiographic studies, and emergency department throughput, improved after primary stroke center certification; however, outcomes such as hospital length of stay (LOS) and mortality were not significantly different. They did not look at functional outcomes of stroke patients.

The results of this investigation may call into question the raison d'être of stroke center certification. They did more studies, faster, but had no decrease in hospital LOS or mortality. Granted, they did not look at stroke residual severity and functional status. Perhaps there was an improvement in patients' functional status and activities of daily living. If that were the case, then maybe stroke center certification is a cost-effective program transformation. If on the other hand, medical system change does not result in an improvement of the human condition or a decrease in costs, then perhaps we should rethink it. I eagerly await more studies in this area.

E. A. Ramoska, MD, MPHE

Effect of Functional Status on Survival in Patients With Stroke: Is Independent Ambulation a Key Determinant?

Chiu H-T, Wang Y-H, Jeng J-S, et al (Natl Taiwan Univ Hosp, Taipei)
Arch Phys Med Rehabil 93:527-531, 2012

Objective.—To investigate the effect of functional status, measured using the Modified Rankin Scale (MRS), at 3 months after stroke on survival in patients with stroke.

Design.—Cohort study.

Setting.—Referral medical center.

Participants.—Patients with stroke (N = 1032).

Interventions.—Not applicable.

Main Outcome Measure.—Survival after stroke.

Results.—The Kaplan-Meier survival curves stratified by the 3-month MRS score showed 2 clear groups of patients with 3-month MRS scores of 0 to 3 (able to walk without assistance) and 4 or 5 (unable to walk without assistance). Accordingly, we grouped the patients into a high function (HF) group (3-month MRS$\leq$3) and a low function (LF) group (3-month MRS$\geq$4). Multiple Cox regression analysis showed that the LF group had significantly poorer survival (adjusted hazard ratio = 4.69; 95% confidence interval [CI], 2.89–7.60; $P < .001$) than the HF group. Other significant risk factors of higher mortality were older age, history of diabetes mellitus, and heart disease.

Conclusions.—This study showed a significant influence of the 3-month MRS score on stroke survival. Moreover, independent ambulation may be a major determinant of a favorable survival prognosis. This finding suggests a potential role of rehabilitation in promoting stroke survival by maximizing ambulation function.

▶ The authors inform us that this study started after they noticed that plots of survival after stroke stratified by modified Rankin Score measured 3 months after a stroke (mRS-3) revealed 2 distinct clusters. The survival curves of those patients with mRS-3 $\leq$3 appeared to have a similar and distinctly better survival pattern than those patients with mRS-3 $\geq$4.

A key difference between the 2 groups of patients identified this way is that those with mRS-3 $\leq$3 are able to walk independently. In fact, the mRS-3 values, when used individually or dichotomized to describe independent walking, are statistically significant factors for predicting the likelihood of death. The authors report that the dichotomized mRS-3 values performed better in the hazards model.

This is a limited study and further work is needed, but the fact that it is possible to communicate some sense of risk of death beyond 3 months (from the time of a stroke) to patients and their families makes this work valuable. However, patients and families would likely want to know about chances to survive and have a level of function at the time of the acute stroke.

N. B. Handly, MD, MSc, MS

Effects of microbubbles on transcranial Doppler ultrasound-assisted intracranial urokinase thrombolysis
Liu W-S, Huang Z-Z, Wang X-W, et al (First Affiliated Hosp of Harbin Med Univ, China; et al)
Thromb Res 130:547-551, 2012

Introduction.—To evaluate the efficacy of microbubbles in transcranial Doppler ultrasound (TCD)-assisted urokinase thrombolysis.

Materials and Methods.—Male New Zealand white rabbits (N = 32) were randomly divided into 2 groups, a urokinase group and a combined urokinase plus microbubble group. The middle cerebral artery (MCA) was occluded by injecting autologous blood clots through the carotid artery. In the urokinase plus microbubble group, sulfur hexafluoride (SonoVue) microbubbles were injected intravenously immediately after intravenous injection of urokinase. The 2 groups were monitored by TCD from before until 2 h after thrombolysis, and the hemodynamic changes and infarct size were recorded.

Results.—The urokinase alone group had 1 case of complete recanalization and 4 cases of partial recanalization (recanalization rate, 31.3%). The urokinase plus microbubble group had 3 cases of complete recanalization and 6 cases of partial recanalization (recanalization rate, 56.3%). The average size of the infarction foci was 13.9% in the urokinase group and 9.1% in the urokinase plus microbubble group ($P = 0.025$). Pathological examination revealed no cerebral hemorrhage in either group.

Conclusions.—The addition of microbubbles enhanced the effects of transcranial Doppler ultrasound-assisted urokinase thrombolysis.

▶ Several years ago, I attended a research presentation that demonstrated that transcranial Doppler (TD) ultrasound could enhance the activity of tissue plasminogen activator (t-PA) in a manner that was distinct from the heating that would result from the ultrasound exposure.

I thought at the time this would be very interesting because the TD ultrasound could be used to both assess middle cerebral artery blood flow and enhance the treatment of occlusion with lower levels of t-PA.

Moving forward in time, there is a large body of work demonstrating the effects of TD ultrasound with thrombolysis with t-PA. It appears that the nonheating effect of TD ultrasound on lysis is due to enhanced structural changes to the clot that increases the access of the t-PA molecule to its binding sites on the clot.

However, the authors note that t-PA is of significant cost such that a lower cost agent, urokinase, is used in much of the world, although it is less effective when compared with t-PA. Because ultrasound contrast bubbles can be made to expand and contract with ultrasound pulses, one of the drivers for this study was to determine if the forces resulting from bubble activation by ultrasound could further enhance thrombolysis by urokinase.

Ultrasound is not without some risk when used on the brain. There are risks of hemorrhage likely resulting from damage to the blood—brain barrier. An ultrasound power setting was chosen to minimize this possibility and no gross hemorrhage was detected.

This work should stimulate further work in this area. If we in the emergency department start using TD ultrasound on our stroke patients, we might be able to both diagnose and treat more effectively. Ultrasound contrast would also help both in identifying the intracranial vessels as well as enhance thrombolysis.

N. B. Handly, MD, MSc, MS

Neuroprotective Effect of Curcumin in an Experimental Rat Model of Subarachnoid Hemorrhage

Kuo C-P, Lu C-H, Wen L-L, et al (Duke Univ Med Ctr, Durham, NC; Natl Defense Med Ctr and Tri-Service General Hosp, Taipei, Taiwan, Republic of China; En Chu Kong Hosp, Taipei, Taiwan, Republic of China; et al)
Anesthesiology 115:1229-1238, 2011

Background.—Subarachnoid hemorrhage (SAH) causes a high mortality rate and morbidity. It was suggested that oxidant stress plays an important role in neuronal injury after SAH. Therefore, we assessed the effect of curcumin on reducing cerebral vasospasm and neurologic injury in a SAH model in rat.

Methods.—A double-hemorrhage model was used to induce SAH in rats. Groups of animals were treated with intraperitoneal injection of 20 mg/kg curcumin (curcumin group, n = 24) or dimethyl sulfoxide (vehicle group, n = 33), normal saline (SAH group, n = 34) or normal saline (sham group, n = 22), 3 h after SAH induction and daily for 6 days. Glutamate was measured before SAH induction and once daily for 7 days. Glutamate transporter-1, wall thickness and the perimeter of the basilar artery, neurologic scores, neuronal degeneration, malondialdehyde, superoxide dismutase, and catalase activities were assessed.

Results.—Changes of glutamate levels were lower in the curcumin group *versus* the SAH and vehicle groups, especially on day 1 (56 folds attenuation *vs.* vehicle). Correspondingly, glutamate transporter-1 was preserved after SAH in curcumin-treated rats. In the hippocampus and the cortex, malondialdehyde was attenuated (30% and 50%, respectively). Superoxide dismutase (35% and 64%) and catalase (34% and 38%) activities were increased in the curcumin rats compared with the SAH rats. Mortality rate (relative risk: 0.59), wall thickness (30%) and perimeter (31%) of the basilar artery, neuron degeneration scores (39%), and neurologic scores (31%) were improved in curcumin-treated rats.

Conclusions.—Curcumin in multiple doses is effective against glutamate neurotoxicity and oxidative stress and improves the mortality rate in rats with SAH.

▶ It is not unusual for us to learn how to recognize a disease and then pass off that patient to a specialist. But when we cannot get the patient to the specialist immediately, emergency physicians are responsible for initiating treatments. This is typical in the case of a subarachnoid hemorrhage (SAH). As our understanding of the processes that are initiated after subarachnoid hemorrhage improve, we can more effectively participate in the treatment process.

Some SAH models have suggested that some of the changes after the injury are mediated by inflammation. Extracellular glutamate rises in the brain after SAH. Additionally, oxidative stress with free radical levels increases. It is not known if these 2 steps occur independently or are sequential. However, it is thought that each of these steps leads to neuronal injury and death.

The results from this study are not ready for immediate use. The study used a mouse model for SAH. The numbers of mice studied were small. We are not likely to be dosing humans with intraperitoneal turmeric. However, the value of this study is that we can become more aware that oxidative stress likely plays some role in the damage after SAH and that it may be possible to enhance our ability to prevent some of the damage of SAH by diet or refined products based on curcumin.

N. B. Handly, MD, MSc, MS

Variables Associated With Discordance Between Emergency Physician and Neurologist Diagnoses of Transient Ischemic Attacks in the Emergency Department

Schrock JW, Glasenapp M, Victor A, et al (MetroHealth Med Ctr, Cleveland, OH; Case Western Reserve Univ, Cleveland, OH)
Ann Emerg Med 59:19-26, 2012

Study Objective.—Transient ischemic attack is a common clinical diagnosis in emergency department (ED) patients with acute neurologic complaints. Accurate diagnosis of transient ischemic attack is essential to help guide evaluation and avoid treatment delays. We seek to determine the prevalence of discordant diagnosis for patients receiving an ED diagnosis of transient ischemic attack compared with neurologist final diagnosis. Secondary goals are to evaluate the influence of atypical transient ischemic attack symptoms, the ABCD2 score, and emergency physician experience on discordant diagnoses.

Methods.—We performed a retrospective cohort study evaluating all ED patients receiving a diagnosis of transient ischemic attack during a 4-year period. The emergency physician diagnosis was compared with that of the neurologist. The neurologist's final diagnosis was considered the criterion standard diagnosis. Subject demographic and clinical information was collected with a structured instrument. The following atypical symptoms present at the ED evaluation were evaluated with logistic regression: headache, tingling, involuntary movement, seeing flashing lights or wavy lines, dizziness, confusion, incontinence, and ABCD2 score of 4 or greater. Bivariate analysis was used to evaluate the influence of emergency physician experience (≤ 6 years versus > 6 years) on discordant diagnosis. Odds ratios (ORs) and proportions are reported with 95% confidence intervals (CIs), interquartile range was used where appropriate.

Results.—We evaluated 436 subjects, of whom 7 were excluded, allowing 429 subjects for evaluation. Of these individuals, 156 (36%; 95% CI 32% to 41%) received a discordant diagnosis. The median emergency physician time in clinical practice was 6 years (interquartile range 2 to 12 years). Features associated with a discordant transient ischemic attack diagnosis included headache (OR 2.52; 95% CI 1.59 to 3.99), involuntary movement (OR 3.19; 95% CI 1.35 to 7.54), and dizziness (OR 1.92; 95% CI 1.22 to 3.02). Incontinence, confusion, and seeing wavy lines or flashing lights were not significantly associated with a discordant diagnosis. Patients with tingling and a high ABCD2 score had an increased odds of concordant transient ischemic attack diagnosis (OR 0.54, 95% CI 0.32 to 0.92; OR 0.53, 95% CI 0.35 to 0.82, respectively).

Conclusion.—Discordant diagnoses between emergency physicians and neurologists were observed in 36% of patients. The presence of headache, involuntary movement, and dizziness predicted discordant diagnoses, whereas the presence of tingling and an increased ABCD2 score predicted concordant transient ischemic attack diagnosis.

▶ The attached article references the importance of timely diagnosis of transient ischemic attacks (TIAs) in patients with acute neurological deficits based on the relative frequency that these transient events return and become the more permanent cerebrovascular accidents (CVAs). The authors state that discordance in the final diagnosis between emergency physicians and neurologists may lead to ineffective patient care or unnecessary testing. In this study, the newer TIA timeframe of less than 1 hour was the standard, and the authors used the ABCD2 score as a guide. Although this is from the facility's department of emergency medicine, the article has a negative emergency medicine slant. The authors report that 36% of the included patients ultimately received an alternative diagnosis and referenced a rate as high as 60%, but fail to realize that the vast majority of emergency medicine diagnoses are presumptive. The discordant diagnoses may be related to the luxury of time and testing. The emergency physician has minutes to hours with the patient and access to screening tests (computed tomography), whereas the neurologist has hours to days and the more definitive tests (magnetic resonance imaging). Last, 1 category, migraine, is a known stroke mimic, and would be a diagnosis of exclusion after TIA and cerebrovascular accident have been ruled out.

E. C. Bruno, MD

Stroke Mimics and Intravenous Thrombolysis
Artto V, Putaala J, Strbian D, et al (Helsinki Univ Central Hosp, Finland)
Ann Emerg Med 59:27-32, 2012

Study Objective.—The necessity for rapid administration of intravenous thrombolysis in patients with acute ischemic stroke may lead to treatment of patients with conditions mimicking stroke. We analyze stroke patients treated with intravenous thrombolysis in our center to characterize cases classified as stroke mimics.

Methods.—We identified and reviewed all cases with a diagnosis other than ischemic stroke in our large-scale single-center stroke thrombolysis registry. We compared these stroke mimics with patients with neuroimaging-negative and neuroimaging-positive ischemic stroke results.

Results.—Among 985 consecutive intravenous thrombolysis—treated patients, we found 14 stroke mimics (1.4%; 95% confidence interval 0.8% to 2.4%), 694 (70.5%) patients with neuroimaging-positive ischemic stroke results, and 275 (27.9%) patients with neuroimaging-negative ischemic stroke results. Stroke mimics were younger than patients with neuroimaging-negative or -positive ischemic stroke results. Compared with patients with neuroimaging-positive ischemic stroke results, stroke mimics had less severe symptoms at baseline and better 3-month outcome. No differences appeared in medical history or clinical features between stroke mimics and patients with neuroimaging-negative ischemic stroke results. None of the stroke mimics developed symptomatic intracerebral hemorrhage compared with 63 (9.1%) among patients with neuroimaging-positive ischemic stroke results and 6 (2.2%) among patients with neuroimaging-negative ischemic stroke results.

Conclusion.—Stroke mimics were infrequent among intravenous thrombolysis—treated stroke patients in this cohort, and their treatment did not lead to harmful complications.

▶ Emergency physicians are under pressure to rapidly assess patients with acute neurological deficits who may be candidates for aggressive measures, specifically intravenous thrombolytics for the treatment of presumed cerebrovascular accidents (CVA). With such critical time restraints in place, clinical presentations that mimic acute CVAs are bound to fall into the treatment group, particularly those medical conditions that present with acute neurological deficits. The authors to this retrospective cohort study assessed the percentage of stroke mimics that are treated with thrombolytics and determined if this intervention resulted in adverse events. A chart review of those patients receiving intravenous thrombolytics demonstrated that 1.4% of the treated group was ultimately determined to be stroke mimics. This group tended to be younger and female, possibly suggesting hemiplegic migraines. Fortunately, no patient who errantly received the thrombolytics experienced a bleeding complication, whereas 2.2% of those with CVA suffered an adverse bleeding event. With the current diagnostic testing standard, stroke impersonators will likely continue to receive thrombolytics, but these results (low incidence and low complication rate) support the aggressive approach.

E. C. Bruno, MD

7   Psychiatry

Can Activation of Coagulation and Impairment of Fibrinolysis in Patients With Anxiety and Depression Be Reversed After Improvement of Psychiatric Symptoms? Results of a Pilot Study
Geiser F, Gessler K, Conrad R, et al (Univ of Bonn, Germany; et al)
J Nerv Ment Dis 200:721-723, 2012

Anxiety and depression are associated with an activation of coagulation and impairment of fibrinolysis. This study addresses the question whether these findings are reversed after psychotherapy and improvement of psychiatric symptoms. Three factors of coagulation and fibrinolysis as well as level of anxiety and depression were reassessed in 12 patients 1 to 3 years after intensive inpatient psychotherapy. The patients showed a substantial improvement of their severe anxiety disorder and comorbid depressive disorder. Simultaneously, we found a significant decrease in factor VII and plasminogen activator inhibitor. We conclude that reduction of severe anxiety and depression may be associated with a reversal of the procoagulant effect (activation of coagulation and impairment of fibrinolysis) of these psychological states. Because of the small sample size of this pilot study, further research is needed.

▶ We often think that anxiety in acute myocardial infarct needs treatment to reduce myocardial demand. But here is an article that suggests that we need to think that anxiety might increase the risk for clot formation, so treatment of anxiety is critical for another reason.

Prior work had found that among individuals with anxiety and depression, levels of procoagulants were increased when compared with matched controls. In this study it was found, although in a small sample, that as depression and anxiety were improved, the amount of hypercoagulopathy decreased as well. If causality is present, then we should consider that anxiety and depression are the stimuli and hypercoagulopathy is the effect. It would be nice to follow more individuals longitudinally as they pass through ups and downs of treatment of their disease. Perhaps patients with bipolar disease may also be good candidates in which to observe the link between stimulus and effect.

We should consider this study as support for further work. So far we can say there is an association. To show causality will take a lot more effort. It may be that there is a stimulus that triggers both what we see in patients with anxiety and depression and hypercoagulopathy. Or it could be that hypercoagulopathy triggers anxiety and depression.

We also would want to know how fast changes in one can yield changes in the other; for myocardial ischemia, we want to be sure we minimize the risks as fast as we can.

N. B. Handly, MD, MSc, MS

8 Gastrointestinal

Eliminating routine oral contrast use for CT in the emergency department: impact on patient throughput and diagnosis
Levenson RB, Camacho MA, Horn E, et al (Beth Israel Deaconess Med Ctr, Boston, MA)
Emerg Radiol 2012 [Epub ahead of print]

This study aimed to assess the effect of eliminating routine oral contrast use for abdominopelvic (AP) computed tomography (CT) on emergency department (ED) patient throughput and diagnosis. Retrospective analysis was performed on patients undergoing AP CT during 2-month periods prior to and following oral contrast protocol change in an urban, tertiary care ED. Patients with inflammatory bowel disease, prior gastrointestinal tract-altering surgery, or lean body habitus continued to receive oral contrast. Oral contrast was otherwise eliminated from the AP CT protocol. Patients were excluded if they would not have typically received oral contrast, regardless of the intervention. Data recorded include patient demographics, ED length of stay (LOS), time from order to CT, 72-h ED return, and repeat imaging. Two thousand and one ED patients (1,014 before and 987 after protocol change) underwent AP CT during the study period. Six hundred seven pre-intervention and 611 post-intervention were eligible for oral contrast and included. Of these, 95% received oral contrast prior to the intervention and 42% thereafter. After the intervention, mean ED LOS among oral contrast eligible patients decreased by 97 min, $P < 0.001$. Mean time from order to CT decreased by 66 min, $P < 0.001$. No patient with CT negative for acute findings had additional subsequent AP imaging within 72 h at our institution that led to a change in diagnosis. Eliminating routine oral contrast use for AP CT in the ED may be successful in decreasing LOS and time from order to CT without demonstrated compromise in acute patient diagnosis.

▶ Conversations have undoubtedly occurred between emergency physicians (EPs) and radiologists over the merits of oral contrast in conjunction with computed tomography (CT) imaging in the evaluation of patients presenting with abdominal pain. When oral contrast was the standard, patients had their emergency department length of stay increase to permit the contrast to "get downstream" to enhance the more distal caudal gastrointestinal structures. More recently, a compromise has resulted in less oral contrast in acceptable patient populations. The authors of this retrospective study sought to determine if the elimination of oral contrast would result in a decreased length of stay for patients receiving CT imaging as part of their abdominal pain workup. Comparing similar patients, the removal of oral contrast resulted in an average decrease in the emergency department stay of 97 minutes and a 66-minute decrease to get the imaging procedure. Additionally, a negative CT report in the emergency department did not result in a statistically significant increase (2.6% vs 5.3%) in return visits within 72 hours of the first visit. The results further support the practice of nonoral contrast-enhanced CTs for the evaluation of patients with abdominal pain, but EPs must continue to give the discharged patients informative instructions and expectations.

E. C. Bruno, MD

Clinical triage decision vs risk scores in predicting the need for endotherapy in upper gastrointestinal bleeding

Farooq FT, Lee MH, Das A, et al (Gastro One, Memphis, TN; Univ Hosps Case Med Ctr, Cleveland, OH; Mayo Clinic, Scottsdale, AZ)
Am J Emerg Med 30:129-134, 2012

Background.—Acute upper gastrointestinal hemorrhage (UGIH) is a common reason for hospitalization with substantial associated morbidity, mortality, and cost. Differentiation of high- and low-risk patients using established risk scoring systems has been advocated.

The aim of this study was to determine whether these scoring systems are more accurate than an emergency physician's clinical decision making in predicting the need for endoscopic intervention in acute UGIH.

Methods.—Patients presenting to a tertiary care medical center with acute UGIH from 2003 to 2006 were identified from the hospital database, and their clinical data were abstracted. One hundred ninety-five patients

TABLE 1.—Rockall Score

	Score			
	0	1	2	3
Age (y)	<60	60-79	≥80	
Shock	SBP ≥ 100 mm Hg, P < 100 beats/min	SBP ≥ 100 mm Hg, P ≥ 100 beats/min	SBP < 100 mm Hg	
Comorbidity	None		CHF, CAD, and other major diseases	Renal or liver failure and cancer
Diagnosis	MW tear, no lesion	All other	UGI cancer	
Major SRH	None, flat spot		Fresh blood, adherent clot, visible or spurting vessel	

Rockall scoring system: scores for age, shock, and comorbidity comprise the cRS. Scores for diagnosis and major stigmata of recent hemorrhage + cRS equals the complete Rockall score. SBP indicates systolic blood pressure; P, pulse rate; CHF, congestive heart failure; CAD, coronary artery disease; MW, Mallory-Weiss; UGI, upper GI; SRH, stigmata of recent hemorrhage.

TABLE 2.—Blatchford Score

Admission Risk Marker		Score
BUN (mmol/L)		
6.5-8.0		2
8.0-10.0		3
10.0-25.0		4
>25		6
Hgb (g/L), male	Hgb (g/L), female	
120-130	100-120	1
100-120		3
<100	<100	6
Systolic blood pressure (mm Hg)		
100-109		1
90-99		2
<90		3
Other markers		
Pulse ≥100 beats/min		1
Melena		1
Syncope		2
Liver disease		2
Cardiac failure		2

Blatchford score: note that unit conversion is necessary before score calculation (BUN typically reported as milligrams per deciliter, and hemoglobin level as grams per deciliter in the United States). BUN indicates blood urea nitrogen; Hgb, hemoglobin.

met the inclusion criteria and were included in the analysis. The clinical Rockall score and Blatchford score (BS) were calculated and compared with the clinical triage decision (intensive care unit vs non—intensive care unit admission) in predicting the need for endoscopic therapy.

Results.—Clinical Rockall score greater than 0 and BS greater than 0 were sensitive predictors of the need for endoscopic therapy (95% and 100%) but were poorly specific (9% and 4%), with overall accuracies of 41% and 39%. At higher score cutoffs, clinical Rockall score greater than 2 and BS greater than 5 remained sensitive (84% and 87%) and were more specific (29% and 33%), with overall accuracies of 48% and 52%. Clinical triage decision, as a surrogate for predicting the need for endoscopic therapy, was moderately sensitive (67%) and specific (75%), with an overall accuracy (73%) that exceeded both risk scores.

Conclusions.—The clinical use of risk scoring systems in acute UGIH may not be as good as clinical decision making by emergency physicians (Tables 1 and 2).

▶ Upper gastrointestinal bleeding (UGIB) may represent a life-threatening condition and generally warrants further inpatient management, specifically endoscopy. Advocates for outpatient management attempt to optimize clinical outcomes in patients stable for discharge. Identification of those patients who require inpatient management may be based on gestalt, clinical assessment tools, or both. The authors of this review compared clinical decision rules with 2 scoring systems: Blatchford (Table 2) and Rockall (Table 1). Patients were included in the study if they had emergency department—identified UGIB based on observed hematemesis, melena, or nasogastric tube aspirate. The results demonstrated that clinical decisions were more effective in determining the need for intensive care admission and emergent endoscopy when compared with both scoring systems. Application of the Rockall system has an inherent disadvantage by inclusion of 2 points based on the endoscopy results. Emergency physicians will not have this information at the outset, unless the patient had a recent scope.

E. C. Bruno, MD

Adult intussusception: presentation, management, and outcomes of 148 patients

Lindor RA, Bellolio MF, Sadosty AT, et al (Mayo Clinic College of Medicine, Rochester, MN; Mayo Clinic, Rochester, MN)
J Emerg Med 43:1-6, 2012

Background.—Intussusception is a predominantly pediatric diagnosis that is not well characterized among adults. Undiagnosed cases can result in significant morbidity, making early recognition important for clinicians.

Study Objectives.—We describe the presentation, clinical management, disposition, and outcome of adult patients diagnosed with intussusception during a 13-year period.

Methods.—A retrospective study of consecutive adult patients diagnosed with intussusception at a tertiary academic center was carried out from 1996 to 2008. Cases were identified using International Classification of Diseases, 9th Revision codes and a document search engine. Data were abstracted in duplicate by two independent authors.

Results.—Among 148 patients included in the study, the most common symptoms at presentation were abdominal pain (72%), nausea (49%), and vomiting (36%). Twenty percent were asymptomatic. Sixty percent of cases had an identifiable lead point. Patients presenting to the emergency department (ED) (31%) had higher rates of abdominal pain (relative risk [RR] 5.7) and vomiting (RR 3.4), and were more likely to undergo surgical intervention (RR 1.8) than patients diagnosed elsewhere. There were 77 patients who underwent surgery within 1 month; patients presenting with abdominal pain (RR 2.2), nausea (RR 1.7), vomiting (RR 1.4), and bloody stool (RR 1.9) were more likely to undergo surgery.

Conclusions.—Adult intussusception commonly presents with abdominal pain, nausea, and vomiting; however, approximately 20% of cases are asymptomatic and seem to be diagnosed by incidental radiologic findings. Patients presenting to an ED with intussusception due to a mass as a lead point or in an ileocolonic location are likely to undergo surgical intervention.

▶ Emergency departments are seemingly filled with patients with recurrent abdominal pain, and many times radiological imaging is included in the diagnostic workups. Occasionally, these workups reveal the less common surgical diagnosis. Traditionally seen in the pediatric population, adult intussusception is a recognized condition that may need surgical intervention. The attached article represents a retrospective review of 148 cases of adult intussusception encompassing a 12-year period. Patients most often presented with abdominal pain (72%); however, up to 20% were asymptomatic and an incidental finding. The authors also describe factors that predict the need for surgical intervention and the more common location for the intussusception. Patients were more likely to need surgical management when a mass or leading edge was identified on the diagnostic imaging. No gender difference was identified, and the location of the intussusception was most often enteroenteric. This is a rare condition, but knowledge of the management is important for proper initial management. With increasing use of computed tomography, this diagnostic entity may be discovered more frequently.

E. C. Bruno, MD

Ondansetron Use in the Pediatric Emergency Room for Diagnoses Other Than Acute Gastroenteritis

Sturm JJ, Pierzchala A, Simon HK, et al (Emory Univ, Atlanta, GA)
Pediatr Emerg Care 28:247-250, 2012

Background.—Ondansetron is widely used in the pediatric emergency department (PED) for vomiting and acute gastroenteritis (GE). Little is known about the spectrum of its use in diagnoses other than acute GE.

Objective.—The objective of this study was to evaluate the spectrum of diagnoses for which ondansetron is used in the PED.

Methods.—Medical records from 2 tertiary care PEDs from January 2006 to December 2008 were retrospectively reviewed. Patients 3 months to 18 years of age given ondansetron in the PED were identified. Patients without a primary discharge diagnosis (based on *International Classification of Diseases, Ninth Revision* code) of vomiting or GE were defined as non-GE. Patient age, initial triage level (1 = lowest acuity, 5 = highest), route of administration (enteral vs parenteral), primary diagnosis, disposition, and prescription for ondansetron at discharge were recorded; GE and non-GE patients were compared based on age and triage acuity.

Results.—There were 32,971 patients who received ondansetron in the PED; 12,620 (38%) were non-GE patients. Non-GE patients were older (8.3 vs 4.3 years, $P < 0.001$) and of higher average initial triage level (2.95 vs 2.33, $P < 0.001$) compared with GE patients. Within non-GE patients, 79% received ondansetron enterally, 71% were discharged, and 37% of those discharged received an ondansetron prescription. The most common primary diagnoses for non-GE discharged patients were fever (15%), abdominal pain/tenderness (13%), head injury/concussion (7%), pharyngitis (6%), viral infection (6%), migraine variants (5%), and otitis media (5%). The most common diagnoses of patients admitted were appendicitis (11%), asthma (6%), pneumonia (4%), and diabetes (4%).

Conclusions.—Although ondansetron is a widely accepted treatment for GE in children, this study identifies a broader spectrum of primary diagnoses for which ondansetron is being used.

▶ Once available in a generic form, ondansetron has become more ubiquitous in emergency medicine. Additionally, emergency physicians (EPs) have expanded their use of ondansetron for medical and traumatic conditions other than acute gastroenteritis (AGE). The authors of this retrospective review analyzed which pediatric patients were receiving ondansetron for diagnoses other than AGE, though this remained the majority (62%).

The authors demonstrated increased ondansetron use with the study period, especially in the non-AGE cohort. The data received numerous diagnoses, including fever, abdominal pain/tenderness, head injury/concussion, and migraine variants. The results do not suggest that ondansetron is being administered in a frivolous manner. A more appropriate cohort division would be nausea/vomiting versus non—nausea/vomiting, as one could extrapolate that the increased use is related to the treatment of vomiting, regardless of the etiology (ie, viral syndrome, acute pancreatitis, pneumonia). EPs are focusing on the cessation of the nausea and vomiting while continuing to search for the primary cause of the signs and symptoms.

E. C. Bruno, MD

9 Endocrinology

Prevalence of hypokalemia in ED patients with diabetic ketoacidosis

Arora S, Cheng D, Wyler B, et al (Univ of Southern California, Los Angeles, CA)
Am J Emerg Med 30:481-484, 2012

Objective.—Although patients with diabetic ketoacidosis (DKA) are expected to have total body potassium depletion, measured levels may be normal or elevated due to extracellular shifts of potassium secondary to acidosis. Because insulin therapy decreases serum potassium levels, which creates potential to precipitate a fatal cardiac arrhythmia in a patient with hypokalemia, the American Diabetes Association (ADA) recommends obtaining a serum potassium level before giving insulin. Although the ADA guidelines are clear, the evidence on which they are based is largely anecdotal. The purpose of this study was to estimate the prevalence of hypokalemia in patients with DKA before initiation of fluid resuscitation and insulin therapy.

Methods.—This is a prospective cross-sectional descriptive study of patients with a capillary blood glucose level of 250 mg/dL or higher (at risk for DKA) seen in an urban county emergency department over a 1-year period. Those who consented provided basic demographic information and had a venous blood gas and chemistry panel drawn. Diabetic ketoacidosis and hypokalemia were defined using ADA recommendations.

Results.—The mean age in our sample was 40.2 years, and 81% of patients were Hispanic. Of 503 analyzable patients with hyperglycemia, 54 (10.7%) met all criteria for DKA. Of patients with DKA, 3 (5.6%) of 54 (95% confidence interval, 1.2%-15.4%) had hypokalemia. Two of these patients had values of 3.0 mmol/L, and 1 had a value of 2.8 mmol/L.

Conclusion.—Hypokalemia was observed in 5.6% of patients with DKA. These findings support the ADA recommendation to obtain a serum potassium before initiating intravenous insulin therapy in a patient with DKA.

▶ Potassium levels in the patient suffering from diabetic ketoacidosis (DKA) are of critical importance, considering the complications related to both hyperkalemia and hypokalemia. Although the potassium on the initial chemistry panel may be normal or even elevated, the total body potassium is depleted. Initiation of treatment for DKA, specifically insulin management, is likely to exacerbate this potassium deficiency further by driving the potassium to the intracellular space. The authors of this prospective cross-sectional study looked to quantify the prevalence of hypokalemia in patients suffering from DKA with hyperglycemia. The authors excluded patients with blood sugars below 250 mg/dL, even though patients with lower blood sugars than 250 mg/dL could still be in DKA. They were able to identify that 5.6% of patients with DKA were hypokalemic on the presenting laboratory diagnostic testing, and concluded that compliance with the American Diabetes Association's direction to obtain a serum potassium before starting the insulin drip is optional. With insulin boluses for DKA falling out of favor, the treating physician is truly in no rush to start the insulin infusion. Volume resuscitation is the priority and the insulin drip can wait until the chemistry panel results are complete.

E. C. Bruno, MD

Emergency Department Patients With Diabetes Have Better Glycemic Control When They Have Identifiable Primary Care Providers
Horwitz DA, Schwarz ES, Scott MG, et al (Maricopa Med Ctr, Phoenix, AZ; Barnes Jewish Hosp and Washington Univ School of Medicine, St Louis MO)
Acad Emerg Med 19:650-655, 2012

Objectives.—The objective was to determine if emergency department (ED) patients with diabetes mellitus (DM) who have primary care providers (PCPs) have better control of their DM than patients with no PCPs.

Methods.—This was a prospective, cross-sectional, observation study at a large, adult, urban, academic ED with 85,000 annual visits. ED patients with a history of DM were eligible. Patients with severe systemic disease, diabetic ketoacidosis (DKA), sepsis, active steroid use, pregnancy, or cognitive impairment were excluded. Consenting patients had hemoglobin A1c (HgbA1c) analysis and completed a questionnaire regarding demographics, lifestyle, medication usage, educational level attained, and health care access, including whether or not they had PCPs. HgbA1c levels were compared between subjects with and without PCPs using medians with interquartile ranges (IQRs). A continuous plot was developed to demonstrate the proportion of patients without PCPs (PCP−) compared to those with PCPs (PCP+) at every level of %HgbA1c across the entire measured range. Multivariate logistic regression analysis was used to determine which clinical and demographic factors obtained from the questionnaire were associated with improved glycemic control (increased relative risk [RR] of having a %HgbA1c < 8%).

Results.—A total of 284 patients were screened; 227 were enrolled, had HgbA1c analysis performed, and had complete PCP, race, and sex information. Complete demographic data (insurance status, employment status, etc.) were available on 209 subjects. Sixty-four of the 227 patients (28.2%) denied having PCPs. Median HgbA1c was 7.7% (IQR = 6.5% to 9.68%) in PCP+ versus 8.9% (IQR = 6.8% to 11.3%) in PCP− patients (p = 0.01). Ninety-one of 163 (55.8%) PCP+ subjects had a median HgbA1c < 8% versus 25 of 64 (39.1%) in the PCP− group (p = 0.02). After adjusting for multiple clinical and demographic variables, having a PCP remained significantly associated with a median HgbA1c value less than 8% (RR = 1.43; p = 0.04).

Conclusions.—Diabetes control was significantly better in patients with PCPs, even after adjusting for a number of potentially confounding social and demographic factors.

▶ Power analysis suggested that approximately 220 subjects would be needed to detect a 1% difference in glycosylated hemoglobin A1c (g-Hgb) between patients with and without a primary care physician (PCP). Unfortunately, we do not know over what time period the recruitment ran. Without this information, it might not be possible to be assured that there could not be seasonal variation to the difference (not likely, however). Additionally, we do not know how many potential subjects were not screened over the course of the study to determine if this sample actually is representative of the patients served by the emergency department. How many patients would present to the emergency department outside of the hours of the study?

Nevertheless, the authors found that patients who said that they had a PCP did have lower g-Hgb levels that those patients who did not. Consider the following: if patients do have a PCP, then at some point, the PCP is going to prescribe a measurement of g-Hgb (if for no other reason to meet quality measures for Medicare). Having a g-Hgb level, the PCP can talk to the patient about this result and what needs to be done about it. Adjustments to medical management could be made. Unfortunately, it is not possible to determine if the patients without PCPs had recent g-Hgb testing in this study, so it is not possible to show that knowledge about this interaction with PCPs might be the critical component.

Certainly, though, the health burden of poorly controlled diabetes among many patients using the emergency department is a problem and directing an intervention appropriately whether via a PCP or not depends on our better understanding this phenomenon.

N. B. Handly, MD, MSc, MS

10 Pediatric Emergency Medicine

General Issues

Reasons for Nonurgent Pediatric Emergency Department Visits: Perceptions of Health Care Providers and Caregivers

Salami O, Salvador J, Vega R (Bronx Lebanon Hosp Ctr Affiliated with Albert Einstein College of Medicine, Bronx, NY)
Pediatr Emerg Care 28:43-46, 2012

Objectives.—This study aimed to determine the most important reasons for pediatric nonurgent (NU) emergency department (ED) visits as perceived by caregivers, primary care pediatricians (PCPs), and ED personnel and to assess the differences among these 3 groups in perceived reasons and solutions to NUED visits.

Methods.—This study is a cross-sectional survey, with self-administered questionnaires given to caregivers, PCPs, and ED personnel. Responders were asked to rank reasons for NUED visits in order of perceived importance. Opinions on NUED use reduction strategies were also queried.

Results.—Although almost 80% of PCPs expected to be called by caregivers before ED visits, fewer than 30% of caregivers were aware of this expectation. The most important reasons for NUED visits from the caregivers' perspective were need for medical attention outside PCP working hours, lack of health insurance, and better hospitality in the ED. For PCPs and ED personnel, the most important reason was the caregivers' lack of knowledge on what constitutes a true emergency. More than 70% of ED personnel and PCPs recommended caregiver education as the solution to NUED visits. Caregivers were more likely to recommend more PCPs with longer working hours (41%) and more EDs (31%).

Conclusions.—Misconceptions exist among caregivers, PCPs, and ED personnel on NUED visits. Our findings underscore the need to foster understanding and provide concrete areas for intervention.

▶ This survey from the Division of Pediatric Emergency Medicine in Bronx Lebanon Hospital (New York) reveals just what you would expect: that we in medicine and our patients have a communication problem. The vast majority of primary care providers (PCPs; 80%) expected to be called before a trip to the emergency department (ED), whereas less than one-third of caregivers (30%) were aware of this expectation. Because satisfaction is a measure of how close reality comes to our expectations, no wonder we are all so dissatisfied with the state of emergency care. We all have different expectations.

Just over half of caregivers (51%) thought that there was better hospitality in the ED and about 40% of both caregivers and ED personnel thought that there was less waiting time in the ED. Contrast this with the fact that only 9% of PCPs thought there was better hospitality in the ED and only about 7% thought the waiting time was less in the ED. It is apparent that PCPs (at least, in this setting) are not attuned to their patients' perceptions of an office visit as compared with an ED visit.

The one troubling statistic that I noticed in this study was that two-thirds of ED personnel thought that nonurgent ED use was due to caregivers' "exploitation of the system." It seems to me that this is a cynical view of our patients. If we believe that they come to the ED because of "lack of caregiver knowledge of what constitutes a true emergency," then we have a duty to impart that knowledge to them in a nonjudgmental, nonconfrontational manner. Moreover, we also need to work with the PCPs in our area to make sure that patients/caregivers have adequate access to care.

In a way, we may be a victim of our own success. Emergency services have become an efficient and effective mode of delivering medical care. We are open 24/7 and there is no need to make an appointment. We apparently have less waiting time and offer better hospitality than some offices and clinics. Finally, we have access to a vast array of medical technology that may not be available at a private doctor's office or clinic. Is it any wonder that patients preferentially choose us for their medical needs?

E. A. Ramoska, MD, MPHE

Pediatric clavicular fractures: assessment of fracture patterns and predictors of complicated outcome
Strauss BJ, Carey TP, Seabrook JA, et al (Univ of Western Ontario, London, Canada)
J Emerg Med 43:29-35, 2012

Background.—Clavicular fractures are the most common pediatric long-bone fracture, and although the vast majority heal with supportive treatment, complications do occur and can lead to pain and disability. Although many studies have characterized adult complication rates and risk factors, to our knowledge no comparable studies to date have looked at clavicular fractures in the pediatric population.

Study Objectives.—The study aim was to identify the radiological and clinical variables that increase the complication rate of clavicular fractures. Identification of these variables would help emergency physicians identify patients who require more thorough follow-up or surgical intervention.

Methods.—We analyzed radiographs of 537 clavicular fractures on initial presentation to the Pediatric Emergency Department at the Children's Hospital at London Health Sciences Center over a 4-year period, collecting data on variables such as displacement, angulation, and comminution, as well as demographic data such as age and gender. We then determined the outcome of each fracture by reviewing each patient's chart, and through a logistic regression analysis, determined the variables associated with complications.

Results.—Of all the fractures treated supportively (i.e., non-operatively), only 2.5% resulted in a complication. Our analysis determined that patient age was an independent predictor of complications, with each year past zero conferring an 18.1% increase in risk of complication. Furthermore, completely displaced fractures were shown to increase the odds of complication by a factor of 3.2.

Conclusion.—These findings help the emergency physician identify a group of high-risk pediatric patients with clavicular fractures for which more thorough follow-up should be considered.

▶ Clavicular fractures heal without complications and are more commonly found in children. This study included 537 clavicular fractures with bimodal presentation. The younger peak at age 3 years, and the older, between the ages of 13 and 15 years. The majority of clavicular fractures healed normally, with 3.7% have complications. These complications were found in the older age group. Thirty-five percent required open reduction, 6 were refractures, 3 had delayed union, 3 had chronic skin irritation resulting from a bony protrusion, and only 1 had nonunion. This study found that these factors required close orthopedic follow-up: increasing age in a pediatric patient, complete displacement of the fracture, and, possibly, male gender. This may offer a subgroup that would warrant closer follow-up than most.

E. C. Quintana, MD, MPH

Epidemiology of pediatric hand injuries presenting to United States emergency departments, 1990 to 2009
Shah SS, Rochette LM, Smith GA (The Res Inst at Nationwide Children's Hosp, Columbus, OH)
J Trauma Acute Care Surg 72:1688-1694, 2012

Background.—The goal of this study is to describe the epidemiology of hand injuries among children treated in US emergency departments (EDs), including the consumer products and activities most commonly associated with these injuries.

Methods.—A retrospective analysis was conducted of data from the National Electronic Injury Surveillance System for patients younger than 18 years, who were treated in an ED for hand injuries from 1990 through 2009. Sample weights were applied to calculate national estimates, and US Census Bureau data were used to determine injury rates.

Results.—An estimated 16,373,757 (95% confidence interval: 14,082,965–18,664,551) children younger than 18 years were treated in EDs for hand injuries from 1990 through 2009 with a mean annual injury number of 818,688 and rate of 11.6 per 1,000 population. There was a statistically significant decrease in the annual number (by 20.5%) and rate (by 31.5%) of hand injuries during the 20-year study period. Males accounted for 65.3% of hand injuries. Injuries most commonly occurred in the home (57.7%) and were most frequently diagnosed as lacerations (31.3%). Patients aged 10 years to14 years were most frequently diagnosed with fractures (26.7%) and were 1.71 (95% confidence interval: 1.68–1.75) times more likely to be diagnosed with a fracture than patients in other age groups. Hand injuries commonly occurred with products/activities associated with sports/recreational activities (36.4%).

Conclusion.—Hand injuries are a common and preventable source of pediatric morbidity. Prevention efforts should target the home environment and sport/recreational activities.

Level of Evidence.—Epidemiological study, level III.

▶ This study evaluated the epidemiology of hand injuries, including the role of specific consumer products and activities, over a 20-year study period. Hand injury cases in this study included children younger than 18 years treated for an injury to the hand or finger from 1990 through 2009. Of the 1 103 118 cases of hand injuries reported, children younger than age 18 represented 40.1% (442 043 cases). The mean annual pediatric hand injury rate was 11.6 per 1000 population. Patients aged 10 to 14 years sustained the largest number of injuries (39.3%), followed by 15- to 17-year-olds (23.5%), 0- to 4-year-olds (18.7%), and 5- to 9-year-olds (18.5%). Almost 99% of patients were treated and discharged from the emergency department. Sports or recreational activities (basketball, 28.2%, and football, 22.7%) had the most hand injuries, followed by doors/windows (14.2%). Laceration was the most frequent diagnosis among patients aged 0 to 4 years (37.7%), 5 to 9 years (35.7%), and 15 to 17 years (33.3%), and the second most common diagnosis for patients aged 10 to 14 years (25.0%). Patients aged 10 to 14 years were most frequently diagnosed with a fracture (26.7%). Patients aged 0 to 4 years were 3.05 times more likely to be injured by doors than those aged 5 to 17 years. These results could be used for the creation of prevention strategies that focus on the home environment and sport/recreational activities.

E. C. Quintana, MD, MPH

Cardiac Troponin T as a Screening Test for Myocarditis in Children
Eisenberg MA, Green-Hopkins I, Alexander ME, et al (Children's Hosp Boston, MA)
Pediatr Emerg Care 28:1173-1178, 2012

Objective.—The objective of this study was to define the test characteristics of cardiac troponin T (cTnT) in pediatric patients who presented with suspected myocarditis.

TABLE 2.—Diagnostic Testing Results and Outcomes of Myocarditis Patients

Method of Diagnosis	Pathology (n = 4)	MRI (n = 6)	Clinical (n = 8)	Total (% Abnormal) (n = 18)
Mean cTnT, ng/mL	0.43	0.71	2.81	1.30
ECG findings				
ECG performed	4	6	8	18
ECG abnormal	4	5	5	15 (83)
ST-Twave changes	0	4	3	7 (39)
Decreased voltage	3	0	2	5 (28)
Axis deviation	1	0	1	2 (11)
Infarct pattern	0	0	1	1 (6)
Other abnormality*	0	1	3	4 (22)
Echo findings				
Echo performed	4	6	8	18
Echo abnormal	4	5	5	14 (78)
Decreased systolic function	4	4	5	13 (72)
Ventricular dilation	3	1	1	5 (28)
Valvar dysfunction	1	1	1	3 (17)
Pericardial effusion	1	1	1	3 (17)
Atrial dilation	0	0	1	1 (6)
MRI findings				
MRI performed	1	6	1	8
MRI abnormal	0	6	0	6 (75)
Delayed gadolinium enhancement	0	5	0	5 (63)
Abnormal water signal	0	2	0	2 (25)
Path findings				
Path performed	4	1	2	7
Path consistent with myocarditis	4	0	0†	4† (57)
Outcome at discharge				
Recovery	2	5	6	13 (72)
CHF	2	1	1	4 (22)
Death	0	0	1	1 (6)

CHF was defined as ventricular dysfunction requiring the use of any combination of mechanical support, inotropic agents, afterload reduction or diuretics by the treating team
*Atrial enlargement, ventricular hypertrophy, arrhythmia, and conduction abnormalities each occurred once.
†Path inconclusive in 2 patients.

TABLE 4.—Test Characteristics of cTnT

Test Characteristic	Value	95% CI
Sensitivity	100%	0.78−1
Specificity	85%	0.79−0.89
PPV	37%	0.24−0.52
NPV	100%	0.97−1
Positive likelihood ratio	6.55	4.54−8.77
Negative likelihood ratio	0.00	0.00−0.48

Methods.—We performed a retrospective cohort study of all patients at a large urban children's hospital 21 years or younger who had a cTnT test sent for evaluation for myocarditis over a 13-month period. Patients were excluded if they had any history of heart disease or cardiac arrest before presentation, or the cTnT was sent for reasons other than concern for myocarditis. Positive cases of myocarditis were defined by characteristic pathology findings, magnetic resonance imaging results, or diagnosis of the attending cardiologist at time of discharge.

Results.—Six hundred fifty-two patients had cTnT sent during the study period. Two hundred sixty were excluded because of prior history of heart disease, and 171 had the test sent for reasons other than concern for myocarditis. Of the 221 patients included in the study, 49 had an initial positive cTnT ($\geq$ 0.01 ng/mL), whereas 172 had a negative test result. Eighteen cases of myocarditis were identified. All patients with myocarditis had an elevated cTnT at presentation. Using a cutoff value of 0.01 ng/mL or greater as a positive test, cTnT had a sensitivity of 100% (95% confidence interval [CI], 78%−100%), with a negative predictive value of 100% (CI, 97%−100%), and a specificity of 85% (CI, 79%−89%), with positive predictive value of 37% (CI, 24%−52%), in the diagnosis of myocarditis.

Conclusions.—In children without preexisting heart disease, a cTnT level of less than 0.01 ng/mL can be used to exclude myocarditis (Tables 2 and 4).

▶ Myocarditis, a rare disease in children, is a challenging diagnostic dilemma because of its nonspecific presentation. Classic cardiac symptoms for myocarditis are uncommon. This retrospective study was conducted to determine the test characteristics of cardiac troponin T (cTnT) in pediatric patients with clinical concern for myocarditis and assess the ability of cTnT to rule out myocarditis at the time of initial evaluation. A total of 18 patients had myocarditis diagnosed, 4 on pathologic specimen, 6 on magnetic resonance imaging findings, and 8 clinically (Table 2). A lower cTnT cut off, due to a lower cardiac muscle mass of children, provided a higher sensitivity and negative predictive value (Table 4). This may be used as a screening test to exclude the disease.

E. C. Quintana, MD, MPH

Accuracy of plain radiographs to exclude the diagnosis of intussusception
Roskind CG, Kamdar G, Ruzal-Shapiro CB, et al (Columbia Univ College of Physicians and Surgeons, NY; et al)
Pediatr Emerg Care 28:855-858, 2012

Objectives.—To prospectively determine the test characteristics of the 3-view abdominal radiograph to decrease the likelihood of ileocolic intussusception.

Methods.—We conducted a prospective cross-sectional study of children aged 3 months to 3 years suspected of having intussusception at a children's hospital emergency department. Clinicians obtained supine, prone, and left lateral decubitus radiographs. We determined the presence or absence of intussusception by air enema, ultrasound, operative report, or clinical follow-up. A masked pediatric radiologist reviewed all radiographs. The criteria evaluated were whether air was visualized in the ascending colon on each view and in the transverse colon on the supine view.

TABLE 3.—Test Characteristics of 3-View Abdominal Radiography in the Diagnosis of Intussusception When 2 or More of the 3 Views Have Air in the Ascending Colon

	Intussusception	No Intussusception	
Air noted in the ascending colon on <2 views	17	60	77
Air in the ascending colon noted on ≥2 of 3 views	2	49	51
	19	109	128

Sensitivity, 89.5% (95% CI, 75.7−100).
Specificity, 45.0% (95% CI, 35.6−54.3).
Negative predictive value, 96.1 (95% CI, 90.8−100).
LR(−), 0.23 (0.06−0.88).

TABLE 5. Sensitivity of Specific Radiographic Criteria

Criterion	Sensitivity (n =19 With Intussusception), %
Soft tissue mass	26.3
Small-bowel obstruction	15.8
Target sign	0
Meniscus sign	0

Results.—Nineteen (14.8%) of 128 patients had intussusception. Using air in the ascending colon on all 3 views as the diagnostic criteria, the test characteristics of the 3-view radiograph were sensitivity, 100% (95% confidence interval [CI], 79.1−100); specificity, 17.4% (95% CI, 11.1−26.1); negative predictive value, 100% (95% CI, 79.1−100); and likelihood ratio of a negative test, 0. When 2 or more of 3 views had air in the ascending colon, sensitivity decreased to 89.5% (95% CI, 75.7−100) and specificity improved to 45.0% (95% CI, 35.6−54.3). Air in the transverse colon had moderate sensitivity, 84.2% (95% CI, 67.8−100), but further improved specificity, 63.3% (95% CI, 54.2−72.4).

Conclusions.—The presence of air in the ascending colon on the 3-view abdominal radiograph can decrease the likelihood of or exclude intussusception. When clinical suspicion is low, the presence of specific criterion on a 3-view abdominal radiograph series may obviate the need for further studies (Tables 3 and 5).

▶ A common cause of pediatric intestinal obstruction is intussusception, primarily ileocolic. The classic triad of colicky abdominal pain, palpable abdominal mass, and currant jelly stools is not a common finding. Despite the increasing use of ultrasound scan, plain abdominal radiographs have long been used as a diagnostic test to evaluate ileocolic intussusception. This prospective cross-sectional study at a single tertiary care university-affiliated children's hospital emergency department found that air in the ascending colon on all 3 views had 100% sensitivity to detect ileocolic intussusceptions; the specificity was low. When using air in the ascending colon on 2 or more of the 3 views, the sensitivity was somewhat lower but with improved specificity (Table 3). Additional radiologic criteria were evaluated in the study (soft tissue mass, small bowel obstruction, target sign, and meniscus sign), yielding low sensitivity (Table 5). These results suggest that the use of the 3-view abdominal x-rays in those children with low pretest probability of intussusception based on clinical criteria alone may reduce additional diagnostic testing. This may be important in those emergency departments in which pediatric radiologists are not readily available.

E. C. Quintana, MD, MPH

A Clinical Decision Rule to Identify Infants With Apparent Life-Threatening Event Who Can Be Safely Discharged From the Emergency Department
Mittal MK, Sun G, Baren JM (The Children's Hosp of Philadelphia, PA; CHOP-Westat Biostatistics and Data Management Core, Philadelphia, PA)
Pediatr Emerg Care 28:599-605, 2012

Objective.—This study aimed to formulate a clinical decision rule (CDR) to identify infants with apparent-life threatening event (ALTE) who are at low risk of adverse outcome and can be discharged home safely from the emergency department (ED).

Methods.—This is a prospective cohort study of infants with an ED diagnosis of ALTE at an urban children's hospital. Admission was considered warranted if the infant required significant intervention during the hospital stay. Logistic regression and recursive partitioning were used to develop a CDR identifying patients at low risk of significant intervention and thus suitable for discharge from the ED.

Results.—A total of 300 infants were enrolled; 228 (76%) were admitted; 37 (12%) required significant intervention. None died during hospital stay or within 72 hours of discharge or were diagnosed with serious bacterial infection. Logistic regression identified prematurity, abnormal result in the physical examination, color change to cyanosis, absence of symptoms of upper respiratory tract infection, and absence of choking as predictors for significant intervention. These variables were used to create a CDR, based on which, 184 infants (64%) could be discharged home safely from the ED, reducing the hospitalization rate to 102 (36%). The model has a negative predictive value of 96.2% (92%–98.3%).

Conclusions.—Only 12% of infants presenting to the ED with ALTE had a significant intervention warranting hospital admission. We created a CDR that would have decreased the admission rate safely by 40% (Table 5).

▶ An apparent life-threatening event (ALTE) affecting young infants causes much concern among caregivers and medical providers. Multiple studies have demonstrated that despite a high admission rate, there was a low rate of inpatient intervention. This prospective cohort study showed the median age of infants in the cohort was 50 days; 33% of the infants were born preterm. Of the 300 infants enrolled, 228 (76%) were admitted to the hospital. Of these, 37 met criteria for significant intervention. None of the 72 infants discharged home from the

TABLE 5.—Bivariate Analysis Showing Predictors for Significant Intervention

Variables	Significant Intervention, n (%)		P
	No	Yes	
Sex			0.0436
Female	139 (52.85)	13 (35.14)	
Male	124 (47.15)	24 (64.86)	
Ethnicity			0.0107
Black	141 (53.61)	13 (35.14)	
White	94 (35.74)	14 (37.84)	
Other	28 (10.65)	10 (27.03)	
Color			0.0058
Blue	98 (38.28)	23 (62.16)	
Other	158 (61.72)	14 (37.84)	
Choking			0.009
No	82 (31.91)	19 (54.29)	
Yes	175 (68.09)	16 (45.71)	
Cough			0.0672
No	182 (69.2)	31 (83.78)	
Yes	81 (30.8)	6 (16.22)	
Runny nose			0.0667
No	218 (82.89)	35 (94.59)	
Yes	45 (17.11)	2 (5.41)	
Gestation			<0.0001
Preterm	77 (29.28)	23 (62.16)	
Full term	186 (70.72)	14 (37.84)	
Exam			0.0042
Normal	206 (78.33)	21 (56.76)	
Abnormal	57 (21.67)	16 (43.24)	

emergency department (ED) returned to the ED or had a death or other major event during the next 72 hours. The final diagnoses from the ALTE admissions were gastroesophageal reflux (49%), infections (viral), and laryngotracheal malacia. In the neurologic category, 1 patient was found to have seizures and 1 had a nonaccidental subdural hematoma. The overall rate of significant intervention was thus 37 (12%) of 300. No infant was found to have a serious bacterial infection (ie, bacterial meningitis, bacteremia, or urinary tract infection). Bivariate analysis showed that male sex, race, color change to cyanosis, absence of history of choking, absence of history of cough during the previous 24 hours, absence of history of runny nose during the previous 24 hours, premature birth (< 37 weeks of gestation), and abnormal result in the examination in the ED as predictors for significant intervention (Table 5). Logistic regression showing predictors for significant intervention were as following: prematurity, abnormal result in the examination, color change to cyanosis, no history of upper respiratory infection symptoms in the previous 24 hours, and no history of choking during the episode. Use of these clinical decision rules (CDRs) would thus have reduced hospitalization by 40% with a negative predictive value of 96.2% and a specificity of 70.5%. The CDRs wrongly classified 7 of the 184 infants. These promising findings warrant further testing.

E. C. Quintana, MD, MPH

Age variability in pediatric injuries from falls

Unni P, Locklair MR, Morrow SE, et al (Monroe Carell Jr Children's Hosp at Vanderbilt, Nashville, TN)
Am J Emerg Med 30:1457-1460, 2012

Objective.—The objective of this study is to examine the nature and circumstances surrounding pediatric fall-related injuries for specific age groups and their implications for age-appropriate injury prevention efforts.

Methods.—This is a retrospective analysis of data (October 2006 to April 2009) from the trauma registry of a level 1 pediatric trauma center. Inclusion criteria are patients admitted because of fall-related injury younger than 15 years (n = 675). Injury mechanism specifics were obtained from medical records.

Results.—Falls were the leading cause of admissions and accounted for 37% of all cases during this period. Most pediatric fall-related injuries (73%) occurred between 1 and 9 years of age. Although infants accounted for only 8% of fall injuries, a greater proportion of these children were more severely injured. The mean Injury Severity Score for infants was significantly greater than the overall average ($P < .001$). Causes of fall injuries vary by age and have been discussed.

Conclusions.—The high incidence of pediatric fall injuries warrants dedicated injury prevention education. Injury prevention efforts need to be age appropriate in terms of focus, target audience, and setting. Recommendations for injury prevention are discussed (Table 2).

▶ Falls are a common presenting complaint for emergency department evaluation. In this 31-month study, unintentional falls were the leading cause of injuries for all age groups. Most injuries were of moderate severity, except for those in the younger-than-1-year group, which were significantly more severe ($P < .001$, Table 2). In infants, falls resulted from the infant (younger than 6 months old) slipping out of a parent's, sibling's, or caregiver's arms (46%). This typically happened when the person carrying the infant slipped or fell. In infants older than 6 months, a major fall type in this group was from furniture, kitchen countertops, or tables. In the 1- to 4-year-old group, 34% of fall injuries were from this age group, primarily falls from furniture (23%), playground equipment (18%), and slipping or tripping (17%). Falls from 1 level to another (falls from trampolines, windows, decks, and toy vehicles) comprised 19% of fall injuries in this 1- to 4-year-old group. The 5- to 9-year-old group accounted for the highest number

TABLE 2.—Injury Severity Score by Age

ISS	<1 y	1-4 y	5-9 y	10-14 y
Mild (< 9)	12 (21%)	27 (12%)	31 (12%)	29 (23%)
Moderate (9-15)	22 (39%)	190 (82%)	224 (86%)	77 (62%)
Severe (> 15)	22 (39%)	14 (6%)	7 (3%)	19 (15%)
Total	56 (100%)	232 (100%)	262 (100%)	125 (100%)

of fall-related hospitalizations (39%). Almost a third of these injuries were caused by falls from playground equipment, monkey bars, and slides. The 10- to 14-year-old group accounted for 19% of fall hospitalizations, with the leading cause reported as falls from skateboards (24%). This information is important to keep in mind when evaluating pediatric falls, because most age-appropriate prevention education for parents and caregivers.

E. C. Quintana, MD, MPH

Emergency Department Transport Rates of Children From the Scene of Motor Vehicle Collisions: Do Booster Seats Make a Difference?

House DR, Huffman G, Walthall JDH (Indiana Univ School of Medicine, Indianapolis)
Pediatr Emerg Care 28:1211-1214, 2012

Background.—Motor vehicle collisions (MVCs) are the leading cause of death and disability among children older than 1 year. Many states currently mandate all children between the ages of 4 and 8 years be restrained in booster seats. The implementation of a booster-seat law is generally thought to decrease the occurrence of injury to children. We hypothesized that appropriate restraint with booster seats would also cause a decrease in emergency department (ED) visits compared with children who were unrestrained. This is an important measure as ED visits are a surrogate marker for injury.

Objective.—The main purpose of this study was to look at the rate of ED visits between children in booster seats compared with those in other or no restraint systems involved in MVCs. Injury severity was compared across restraint types as a secondary outcome of booster-seat use after the implementation of a state law.

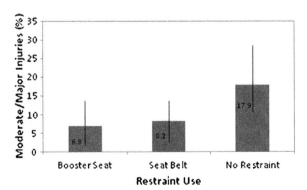

FIGURE 2.—Moderate/major injuries by restraint use. (Reprinted from House DR, Huffman G, Walthall JDH. Emergency department transport rates of children from the scene of motor vehicle collisions: do booster seats make a difference? *Pediatr Emerg Care.* 2012;28:1211-1214, with permission from Lippincott Williams & Wilkins.)

TABLE 2.—Booster Seat and Seatbelt Use by Demographics

	% Booster Seat	% Seatbelt	% No Restraint	P
Male (n = 75)	37.3	44.0	18.7	0.891
Female (n = 84)	35.7	47.6	16.7	
White (n = 61)	52.5	37.7	9.8	0.004
African American (n = 83)	28.9	45.0	24.1	
Other (n = 15)	13.3	73.3	13.3	
4 y (n = 40)	52.5	35.0	12.5	0.020
5 y (n = 32)	40.6	31.2	28.1	
6 y (n = 29)	41.4	41.4	17.2	
7 y (n = 33)	27.3	57.6	15.1	
8 y (n = 25)	12.0	72.0	16.0	

TABLE 3.—Secondary Outcomes by Restraint Use

	Booster Seat	Seatbelt	No Restraint	P
% Died (n)	0.0 (0)	1.4 (1)	3.6 (1)	0.377
% Major/moderate injury (n)	6.9 (5)	8.2 (6)	17.9 (5)	0.236
Mean GCS score (SD)	14.97 (0.18)	14.71 (1.68)	14.50 (2.27)	0.363

Methods.—A prospective observational study was performed including all children 4 to 8 years old involved in MVCs to which emergency medical services was dispatched. Ambulance services used a novel on-scene computer charting system for all MVC-related encounters to collect age, sex, child-restraint system, Glasgow Coma Scale score, injuries, and final disposition.

Results.—One hundred fifty-nine children were studied with 58 children (35.6%) in booster seats, 73 children in seatbelts alone (45.2%), and 28 children (19.1%) in no restraint system. 76 children (47.7%), 74 by emergency medical services and 2 by private vehicle, were transported to the ED with no significant difference between restraint use (P = 0.534). Utilization of a restraint system did not significantly impact MVC injury severity. However, of those children who either died (n = 2) or had an on-scene decreased Glasgow Coma Scale score (n = 6), 75% (6/8) were not restrained in a booster seat.

Conclusions.—The use of booster-seat restraints does not appear to be associated with whether a child will be transported to the ED for trauma evaluation (Fig 2, Tables 2 and 3).

▶ This prospective observational study evaluated booster seat—restrained 4- to 8-year-old children with the hypothesis that they will have fewer emergency department (ED) visits and injuries from motor vehicle collisions (MVC) than unrestrained or improperly restrained children. Only 58 children (36.5%) were in booster seats, 73 (45.9%) were in seatbelts, and 28 (17.6%) were not restrained. White children were more likely to be in a booster seat; moreover, younger-aged children were associated with increased booster seat use (Table 2). There were no significant differences among injury severity and restraint use; however, there was a trend in the 42% of children involved in MVCs toward increasing injury severity in those unrestrained compared with those restrained in a seatbelt or booster seat (Fig 2). There were 2 deaths out of 159 children. Similarly, other secondary outcomes, Glasgow Coma score and death, showed no significant differences across booster seat use or any restraint use (Table 3). Based on continued emergency medical services transport of uninjured or minorly injured children, ED transport could not be used as a marker to best determine booster seat effect on health care cost or injury severity. At best, it is reflective of the parental concerns regarding their small children.

E. C. Quintana, MD, MPH

Utilization of a Pediatric Observation Unit for Toxicologic Ingestions
Plumb J, Dudley NC, Herman BE, et al (Univ of Utah School of Medicine, Salt Lake City)
Pediatr Emerg Care 28:1169-1172, 2012

Objectives.—The objectives of this study were to evaluate the efficacy and utilization of an observation unit (OU) for admission of pediatric patients after a toxicologic ingestion; compare the characteristics and outcomes of patients admitted to the pediatric OU, inpatient (IP) service, and intensive care unit (ICU) after ingestions using retrospective chart review; and attempt to identify factors associated with unplanned IP admission after an OU admission.

Methods.—This was a retrospective chart review of children seen in the emergency department (ED) after potentially toxic suspected ingestions and then admitted to the OU, IP service, or ICU from June 2003 to September 2007.

Results.—One thousand twenty-three children were seen in the ED for ingestions: 18% were admitted to the OU, 15% to the IP service service, and 6% to the ICU. Observation unit patients had less mental status changes reported and were less frequently given medications while in the ED. Eighty-one percent of OU patients were admitted with poison center recommendation. Ninety-four percent of OU patients were discharged within 24 hours, and less than half of IP service/ICU patients were discharged that quickly.

TABLE 1.—ED Findings for Patients Admitted After Suspected Toxicologic Ingestions, by Admission Location*

In ED	OU (n = 183)	IP Unit (n = 153)	ICU (n = 61)
Mental status change	30% (55)	45% (69)	74% (45)
Vital sign abnormality	18% (33)	22% (34)	48% (29)
Medication given as treatment	10% (19)	41% (62)	72% (44)

*Number of patients reported in parentheses.

TABLE 2.—Most Common Substances Ingested, or Suspected of Ingestion, for Admitted Patients*

Substance Ingested	OU	IP Unit	ICU
Acetaminophen	3%	22%	21%
CNS/psychiatric	32%	37%	46%
Cardiac/anti-HTN	16%	5%	8%
Cough/cold	10%	14%	8%
Detergent/caustic	2%	6%	2%
Hydrocarbon	10%	3%	7%
Hypoglycemic	8%	1%	0%
Opioid	7%	5%	12%
Stimulant	8%	9%	8%

*All reported/suspected substances were documented; these are the most common. In the case of suspected polypharmacy ingestion, each drug was listed. Totals will be greater than 100%.

TABLE 3.—Reasons Given for Admission From the ED*

Reason	OU	IP Unit	ICU
Poison center recommendation	81%	39%	34%
Mental status change	21%	38%	38%
Vital sign abnormality	8%	11%	20%
Psychiatric consult	2%	75%	16%
Child abuse/neglect consult	0.3%	9%	0%
NAC	0%	20%	16%
Telemetry/arrhythmia	0%	16%	10%
Respiratory distress/failure	0%	5%	20%

*All reasons given by admitting ED physician for admission; individual patients had between 1 and 6 reasons given for admission. Totals will be greater than 100%.

TABLE 4.—Reasons for UIA for OU Patients

Patient No.	Age, y	Reason for UIA
1	2.1	Increased acetaminophen level and NAC administration
2	3.4	Mental status change and social work involvement
3	1.3	Hypoxia
4	15	Mental status change and psychiatry involvement
5	1.8	Bradycardia and intravenous fluids
6	0.8	Hypoxia and repeat naloxone administration
7	14	Continued agitation and lorazepam administration
8	8	Continued ataxia
9	2	Hypoglycemia and frequent glucose checks
10	0.8	Oral burns and need for endoscopy

No significant associations were found between specific historical and physical examination or laboratory characteristics in the ED and the need for unplanned IP admission.

Conclusions.—Observation unit patients admitted after ingestions were young, typically ingested substances found in the home, and required observation according to poison center recommendations. Ninety-four percent were able to be discharged home within 24 hours even after ingesting some of the most concerning substances such as central nervous system depressants, cardiac/antihypertension medications, hypoglycemics, and opiates. All OU patients did well without any adverse events reported. Many patients requiring prolonged observation after an ingestion, and who do not require ICU care, may be appropriate for OU management. This study suggests a potential underutilization of observation units in this setting (Tables 1-4).

▶ Overdoses and toxic ingestion are a common emergency department (ED) presentation in children. Most are nontoxic; however, there is a subset that requires variable observation periods. If that is needed, what should one do? Usually that subset of pediatric patients was admitted to either pediatric ward or intensive care unit (ICU). This study evaluated effectiveness of an observation unit (OU) versus inpatient status. Observation unit patients had less mental status changes reported and were less frequently given medications compared with inpatient service patients while in the ED (Table 1). The most common ingestions with OU admissions were psychotropic/central nervous system medications (32%) and cardiac/antihypertension medications (16%) (Table 2). Poison Control Center recommendations lead to most of the reasons for OU admission (81%, Table 3). The OU patients had fewer laboratory tests, studies, consultations, or pharmacologic treatments in contrast with the inpatient pediatric patients. The discharge percentage from the OU was 94% within 24 hours of admission, whereas there was a discharge rate of less than 50% from inpatient pediatrics. There were no adverse events for OU patients. Only 10 patients had an unplanned admission from OU care (Table 4). Univariate analyses found no significant associations between specific historical, physical examination, or laboratory characteristics in the ED and the need for an unplanned admission. OU management is appropriate for patients requiring prolonged observation after a toxicologic ingestion who do not require intensive care unit admittance.

E. C. Quintana, MD, MPH

Conducted Electrical Weapon (TASER) Use Against Minors: A Shocking Analysis
Gardner AR, Hauda WE II, Bozeman WP (Wake Forest Univ Health Sciences, Winston-Salem, NC; Virginia Commonwealth Univ School of Medicine, Falls Church)
Pediatr Emerg Care 28:873-877, 2012

Objective.—Conducted electrical weapons (CEWs) such as the TASER are often used by law enforcement (LE) personnel during suspect apprehension. Previous studies have reported an excellent safety profile and few adverse outcomes with CEW use in adults. We analyzed the safety and injury profile of CEWs when used during LE apprehension of children and adolescents, a potentially vulnerable population.

Injury Severity Guide

Mild	Moderate	Severe
Outpatient treatment _and_ No or mild disability expected	Inpatient treatment _and / or_ Moderate disability expected	Inpatient treatment _and_ Severe disability expected _or_ Death
Examples: *Contusions, abrasions, minor lacerations*	*Examples:* *Long bone fracture, Hemo/Pneumothorax, Liver / Spleen lacerations, Moderate head Injury*	*Examples:* *Loss of limb or eye, Severe Head Injury, Ventricular fibrillation*

FIGURE 2.—Injury severity classifications. (Reprinted from Gardner AR, Hauda WE II, Bozeman WP. Conducted electrical weapon (TASER) use against minors: a shocking analysis. *Pediatr Emerg Care.* 2012;28:873-877, with permission from Lippincott Williams & Wilkins.)

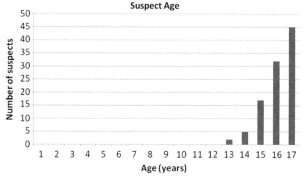

FIGURE 3.—Age of minor suspects. (Reprinted from Gardner AR, Hauda WE II, Bozeman WP. Conducted electrical weapon (TASER) use against minors: a shocking analysis. *Pediatr Emerg Care.* 2012;28:873-877, with permission from Lippincott Williams & Wilkins.)

Methods.—Consecutive CEW uses by LE officers against criminal suspects were tracked at 10 LE agencies and entered into a database as part of an ongoing multicenter injury surveillance program. All CEW uses against minors younger than 18 years were retrieved for analysis. Primary outcomes included the incidence and type of mild, moderate, and severe CEW-related injury, as assessed by physician reviewers in each case. Ultimate outcomes, suspect demographics, and circumstances surrounding LE involvement are reported secondarily.

Results.—Of 2026 consecutive CEW uses, 100 (4.9%) were uses against minor suspects. Suspects ranged from 13 to 17 years, with a mean age of 16.1 (SD, 0.99) years (median, 16 years). There were no significant (moderate or severe) injuries reported (0%; 97.5% confidence interval, 0.0%–3.6%). Twenty suspects (20%; 95% confidence interval, 12.7%–29.1%) were noted to sustain 34 mild injuries. The majority of these injuries (67.6%) were expected superficial punctures from CEW probes. Other mild injuries included superficial abrasions and contusions in 7 cases (7%).

Conclusions.—None of the minor suspects studied sustained significant injury, and only 20% reported minor injuries, mostly from the expected probe puncture sites. These data suggest that adolescents are not at a substantially higher risk than adults for serious injuries after CEW use (Figs 2 and 3).

▶ A conducted electrical weapon (CEW) is a tool used by law enforcement officer as a less lethal force option toward suspect apprehension. The primary outcome measure in this study, in those younger than 18 years old, was significant injuries, with a composite of moderate and severe injuries. The ages of minor suspects ranged from 13 to 17 years (Fig 3). The mean age was 16.1 years (SD, 0.99; median, 16 years). The mean recorded height was 5 ft 8 in or 68 in (SD, 3.55; median, 68 in), and the mean weight was 168 lb (SD, 40.64; median, 156 lb). Ninety-two (92%) of the suspects were male. Alcohol or other drug intoxication was known or suspected by police in 30 cases (30%). Alcohol was noted to be the predominant cause of intoxication in 17 (56%) of these, followed by marijuana in 6 cases (19.4%). Sixty-four percent of the injuries were in the torso, followed by 55 (32%) in the extremities or buttocks, and 6 (4%) in the head or neck. There were no cases of significant (moderate or severe, Fig 2) injuries reported (0%; 97.5% CI, 0.0-3.6%) among the 100 suspects. The majority, 23 (67.6%) of 34, of these were superficial puncture wounds that were an expected result of contact with the CEW probes. Seven patients (7%) sustained 11 unanticipated mild injuries including 8 superficial abrasions (23.5%) in 4 patients, 2 minor lacerations (5.9%) in 2 patients, and 1 episode (2.9%) of epistaxis. An electrocardiogram (ECG) was obtained in 5 suspects (5%); 4 suspects showed a normal sinus rhythm with no abnormalities noted. One subject was a 17-year-old male (height, 6 ft 3 in; weight, 260 lb) with suspected stimulant drug intoxication who sustained 2 discharges of a CEW to the anterior torso lasting approximately 40 seconds. He was noted to have a sinus tachycardia with prolonged PR interval and unifocal premature ventricular contractions. After observation, there was a complete resolution of all the abnormalities. The data in this study support that CEW use during apprehension of adolescents does not seem to pose unacceptable levels of risk, although continued studies are warranted.

E. C. Quintana, MD, MPH

Petechaiae/Purpura in Well-Appearing Infants
Lee MH, Barnett PLJ (Univ of Melbourne, Victoria, Australia)
Pediatr Emerg Care 28:503-505, 2012

Background.—Well infants with petechiae and/or purpura can present to emergency departments, and their management can be difficult. Many will have extensive investigations and treatment that may not be necessary.

Methods.—This was a retrospective and descriptive audit investigating well infants (<8 months of age) presenting with petechiae or purpura in the absence of fever to a pediatric emergency department over a 9½-year period. All presenting problems of petechiae or purpura were reviewed. Patients were excluded if they appeared unwell, were febrile or have a history of fever, or had eccyhmoses on presentation.

Results.—Thirty-six babies were identified. The average age was 3.8 months (range, 1—7 months). The majority of the infants had localized purpura/petechiae to the lower limbs (92%) with two thirds of these patients having bilateral signs. None had generalized signs. Most infants had a full blood count (94%), coagulation profile (59%) and C-reactive protein (59%), and blood cultures (59%), with all being normal (except for mild elevation in platelets). Nine patients were admitted for observation, with only 1 patient having progression of signs. This patient had a diagnosis of acute hemorrhagic edema of infancy. The rest of the patients were thought to have either a mechanical reason for their petechiae/purpura (tourniquet phenomena) or a formal diagnosis was not specified.

Conclusions.—Well infants with localized purpura and/or petechiae with an absence of fever are more likely to have a benign etiology. Further study is required to determine if a full blood count and coagulation profile is necessary, or a period of observation (4 hours) is all that is required. If there is no progression of signs, it is likely that they can be safely discharged. The likely cause may be due to a tourniquet phenomenon (eg, diaper).

▶ The presence of petechiae/purpura (P/P) prompts the treating emergency physician to consider meningococcal disease, whether the patient is well-appearing or not. With such catastrophic outcomes associated with meningococcemia, patients will routinely get diagnostic testing, including a complete blood count with platelets and a period of observation. The authors of this study believe that much of this testing is unnecessary and advocate for a less invasive approach for afebrile patients with P/P. In this retrospective review, afebrile patients generally had a benign etiology for their skin abnormalities. Great caution should be used when following these recommendations and when considering a rapidly progressing deadly illness. The authors do advocate for more research into the merits of regular diagnostic testing, and further recommend a period of observation (4 hours) to assess for progression of the P/P. Until more robust data with a larger sample size can support the attached results, emergency physicians should probably continue to use their clinical judgment when ordering blood work.

E. C. Bruno, MD

Infectious Disease

Adherence of families to a group a streptococcal pharyngitis protocol used in a pediatric emergency department

Pockett CR, Thompson GC (Univ of Alberta, Edmonton, Canada)
Pediatr Emerg Care 27:374-378, 2011

Objectives.—In an effort to limit inappropriate antibiotic use for children with pharyngitis, our pediatric emergency department (PED) has implemented a strep throat protocol using preprinted prescriptions given to families pending pharyngeal swab results. We sought to determine the rate of adherence of families managed with this protocol and to identify whether clinical features are associated with adherence.

Methods.—We conducted a prospective cohort study of children aged 2 to 17 years presented to the PED with suspected group A streptococcal (GAS) pharyngitis. Prescription-filling activity was tracked using a novel carbon-copy prescription and compared with throat swab result. Health records were reviewed for demographic and clinical information. Adherence was defined as prescriptions being filled after notification of a positive swab result and prescriptions not being filled when throat swab result was negative.

Results.—Three hundred nine children were screened for GAS pharyngitis. One hundred swabs (32.4%) were positive for GAS pharyngitis, of which 15 prescriptions were filled before swab results. No record of prescription filling was found for 37 of the children with positive swab results. Only 9 families (4.3%) filled the prescription when the swab result was negative. Overall, 247 families (80.2%) were adherent to the protocol. Families of children aged 2 to 5 years were more likely to be adherent than those aged 13 to 17 years (odds ratio, 3.5; 95% confidence interval, 1.15-10.66).

Conclusions.—Most families are adherent to our GAS pharyngitis protocol. Very few families filled prescriptions when the swab result was negative. Age was the only factor influencing adherence. Our current GAS pharyngitis protocol is an effective management strategy for children presenting with pharyngitis to the PED.

▶ Physicians cannot rely on just physical examination to diagnose strep pharyngitis. This study evaluated how reliable parents were to following a protocol in which those patients suspected of having group A streptococcal pharyngitis (GAS) had a throat swab culture. Unit clerks would contact the family for those with a positive GAS throat culture and advise the family to fill the given prescription. Negative throat swabs were recorded but the family was not contacted. Families received a copy of an inactivated antibiotic prescription, which the local pharmacist faxed to the ED. The faxed prescription was activated by the unit clerk regardless of time, date, or culture results. This study found that 80% of families followed the strep throat protocol. The largest proportion of non-adherence were patients with positive throat cultures who did not fill their prescriptions.

There were some limitations to these findings: some pharmacies filling out the prescriptions did not follow the protocol or received additional prescriptions from other physicians who were not aware of the current treatment. Only 4.3% of patients filled their prescription despite a negative throat culture. Unfortunately, these results showed that this protocol is unlikely to decrease the inappropriate treatment of viral pharyngitis with antibiotics.

E. C. Quintana, MD, MPH

Delayed Versus Immediate Antimicrobial Treatment for Acute Otitis Media

Tähtinen PA, Laine MK, Ruuskanen O, et al (Turku Univ Hosp, Finland)

Pediatr Infect Dis J 31:1227-1232, 2012

Background.—Watchful waiting with the option of delayed antimicrobial treatment for acute otitis media is recommended in several guidelines. Our aim was to study whether delayed, as compared with immediate, initiation of antimicrobial treatment worsens the recovery from acute otitis media in young children.

Methods.—Children (6—35 months) with acute otitis media received either delayed or immediate antimicrobial treatment with amoxicillin-clavulanate for 7 days. The delayed antimicrobial treatment group (n = 53) consisted of placebo recipients from a randomized-controlled trial to whom antimicrobial treatment was initiated after a watchful waiting period. The immediate antimicrobial treatment group (n = 161) consisted of children allocated to receive antimicrobial treatment immediately.

Results.—Improvement during antimicrobial treatment (which includes both symptoms and otoscopic signs) was observed in 91% and 96% of children in the delayed and immediate antimicrobial treatment groups, respectively ($P = 0.15$). Median watchful waiting period was 48 hours. Delayed initiation of antimicrobial treatment was associated with prolonged resolution of fever, ear pain, poor appetite and decreased activity, but not ear rubbing, irritability, restless sleep or excessive crying. Parents of children in the delayed antimicrobial treatment group missed more work days (mean 2.1 versus 1.2 days, $P = 0.03$). Diarrhea, vomiting and rash were equally common in both groups.

Conclusions.—Our results indicate that delayed initiation of antimicrobial treatment does not worsen the recovery from acute otitis media, as measured by improvement during treatment. However, watchful waiting before the initiation of delayed antimicrobial treatment might be associated with transient worsening of a child's condition, prolongation of symptoms and economic losses.

▶ Because otitis media is both a common diagnosis and a common presentation in the emergency department, the aim of this study was to determine if delayed, as compared with immediate, initiation of antimicrobial treatment worsens the recovery from acute otitis media and what were the sequelae of a watchful waiting period. This was a small prospective follow-up study in a randomized, double-blind, placebo-controlled trial demonstrating that delayed, as compared with immediate, initiation of antimicrobial treatment did not worsen the recovery from acute otitis media. The improvement during antimicrobial treatment was similar in both groups. Delayed initiation of antimicrobial treatment seems to be associated with prolonged resolution of symptoms, especially with the symptom of fever. Prolongation of fever by 2 days is significant for the family because fever causes anxiety and parental absenteeism from work. A limitation of this study is the lack of generalizability to older children because most of the children were younger than 2 years of age in the study. However, the study patients represented the age group with the highest incidence of acute otitis media.

E. C. Quintana, MD, MPH

The management of bite wounds in children—A retrospective analysis at a level I trauma centre
Jaindl M, Grünauer J, Platzer P, et al (Med Univ of Vienna, Austria; et al)
Injury 43:2117-2121, 2012

Introduction.—Animal bite wounds are a significant problem, which have caused several preventable child deaths in clinical practice in the past. The majority of bite wounds is caused by dogs and cats, and also humans have to be considered to lead to those extreme complicated diagnosis in the paediatric patient population. Early estimation of infection risk, adequate antibiotic therapy and, if indicated, surgical treatment, are cornerstones of successful cures of bite wounds. However, antibiotic prophylaxis and wound management are discussed controversially in the current literature. In our study, we retrospectively investigated the bite source, infection risk and treatment options of paediatric bite wounds.

Methods.—A total of 1592 paediatric trauma patients were analysed over a period of 19 years in this retrospective study at a level I trauma centre, Department of Trauma Surgery, Medical University of Vienna, Austria. Data for this study were obtained from our electronic patient records and follow-up visits. In our database, all paediatric patients triaged to our major urban trauma centre have been entered retrospectively.

Results.—During the 19-year study period, 1592 paediatric trauma patients met the inclusion criteria. The mean age was 7.7 years (range 0—18.9), 878 (55.2%) were males and 714 (44.8%) were females. In our study population, a total of 698 dog bites (43.8%), 694 human bites (43.6%), 138 other bites (8.7%) and 62 cat bites (3.9%) have been observed. A total of 171 wounds (10.7%) have been infected. Surgical intervention was done in 27 wounds (1.7%).

Conclusion.—Gender-related incidence in bite wounds for dog and cat could be detected. Second, our findings for originator of bite wounds reflect the findings in the published literature. Total infection rate reached 10.7%, primary antibiotic therapy was administered in 221 cases (13.9%) and secondary antibiotic therapy in 20 (1.3%) cases. Observed infection rate of punctured wounds and wounds greater than 3 cm was 3 times higher than for all other wounds.

Our findings need to be proven in further prospective clinical trials.

▶ Cat and dog bites are a common occurrence in children, especially children younger than 5 years. In this 19-year retrospective study, the mean age was 7.7 years, with 55.2% boys and 44.8% girls. Fourteen percent of dog-bite wounds were infected compared with 37% infected cat bites. The bites were primarily on the lip (32%) followed by the extremities (shoulder, arm, femur, and tibia, 26.1%). Thirteen percent received primary antibiotic therapy. Primary infection rates for dog bites were 8.5% compared with 30.6% in cats. In contrast, secondary infection rate was similar in cats and dogs (6.5% and 6.3%, respectively). Overall infection rates were as follows: for surface wounds, 27.5%; punctured wounds, 19.2%, less than 1 cm, (10%); 1—3 cm 10.3%; and greater than 3 cm, 18.8%. Interestingly, secondary infection rates were significantly higher in patients who received primary antibiotic therapy (14.9% v 3.7% [*P* > .001]). These interesting findings should be kept in mind when treating pediatric domestic animal bites.

E. C. Quintana, MD, MPH

Accuracy of Ultrasonography Versus Computed Tomography Scan in Detecting Parapharengeal Abscess in Children
Kalmovich LM, Gavriel H, Eviatar E, et al (Tel Aviv Univ, Israel)
Pediatr Emerg Care 28:780-782, 2012

Objective.—Significant morbidity and rarely mortality have been described in parapharyngeal space infections in children; hence, the decision on the timing of surgical intervention might be crucial. The aim of this study was to compare the accuracy of plain x-rays, ultrasonography (US), and contrast-enhanced computed tomography (CT) in demonstrating a parapharyngeal abscess.

Methods.—A retrospective study on all patients with parapharyngeal abscess admitted and operated on from January 1996 to December 2000 was carried out. Charts were reviewed for patients' demographics, symptoms and signs, details of workup, intraoperative findings, and culture results. The CT scans were reviewed for the presence of a rim enhancement, a presence of a definable wall, and fluid-fluid level and were correlated with the plain x-rays and US results and intraoperative findings.

Results.—Eighteen patients with proven parapharyngeal infection were included: 10 with proven abscess and 8 with cellulitis. The sensitivity and specificity of lateral neck radiograph and US were low compared with a specificity of 87.5 while evaluating fluid-fluid level seen on the CT scan, sensitivity of 58.3% for the presence of a definable abscess wall, and a sensitivity of 100% for the presence of a prominent wall.

Conclusions.—Our study demonstrates good rates of accuracy of CT scan for diagnosing a parapharyngeal abscess. Our study suggest that it is appropriate to obtain a CT scan upon presentation in all children with suspected parapharyngeal abscess and that a CT scan is proven to be a useful diagnostic tool in establishing a treatment plan.

▶ This retrospective study evaluated the accuracy of different diagnostic testing for retropharyngeal abscess. Eighteen patients with a parapharyngeal infection, 12 boys and 6 girls, with a mean age of 3.6 years were included in this study. Twelve parapharyngeal infections were located on the left side with leukocytosis and fever as the most common findings. The most common isolated pathogen was *Staphylococcus*. All patients underwent a preoperative computed tomography (CT) scan, 4 underwent a lateral neck radiograph, and 8 patients underwent an ultrasound scan before doing the CT scan. The lateral x-rays had a sensitivity of 66.6%, and the ultrasound scan had a sensitivity for the fluid-fluid level of only 33.3% with a PPV of 50%. In contrast, the CT scan had better sensitivity and specificity. These results imply that a contrast-enhanced high-resolution cervical CT scan is indicated after the clinical diagnosis or suspicion of a parapharyngeal abscess, as it is the best imaging modality for the diagnosis of this condition.

E. C. Quintana, MD, MPH

Procalcitonin as a Marker of Bacteremia in Children With Fever and a Central Venous Catheter Presenting to the Emergency Department
Kasem AJ, Bulloch B, Henry M, et al (Phoenix Children's Hosp, AZ)
Pediatr Emerg Care 28:1017-1021, 2012

Objective.—To evaluate the clinical use of procalcitonin (PCT) as a rapid marker for the identification of bacteremia in the emergency department (ED) population of children with fever and a central venous catheter (CVC).

Methods.—Children were identified on presentation to the ED with a chief complaint of fever and who had a CVC. Fever was defined as 38°C or higher orally. Patients were excluded from the study if they had received antibiotics within the previous 24 hours of presenting to the ED, if they had a peripherally inserted central catheter line or by parental refusal. On presentation to the ED, all patients had a complete blood cell count with differential, blood culture from the central line, and PCT levels drawn. All had empiric antibiotics initiated. Blood culture results were recorded, and in the case of positive cultures, time to positive culture was noted.

Results.—Sixty-two patients (aged 5 months—18 y) were enrolled, and 14 (23%) had a positive culture. Mean PCT value in bacteremic patients was 18.47 ± 31.6 ng/mL and 0.65 ± 1.2 ng/mL in nonbacteremic patients ($P < 0.001$). Median PCT for negative blood culture was 0.23 ng/mL (interquartile range, 0.11—0.61) and 1.15 ng/mL for a positive blood culture (interquartile range, 0.45—29.16). The receiver operating characteristic analysis identified a level of PCT of 0.3 ng/mL as the best cutoff point that produced a sensitivity of 93% and a specificity of 63% (area under the curve, 0.82).

Conclusions.—The PCT levels are useful in identifying children with fever and a CVC who are bacteremic in the ED.

▶ Procalcitonin (PCT) is a new marker of systemic inflammatory reactions caused by bacteremia and sepsis. The authors found that patients with central venous lines and fever with an initial PCT less than 0.05 developed a positive blood culture. An analysis of coordinates of the received operating characteristic curve identified a PCT value of 0.3 ng/mL as the optimal threshold, with a corresponding sensitivity and specificity of 93% and 63%, respectively. The mean PCT value in neutropenic patients with a positive blood culture was 19.16 ng/mL compared with 0.65 ng/mL in those who had negative cultures ($P < .001$). This marker shows promise for emergency department management of febrile children with central venous lines.

E. C. Quintana, MD, MPH

Comparison of Amoxicillin/Clavulanic Acid High Dose with Cefdinir in the Treatment of Acute Otitis Media

Casey JR, Block SL, Hedrick J, et al (Legacy Pediatrics, Rochester, NY; Kentucky Pediatric Res, Bardstown; et al)
Drugs 72:1991-1997, 2012

Background.—10 days of amoxicillin/clavulanic acid high dose and 5 days of cefdinir have been the preferred first- or second-line antibiotics for treatment of children with acute otitis media (AOM) since 2004, as recommended by the American Academy of Pediatrics in the USA, but no head-to-head comparison study has been done.

Objective.—The purpose of the study was to compare the clinical efficacy of amoxicillin/clavulanic acid high-dose therapy for 10 days with cefdinir therapy for 5 days for AOM at recommended doses.

Methods.—This was an investigator-blind trial in young children 6—24 months old with no history of recurrent AOM who were randomly assigned to amoxicillin/clavulanic acid (80 mg/kg/day amoxicillin) or cefdinir (14 mg/kg/day), both in two divided doses.

The diagnosis of AOM was based on specific clinical criteria by validated otoscopists at two AOM research centres. The outcome measure for clinical cure was resolution of all symptoms and signs of AOM except for persistence of middle-ear effusion at test-of-cure (TOC) 11—14 days after initiation of antibiotic treatment. Clinical failure was defined as persistence of symptoms and signs of AOM and the need for additional antibiotic therapy. Subjects lost to follow up or who had not taken at least 80% of the prescribed medication were classified as having an indeterminate response. Compliance was monitored using Medical Electronic Monitoring System (MEMS) caps and antibiotic bottle volume measurement at the TOC

TABLE 1.—Clinical Outcomes with Amoxicillin/Clavulanic Acid High Dose versus Cefdinir

Outcome	High-Dose Amoxicillin/Clavulanic Acid $N = 165$	Cefdinir $N = 165$
Clinical cure (no. of pts)	141	115
Clinical failure (no. of pts)	22	47
Indeterminate (no. of pts)	3	3
Cure rate (%)	86.5[a]	71.0

pts = patients.
[a]Chi-square = 10.8, degrees of freedom = 1, p-value = 0.001.

TABLE 2.—Odds Ratios for Clinical Cure per Increasing Month of Age Estimated From a Logistic Regression Model for Amoxicillin/Clavulanic Acid High Dose and Cefdinir Treatment Groups

Treatment	Odds Ratio (95% CI)	p-Value
High-dose amoxicillin/clavulanic acid	0.992 (0.932, 1.056)	>0.05
Cefdinir	0.932 (0.881, 0.986)	0.01

visit. A logistic regression model was used to estimate the association of age with cure rate. Full interactions in terms of age with treatment were included to estimate any age gradient differential.

Results.—A total of 330 children (average age 13.1 months) with AOM were studied. At TOC, 256 children had clinical cure, 69 had clinical failure, and 5 were lost to follow-up. High-dose amoxicillin/clavulanic acid-treated children had a better cure rate (86.5%) than cefdinir-treated patients (71.0%; $p = 0.001$). Cefdinir was correlated with less frequent cure outcomes as children increased in age between 6 and 24 months. The odds ratios for clinical cure per increasing month of age estimated from a logistic regression model for amoxicillin/clavulanic acid high dose and cefdinir treatment groups was 0.992 (95% CI 0.932, 1.056), $p > 0.05$ and 0.932 (95% CI 0.881, 0.986), $p = 0.01$. The differences in the odds ratios are significant at $p < 0.002$, indicating a stable clinical cure rate across the ages of children studied for amoxicillin/clavulanic acid and decreasing clinical cure rates as children increased in age for cefdinir.

Conclusion.—In children with *bona fide* AOM for whom clinical outcomes are assessed by validated otoscopists, 10 days of high-dose amoxicillin/clavulanic acid is significantly more effective than 5 days of cefdinir as therapy for AOM. Because of the identified age effect (correlated to child weight), higher doses of cefdinir may have led to a different conclusion; 10 days of cefdinir may also have led to a different conclusion (Tables 1 and 2).

▶ This was a prospective, randomized, investigator-blinded trial that included 330 children aged 6–24 months with acute otitis media. Antibiotic treatment consisted of amoxicillin/clavulanic acid high dose (80 mg/kg/day amoxicillin divided twice daily) or cefdinir (14 mg/kg/day divided twice daily). High-dose amoxicillin/clavulanic acid was given for 10 days and cefdinir for 5 days. There is a significant difference between the 2 antibiotics ($P < .002$). The difference in efficacy with high-dose amoxicillin/clavulanic acid between the ages of 6 and 24 months in the children treated did not impact the overall cure rate (OR 0.87 [95% CI 0.28, 2.69]; $P = .8$). In contrast, the difference in efficacy with cefdinir between the ages of 6 and 24 months in the children treated did adversely impact the overall cure rate (OR 0.28 [95% CI 0.10, 0.78]; $P = .01$) (Table 1). The odds ratio for cure remained stable for treatment with high-dose amoxicillin/clavulanic acid but significantly declined for treatment with cefdinir ($P = .01$) (Table 2). The better efficacy observed with high-dose amoxicillin/clavulanic acid must be taken in the context that these children were in a clinical trial where compliance was very high (>80%), which may be different in the emergency department population, as amoxicillin/clavulanic has significant gastrointestinal symptoms.

E. C. Quintana, MD, MPH

Neuroscience

The frequency of cerebral ischemia/hypoxia in pediatric severe traumatic brain injury

Padayachy LC, Rohlwink U, Zwane E, et al (Univ of Cape Town, South Africa; Univ of Swaziland, Mbabane)
Child's Nerv Syst 28:1911-1918, 2012

Introduction.—The frequency of adverse events, such as cerebral ischemia, following traumatic brain injury (TBI) is often debated. Point-in-time monitoring modalities provide important information, but have limited temporal resolution.

Purpose.—This study examines the frequency of an adverse event as a point prevalence at 24 and 72 h post-injury, compared with the cumulative burden measured as a frequency of the event over the full duration of monitoring.

Methods.—Reduced brain tissue oxygenation ($PbtO_2$ <10 mmHg) was the adverse event chosen for examination. Data from 100 consecutive children with severe TBI who received $PbtO_2$ monitoring were retrospectively examined, with data from 87 children found suitable for analysis. Hourly recordings were used to identify episodes of $PbtO_2$ less than 10 mmHg, at 24 and 72 h post-injury, and for the full duration of monitoring.

Results.—Reduced $PbtO_2$ was more common early than late after injury. The point prevalence of reduced $PbtO_2$ at the selected time points was relatively low (10% of patients at 24 h and no patients at the 72-h mark post-injury). The cumulative burden of these events over the full duration of monitoring was relatively high: 50% of patients had episodes of $PbtO_2$ less than 10 mmHg and 88% had $PbtO_2$ less than 20 mmHg.

Conclusion.—Point-in-time monitoring in a dynamic condition like TBI may underestimate the overall frequency of adverse events, like reduced $PbtO_2$, particularly when compared with continuous monitoring, which also has limitations, but provides a dynamic assessment over a longer time period.

▶ Posttraumatic cerebral ischemia is an important contributing factor to secondary injury and poor outcome in traumatic brain injury. Although this has been studied more frequently in adults, it is less studied in pediatrics. The aim of the present study is to examine the frequency of cerebral hypoxic/ischemic events in a cohort of children with severe traumatic brain injury, as defined by episodes of $PbtO_2$ (brain tissue oxygen) <10 mm Hg. The results were as follows: The median Glasgow Coma Scale before monitoring was 6 with an average duration of monitoring of 5.8 ± 3.2 days with an intensive care unit stay for 8 ± 4.2 days.

Apart from the poor placement of $PbtO_2$ probes, there were no complications associated with any of the $PbtO_2$ monitors. Patients were monitored for a median of 5.2 days. When the authors compared the results of the early and late periods for patients who had data at both time points, $PbtO_2$ at 24 h was significantly less than $PbtO_2$ at 72 h ($p < .01$). The results from this study show a relatively low prevalence of reduced brain tissue oxygen at selected time points, as defined by $PbtO_2 < 10$ mm Hg, which may be due to ischemia or other causes of tissue hypoxia. In conclusion, cerebral ischemia/hypoxia is not an important factor causing secondary injury in traumatic brain injury.

E. C. Quintana, MD, MPH

Sports-Related Concussions

Upchaw JE, Goccorand JK, Williamo N, ot al (Mod Univ of South Carolina, Charleston)
Pediatr Emerg Care 28:926-935, 2012

During the past decade, awareness of concussions has exploded as both the media and the medical literature have given more focus to this common problem. Concussions after recreational activities, especially athletics, are a frequent complaint in the emergency department. In the past few years, care of these patients has been simplified as grading systems and classifications have been abandoned. However, questions remain as to the best way to rehabilitate these patients to avoid long-term sequelae, especially in children and adolescents. The purpose of this review is to discuss the demographic characteristics, the pathophysiology, definition, clinical characteristics, and management of concussions in children and adolescents (Tables 1 and 2).

▶ Laypersons have been more focused on sport-related concussions. This article reviewed signs and symptoms and appropriate management. Concussions are caused by a direct blow to the head, face, neck, or elsewhere on the body resulting in an "impulsive" force transmitted to the head that results in the rapid onset of short-lived impairment of neurologic function that resolves spontaneously.

TABLE 1.—Signs and Symptoms of Concussion

Headache	Mental "fogginess"
Nausea	Difficulty answering questions
Vomiting	Repetition of questions/statements
Amnesia (anterograde and retrograde)	Difficulty concentrating
	Balance difficulties
Excessive fatigue	Irritability
Dizziness	Nervousness
Loss of consciousness	Increased sadness
Confusion	Insomnia
Phonophobia	Difficulty wakening
Photophobia	
Visual changes ("seeing stars")	

TABLE 2.—RTP Protocol

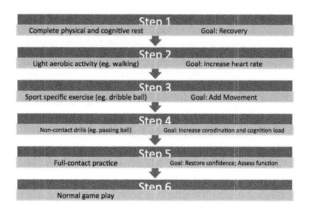

Step 1	
Complete physical and cognitive rest	Goal: Recovery
Step 2	
Light aerobic activity (eg. walking)	Goal: Increase heart rate
Step 3	
Sport specific exercise (eg. dribble ball)	Goal: Add Movement
Step 4	
Non-contact drills (eg. passing ball)	Goal: Increase corodination and cognition load
Step 5	
Full-contact practice	Goal: Restore confidence; Assess function
Step 6	
Normal game play	

A concussion may result in neuropathological changes, with a set of clinical symptoms that may or may not involve loss of consciousness (Table 1). Resolution of the clinical and cognitive symptoms typically follows, but postconcussive symptoms may be present for a long period. No abnormality on standard structural neuroimaging studies is seen in a concussion. Football has contributed the most reported concussions, followed by soccer and basketball. The age range with the highest reported concussion rate is the 10- to 14-year-old age group, followed by 15- to 18-year-olds. Examination, in addition to mental status, could use several other testing tools: balance error scoring system tests postural balance; the standardized assessment of concussion provides a means to better assess not only orientation but also concentration, short-term recall, and memory; sports concussion assessment tool 2 is a combination of multiple tests, including the Glasgow Coma Scale score, that has been used in assessing the concussed patient. Computed tomography scans in concussed patients should be used judiciously where there is a suspicion of clinically significant findings warranting radiation exposure. The return-to-play protocol (Table 2) gives a progression of gradual increase in activity and risk for collision with close physician neurological follow-ups. A feared complication is the second-impact syndrome, which occurs in a player who experiences a first hit then returns to play too soon and may experience a second impact that would in effect build on the pathophysiology of the first. Findings include a loss of autoregulation in the cerebral vessels causing vascular congestion and concurrent increased cerebral blood flow, which together ultimately result in cerebral edema with a mortality rate ranging from 50% to 100%. In the postconcussive syndrome, headache, dizziness, cognitive impairment, and psychological symptoms related to the initial presentation are the most common complaints. Neuropsychological testing is useful in patients with cognitive or psychological complaints.

E. C. Quintana, MD, MPH

Implementation of Adapted PECARN Decision Rule for Children With Minor Head Injury in the Pediatric Emergency Department

Bressan S, Romanato S, Mion T, et al (Univ of Padova, Italy)
Acad Emerg Med 19:801-807, 2012

Objectives.—Of the currently published clinical decision rules for the management of minor head injury (MHI) in children, the Pediatric Emergency Care Applied Research Network (PECARN) rule, derived and validated in a large multicenter prospective study cohort, with high methodologic standards, appears to be the best clinical decision rule to accurately identify children at very low risk of clinically important traumatic brain injuries (ciTBI) in the pediatric emergency department (PED). This study describes the implementation of an adapted version of the PECARN rule in a tertiary care academic PED in Italy and evaluates implementation success, in terms of medical staff adherence and satisfaction, as well as its effects on clinical practice.

Methods.—The adapted PECARN decision rule algorithms for children (one for those younger than 2 years and one for those older than 2 years) were actively implemented in the PED of Padova, Italy, for a 6-month testing period. Adherence and satisfaction of medical staff to the new rule were calculated. Data from 356 visits for MHI during PECARN rule implementation and those of 288 patients attending the PED for MHI in the previous 6 months were compared for changes in computed tomography (CT) scan rate, ciTBI rate (defined as death, neurosurgery, intubation for longer than 24 hours, or hospital admission at least for two nights associated with TBI) and return visits for symptoms or signs potentially related to MHI. The safety and efficacy of the adapted PECARN rule in clinical practice were also calculated.

Results.—Adherence to the adapted PECARN rule was 93.5%. The percentage of medical staff satisfied with the new rule, in terms of usefulness and ease of use for rapid decision-making, was significantly higher (96% vs. 51%, $p < 0.0001$) compared to the previous, more complex, internal guideline. CT scan was performed in 30 patients (8.4%, 95% confidence interval [CI] = 6% to 11.8%) in the implementation period versus 21 patients (7.3%, 95% CI = 4.8% to 10.9%) before implementation. A ciTBI occurred in three children (0.8%, 95% CI = 0.3 to 2.5) during the implementation period and in two children (0.7%, 95% CI = 0.2 to 2.5) in the prior 6 months. There were five return visits (1.4%) postimplementation and seven (2.4%) before implementation ($p = 0.506$). The safety of use of the adapted PECARN rule in clinical practice was 100% (95% CI = 36.8 to 100; three of three patients with ciTBI who received CT scan at first evaluation), while efficacy was 92.3% (95% CI = 89 to 95; 326 of 353 patients without ciTBI who did not receive a CT scan).

Conclusions.—The adapted PECARN rule was successfully implemented in an Italian tertiary care academic PED, achieving high adherence and satisfaction of medical staff. Its use determined a low CT scan rate that was unchanged compared to previous clinical practice and showed an optimal safety and high efficacy profile. Strict monitoring is mandatory to evaluate the long-lasting benefit in patient care and/or resource utilization.

▶ Minor head trauma is a common presentation for evaluation in pediatric emergency departments. It is fine balance in determining those at highrisk versus decreasing radiation exposure from head computed tomography (CT) scans. This study evaluated results before and after implementation of adapted Pediatric Emergency Care Applied Research Network (PECARN) rules. The adaptations were related to the moderate-risk group. In children younger than 2 years old, amnesia was introduced as a predictor and repetitive persistent vomiting. In all children, the recommended observation period for the no-CT was a minimum of 6 hours and at least 12 hours for infants < 6 months from trauma. A total of 644 were included in the study, 356 after and 288 before implementation of adapted PECARN rules. Forty-five percent were younger than 2 years old. Sixty-one percent had a fall as the mechanism of injury. Isolated head trauma occurred in 92% of patients and 637 (99%) had Glasgow Coma Scale scores of 15. Three patients (0.8%) in the postimplementation period and 2 children (0.7%) in the preimplementation period met the definition of clinically important traumatic brain injury. All of them had a hospital admission of 2 nights or more resulting from brain injury. The intracranial injuries identified on CT scan in the postimplementation period were 1 epidural hematoma, 1 subarachnoid bleed, 1 cerebral contusion, and 2 subdural hematomas (all cases but 1 subdural hematoma associated with skull fracture). In the preimplementation period, a case of subdural hematoma and 1 subdural hematoma and cerebral contusion with associated skull fracture were detected on CT. An isolated skull fracture was found in 4 patients. It seems that the adapted PECARN rules were successful in this academic Italian setting. Of note, it is the flexibility of the institution for its observation period. This may not be feasible or have external validity in the US population. Still, it is an interesting proposition that needs long-term investigation.

E. C. Quintana, MD, MPH

Implementation of Adapted PECARN Decision Rule for Children With Minor Head Injury in the Pediatric Emergency Department
Bressan S, Romanato S, Mion T, et al (Univ of Padova, Italy; et al)
Acad Emerg Med 19:801-807, 2012

Objectives.—Of the currently published clinical decision rules for the management of minor head injury (MHI) in children, the Pediatric Emergency Care Applied Research Network (PECARN) rule, derived and validated in a large multicenter prospective study cohort, with high methodologic standards, appears to be the best clinical decision rule to accurately identify children at very low risk of clinically important traumatic brain injuries (ciTBI) in the pediatric emergency department (PED). This study describes the implementation of an adapted version of the PECARN rule in a tertiary care academic PED in Italy and evaluates implementation success, in terms of medical staff adherence and satisfaction, as well as its effects on clinical practice.

Methods.—The adapted PECARN decision rule algorithms for children (one for those younger than 2 years and one for those older than 2 years) were actively implemented in the PED of Padova, Italy, for a 6-month testing period. Adherence and satisfaction of medical staff to the new rule were calculated. Data from 356 visits for MHI during PECARN rule implementation and those of 288 patients attending the PED for MHI in the previous 6 months were compared for changes in computed tomography (CT) scan rate, ciTBI rate (defined as death, neurosurgery, intubation for longer than 24 hours, or hospital admission at least for two nights associated with TBI) and return visits for symptoms or signs potentially related to MHI. The safety and efficacy of the adapted PECARN rule in clinical practice were also calculated.

Results.—Adherence to the adapted PECARN rule was 93.5%. The percentage of medical staff satisfied with the new rule, in terms of usefulness and ease of use for rapid decision-making, was significantly higher (96% vs. 51%, $p < 0.0001$) compared to the previous, more complex, internal guideline. CT scan was performed in 30 patients (8.4%, 95% confidence interval [CI] = 6% to 11.8%) in the implementation period versus 21 patients (7.3%, 95% CI = 4.8% to 10.9%) before implementation. A ciTBI occurred in three children (0.8%, 95% CI = 0.3 to 2.5) during the implementation period and in two children (0.7%, 95% CI = 0.2 to 2.5) in the prior 6 months. There were five return visits (1.4%) postimplementation and seven (2.4%) before implementation ($p = 0.506$). The safety of use of the adapted PECARN rule in clinical practice was 100% (95% CI = 36.8 to 100; three of three patients with ciTBI who received CT scan at first evaluation), while efficacy was 92.3% (95% CI = 89 to 95; 326 of 353 patients without ciTBI who did not receive a CT scan).

Conclusions.—The adapted PECARN rule was successfully implemented in an Italian tertiary care academic PED, achieving high adherence and satisfaction of medical staff. Its use determined a low CT scan rate that was unchanged compared to previous clinical practice and showed an optimal safety and high efficacy profile. Strict monitoring is mandatory to evaluate the long-lasting benefit in patient care and/or resource utilization.

▶ Pediatric patients routinely present for the evaluation and management of minor head injuries. The treating emergency physicians must decide whether to order a computed tomography scan of the head or not. There is a delicate balance between identification of all clinically significant head injuries and minimizing unnecessary exposure to radiation. The Pediatric Emergency Care Applied Research Network (PECARN) has put forward suggested clinical parameters to identify those patients with adequate risks to warrant the imaging.[1] This observational before-and-after study evaluated the effects of implementation of the PECARN clinical practice guidelines in an Italian pediatric emergency department. The authors reference both complex decision rules in the before phase and local adaptations to the rules to better fit their needs. They found a PECARN adherence rate of 93.5%, with nonadherence being attributed to earlier than recommended discharge of patients in the observational phase. Additionally, the authors report an increased computed tomography of the head rate in the after phase (8.4% vs 7.3%), but nowhere near the US rate of 35%. The application also resulted in fewer return visits.

E. C. Bruno, MD

Reference

1. Kuppermann N, Holmes JF, Dayan PS, et al. Identification of children at very low risk of clinically-important brain injuries after head trauma: a prospective cohort study. *Lancet.* 2009;374:1160-1170.

Utility of Plain Radiographs in Detecting Traumatic Injuries of the Cervical Spine in Children
Nigrovic LE, for the Pediatric Emergency Care Applied Research Network (PECARN) Cervical Spine Study Group (Children's Hosp Boston and Harvard Med School, MA; et al)
Pediatr Emerg Care 28:426-432, 2012

Objective.—The objective of this study was to estimate the sensitivity of plain radiographs in identifying bony or ligamentous cervical spine injury in children.

Methods.—We identified a retrospective cohort of children younger than 16 years with blunt trauma-related bony or ligamentous cervical spine injury evaluated between 2000 and 2004 at 1 of 17 hospitals participating in the Pediatric Emergency Care Applied Research Network. We excluded children who had a single or undocumented number of radiographic views or one of the following injuries types: isolated spinal cord injury, spinal cord injury without radiographic abnormalities, or atlantoaxial rotary subluxation. Using consensus methods, study investigators reviewed the radiology reports and assigned a classification (definite, possible, or no cervical spine injury) as well as film adequacy. A pediatric neurosurgeon, blinded to the classification of the radiology reports, reviewed complete case histories and assigned final cervical spine injury type.

Results.—We identified 206 children who met inclusion criteria, of which 127 had definite and 41 had possible cervical spine injury identified by plain radiograph. Of the 186 children with adequate cervical spine radiographs, 168 had definite or possible cervical spine injury identified by plain radiograph for a sensitivity of 90% (95% confidence interval, 85%—94%). Cervical spine radiographs did not identify the following cervical spine injuries: fracture (15 children) and ligamentous injury alone (3 children). Nine children with normal cervical spine radiographs presented with 1 or more of the following: endotracheal intubation (4 children), altered mental status (5 children), or focal neurologic findings (5 children).

TABLE 4.—Characteristics and Injury Types for the 18 Children With Cervical Spine Injuries and Normal and Adequate Cervical Spine Radiographs

Age	Altered Mental Status	Focal Neurologic Findings	Intubated	Injury Mechanism	Cervical Spine Injury	Neurologic Outcome*	Operative Stabilization
1.9	No	No	No	Fall from elevation	Jefferson fracture	Normal	No
2.0	No	No	No	Fall from elevation	Axial single level ligamentous injury	Normal	No
2.7	No	Yes	No	Motor vehicle crash	Atlanta-occipital dislocation	Deficit	Yes
3.0	Yes	Missing	No	Motor vehicle crash	Occipital condyle fracture	Deficit	No
3.8	Yes	Yes	Yes	Motor vehicle crash	Subaxial single level ligamentous injury	Normal	No
4.8	No	No	No	Fall from standing/walking/running	Subaxial unilateral pedicle fracture	Normal	No
5.0	No	No	No	Fall from elevation	C1 arch fracture	Normal	No
5.8	No	Yes	No	Back flip	Os odontoideum	Normal	Yes
5.9	No	No	No	Fall from standing/walking/running	C1 arch fracture	Normal	No
8.6	Yes	No	Yes	Bike rider struck by moving vehicle	Transverse process fracture	Normal	No
9.2	No	No	No	Motor vehicle crash	Spinous process fracture	Normal	No
9.5	No	No	No	Motorized transport crash (eg, motorcycle)	Spinous process fracture	Normal	No
11.2	No	Yes	No	Fall from elevation	Os odontoideum	Normal	Yes
12.1	No	Yes	No	Trampoline	Unilateral facet fracture-dislocation	Normal	Yes
13.0	Yes	No	Yes	Pedestrian struck by moving vehicle	Subaxial compression fracture	Deficit	No
14.9	Missing	No	No	Sports injury	Spinous process fracture	Normal	No
15.3	No	No	No	Sports injury	Subaxial unilateral pedicle fracture	Normal	No
15.7	Yes	No	Yes	Motor vehicle crash	Multilevel vertebral body burst fractures	Normal	No

*Neurologic outcome assessed at the time of hospital discharge.

Conclusions.—Plain radiographs had a high sensitivity for cervical spine injury in our pediatric cohort (Table 4).

▶ Following a principal approach of limiting excessive radiation exposure to pediatric trauma patients, some physicians attempt to minimize the number of unnecessary computer tomography (CT) scans while still trying to not miss clinically relevant injuries. One clinical scenario that is routinely addressed in this manner is cervical spine injuries and the potential for neurologically devastating injuries. Dedicated cervical spine radiographs offer a screening set of images, but cervical spine CTs offer a greater sensitivity with increased radiation directed at vulnerable organs (thyroid gland). The attached report references adult and pediatric studies that demonstrate sensitivities of 80% to 90% but also reference limitations. Using a pediatric research network, the authors attempted to eliminate one limitation, the possibility of facility bias, and searched for a set of generalizable rules to evaluate this subset of pediatric trauma patients.

Patients had to have cervical spine injuries, with or without neurologic deficits. They also had to have adequate cervical spine radiographs. Of those with adequate images, the authors report a 90% sensitivity of identifying the injury on the plain radiographs but failed to identify 18 clinically relevant cervical spine injuries. Patients with neurologic deficits should be eliminated from consideration, as these patients likely would proceed to magnetic resonance imaging for further evaluation, rather than CT. However, 3 patients (17%) with normal images and normal neurologic outcomes required operative stabilization. Once again, the treating emergency physician must maintain vigilance and consider the next step when the mechanism of injury suggests a potentially catastrophic complication.

E. C. Bruno, MD

Procedures

Contact Lens Removal: The "Chopstick" Approach
Stockdale J, El-Shammaa E (The Ohio State Univ and Nationwide Children's Hosp, Columbus)
Pediatr Emerg Care 28:707-708, 2012

A case of adherent soft contact lenses in an apprehensive adolescent patient is described, along with a description of a novel technique for contact lens removal. After topical anesthesia and saline irrigation, the lenses were successfully removed, atraumatically, using a pair of saline-soaked cotton-tipped applicators held in a chopstick fashion (Figs 1 and 2).

▶ Contact lenses are one of the leading causes of eye injuries from consumer products, accounting for approximately 26 490 emergency department visits, and are the leading cause of ocular injury from commercial products. It is always a challenge removing them in adults but a greater challenge in children. Several commercial instruments are available, such as soft lens pincher devices. This author suggested using 2 saline-moistened cotton-tipped applicators (readily available in all EDs) held in a chopstick-like fashion. The patient was

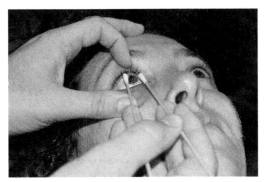

FIGURE 1.—Example of the "chopstick" approach on an adult. (Reprinted from Stockdale J, El-Shammaa E, Contact lens removal: the "chopstick" approach. *Pediatr Emerg Care.* 2012;28:707-708, with permission from Lippincott Williams & Wilkins.)

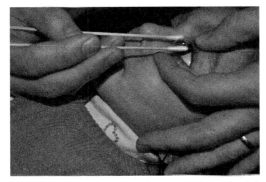

FIGURE 2.—Example of the "chopstick" approach on a child. (Reprinted from Stockdale J, El-Shammaa E, Contact lens removal: the "chopstick" approach. *Pediatr Emerg Care.* 2012;28:707-708, with permission from Lippincott Williams & Wilkins.)

approached from the lower lid to keep the approaching cotton swabs out of her direct line of vision. Then, using the applicators as forceps, the lenses were pinched from each side and removed easily (Figs 1 and 2). This is a great technique to keep in your armamentarium for foreign body removal.

E. C. Quintana, MD, MPH

Etomidate for Short Pediatric Procedures in the Emergency Department
Mandt MJ, Roback MG, Bajaj L, et al (Univ of Colorado Denver Health Science Ctr, Aurora; Univ of Minnesota Med School, Minneapolis)
Pediatr Emerg Care 28:898-904, 2012

Objective.—This study aimed to prospectively determine the etomidate dose associated with adequate sedation and few significant respiratory events for procedures of short duration in children.

Methods.—This is a prospective cohort study in an urban pediatric emergency department of patients 4 to 18 years requiring sedation and analgesia for painful procedures of short duration. Patients received fentanyl 1 μg/kg followed by intravenously administered etomidate 0.1 to 0.2 mg/kg as a loading dose. An additional dose of etomidate 0.1 mg/kg was intravenously administered if needed. The level of sedation was determined by The Children's Hospital of Wisconsin Sedation Score. The primary outcome was to determine the etomidate dose associated with an adequate level of sedation and procedural completion.

Results.—Sixty patients were enrolled. The most frequent procedure was fracture reduction (50/60, 83.3%). Procedures were successfully completed for 59 (98.3%) of 60 patients. The initial dose of etomidate associated with adequate sedation was 0.2 mg/kg intravenously administered for 33 (66.7%) of 50 patients requiring fracture reduction and for 6 (60.0%) of 10 patients receiving a procedure other than fracture reduction. Respiratory depression was noted in 9 (16.4%) of 55 patients, and oxygen desaturation was noted in 23 (39.0%) of 59 patients. Of 58 patients, 21 (36.2%) experienced a respiratory adverse event requiring brief intervention including oxygen supplementation, stimulation, and/or airway repositioning. No patient experienced a significant adverse respiratory event, defined as positive pressure ventilation. Median time to discharge-ready was 21 minutes.

Conclusions.—For short-duration painful emergency department procedures, etomidate 0.2 mg/kg intravenously administered after fentanyl was associated with effective sedation, successful procedural completion, and readily managed respiratory adverse events in children.

▶ No previously published study has directly investigated the optimal etomidate dose for sedation when an opioid analgesic is coadministered for a painful procedure in children. Ninety-eight percent of emergency department (ED) physicians deemed that etomidate sedation was successful. There is no significant difference in proportion of subjects reaching optimal sedation between the 2 etomidate dose levels, 0.2 and 0.3 mg/kg. Respiratory depression occurred in 9 (16.4%) of 55 patients. Breathing cues, including verbal or light tactile stimulus and/or airway repositioning maneuvers, were performed in 27.1%. Oxygen desaturation was noted in 39.0% of patients and supplemental oxygen was administered in 25.4%. The median desaturation level was 86% and the lowest recorded oxygen saturation was 77%. A brief intervention (supplemental oxygen, verbal or tactile stimulus, and/or airway repositioning maneuvers) was performed in 36.2% of patients experiencing a respiratory adverse event such as respiratory depression and/or oxygen desaturation. The respiratory adverse event rate was not significantly associated with an increase in etomidate dose ($P = .52$). Complete procedural amnesia was achieved in most patients with 48 (80.0%) of 60 recalling none of the procedure either immediately after the procedure or at the 72-hour telephone follow-up. The orthopedic providers were not satisfied with etomidate's sedation level. This study suggests that etomidate has a role in pediatric procedural sedation and analgesia for short procedures in the ED. When administered with 1 kg/kg fentanyl intravenously, an initial etomidate dose of

0.2 mg/kg intravenously, with an additional 0.1 mg/kg dose as needed, achieved adequate sedation without significant risk for severe adverse events.

E. C. Quintana, MD, MPH

Diagnosis of Intussusception by Physician Novice Sonographers in the Emergency Department
Riera A, Hsiao AL, Langhan ML, et al (Yale Univ School of Medicine, New Haven, CT)
Ann Emerg Med 60:264-268, 2012

Study objective.—We investigate the performance characteristics of bedside emergency department (ED) ultrasonography by nonradiologist physician sonographers in the diagnosis of ileocolic intussusception in children.

Methods.—This was a prospective, observational study conducted in a pediatric ED of an urban tertiary care children's hospital. Pediatric emergency physicians with no experience in bowel ultrasonography underwent a focused 1-hour training session conducted by a pediatric radiologist. The session included a didactic component on sonographic appearances of ileocolic intussusception, review of images with positive and negative results for intussusceptions, and a hands-on component with a live child model. On completion of the training, a prospective convenience sample study was performed. Children were enrolled if they were to undergo diagnostic radiology ultrasonography for suspected intussusception. Bedside ultrasonography by trained pediatric emergency physicians was performed and interpreted as either positive or negative for ileocolic intussusception. Ultrasonographic studies were then performed by diagnostic radiologists, and their results were used as the reference standard. Test

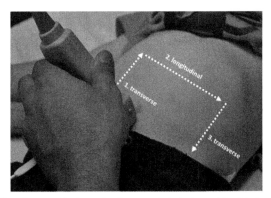

FIGURE 1.—Transducer positioning and trajectory to include views of the right lower quadrant, right upper quadrant, left upper quadrant, and left lower quadrant. (Reprinted from Riera A, Hsiao AL, Langhan ML, et al. Diagnosis of intussusception by physician novice sonographers in the emergency department. *Ann Emerg Med.* 2012;60,3:264-268, Copyright 2012, with permission from American College of Emergency Physicians.)

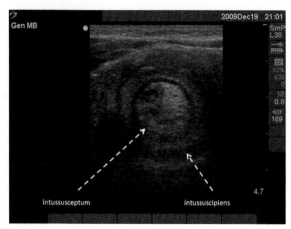

FIGURE 2.—Appearance of typical ileocolic intussusception in transverse orientation as detected by bedside ultrasonography. (Reprinted from Riera A, Hsiao AL, Langhan ML, et al. Diagnosis of intussusception by physician novice sonographers in the emergency department. *Ann Emerg Med.* 2012;60,3:264-268, Copyright 2012, with permission from American College of Emergency Physicians.)

characteristics (sensitivity, specificity, positive and negative predictive values) and likelihood ratios were calculated.

Results.— Six pediatric emergency physicians completed the training and performed the bedside studies. Eighty-two patients were enrolled. The median age was 25 months (range 3 to 127 months). Thirteen patients (16%) received a diagnosis of ileocolic intussusception by diagnostic radiology. Bedside ultrasonography had a sensitivity of 85% (95% confidence interval [CI] 54% to 97%), specificity of 97% (95% CI 89% to 99%), positive predictive value of 85% (95% CI 54% to 97%), and negative predictive value of 97% (95% CI 89% to 99%). A positive bedside ultrasonographic result had a likelihood ratio of 29 (95% CI 7.3 to 117), and a negative bedside ultrasonographic result had a likelihood ratio of 0.16 (95% CI 0.04 to 0.57).

Conclusion.—With limited and focused training, pediatric emergency physicians can accurately diagnose ileocolic intussusception in children by using bedside ultrasonography (Figs 1 and 2).

▶ Bedside ultrasound scan is being used for many diagnoses in the emergency department. This study determined the performance of bedside ultrasonography by pediatric emergency physicians who received a 1-hour limited and focused training in the diagnosis of ileocolic intussusception in children. Bedside ultrasonography was performed with the L38 linear transducer (5 to 10 MHz) and a SonoSite MicroMaxx ultrasonographic system (SonoSite, Bothwell, WA). The technique was as follows: The transducer was placed in the right lower quadrant in a transverse orientation, with the indicator pointing toward the patient's right side. The psoas muscle was identified as a starting landmark. The transducer was then slowly swept superolaterally toward the right upper quadrant, where the liver and gallbladder served as landmarks. After rotating the transducer 90° clockwise, it was swept across the epigastrium toward the left upper quadrant in a longitudinal orientation. From the left upper quadrant, the transducer was rotated 90° counterclockwise to lie in a transverse orientation and swept inferiorly toward the left lower quadrant. A complete bedside scan included views of all 4 quadrants as described, searching for ultrasonographic evidence of intussusception (Figs 1 and 2). The results showed that bedside ultrasonography had a sensitivity of 85%, positive predictive value of 85%, and negative predictive value of 97% for ileocolic intussusception. The likelihood ratio of a positive bedside ultrasonographic result was 29; in contrast, the likelihood ratio of a negative bedside ultrasonographic result was 0.16. These results may support expanding the use of bedside ultrasonography for goal-directed, pediatric-specific emergencies; however, further studies are warranted.

E. C. Quintana, MD, MPH

Children With and Without Developmental Disabilities: Sedation Medication Requirements and Adverse Events Related to Sedation

Kannikeswaran N, Sethuraman U, Sivaswamy L, et al (Wayne State Univ, Detroit, MI)

Pediatr Emerg Care 28:1036-1040, 2012

Objective.—Our objective was to prospectively compare sedation medication requirements and adverse events related to sedation in children with and without developmental disabilities.

Methods.—We conducted a prospective, observational, age-matched, 1:2 case-control study of children (3—10 years) sedated for brain magnetic

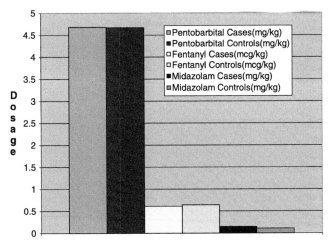

Medications

FIGURE 1.—Sedation medication requirements in children with and without developmental disabilities. (Reprinted from Kannikeswaran N, Sethuraman U, Sivaswamy L, et al. Children with and without developmental disabilities: sedation medication requirements and adverse events related to sedation. *Pediatr Emerg Care.* 2012;28:1036-1040, with permission from Lippincott Williams & Wilkins.)

TABLE 2.—Adverse Events Related to Sedation in Children With and Without Developmental Disabilities

Adverse Event	Cases, n (%)	Controls, n (%)
Hypoxia	7 (10)	13 (9.3)
Airway obstruction/snoring	9 (12.9)	25 (17.9)
Apnea	3 (4.3)	0 (0)
Stridor	1 (1.4)	0 (0)
Emesis	1 (1.4)	5 (3.6)
Emergence/paradoxical reaction	2 (2.9)	3 (2.1)
Sedation failure	0 (0)	5 (3.6)
Oversedation	0 (0)	2 (1.4)

resonance imaging at a tertiary-care children's hospital. Developmental assessment was performed using the Vineland Adaptive Behavioral Scale and by a pediatric neurologist. Patients were sedated according to institutional sedation protocol. Patient demographics, type and dose of sedation medications, depth of sedation, and adverse events were collected. We defined hypoxia as oxygen saturation 90% or less for 30 seconds or longer and requiring airway maneuvers.

Results.—Seventy children were designated as cases (DD) and 140 as controls (DN). DD had a significantly lower mean Vineland Adaptive Behavioral Scale score than did DN (DD: 62.34 ± 9.70, DN: 103.0 ± 13.71; $P < 0.001$). A combination of pentobarbital and fentanyl (DD: 32/70 [45.7%], DN: 60/140 [42.9%]) and combination of pentobarbital and midazolam (DD: 28/70 [40%], DN: 43/140 [30.7%]) were the most common sedatives used in both groups. There was no difference in the mean dose of pentobarbital (DD: 4.68 ± 1.63 mg/kg, DN: 4.67 ± 1.69 mg/kg; $P = 0.9$), fentanyl (DD: 0.61 ± 0.65 µg/kg, DN: 0.64 ± 0.65 µg/kg; $P = 0.7$), and midazolam (DD: 0.15 ± 0.17 mg/kg, DN: 0.11 ± 0.14 mg/kg; $P = 0.1$). There was no difference in the overall adverse events (DD: 30%, DN: 32.9%; $P = 0.7$) as well as hypoxia (DD: 10%; DN: 9.3%, $P = 0.9$).

Conclusions.—When compared with DN children, DD children do not require a higher dose of sedatives and do not have a higher incidence of adverse events (Fig 1, Table 2).

▶ Procedural sedation and analgesia (PSA) is used in children for many reasons, including magnetic resonance imaging (MRI) diagnostic testing. Children with developmental disabilities (DD) are anecdotally believed to be difficult to sedate and have higher sedative medication requirements when compared with typically developing children for PSA. A combination of pentobarbital and fentanyl, and pentobarbital and midazolam were the most common sedative medications used in the 2 groups. Children in both groups were sedated to Ramsay sedation score of 5 (cases, 97.1%; controls, 96.4%). There was no difference in the mean dosages of sedative medications used among the 2 groups (Fig 1). There was significant positive correlation between presedation agitation and mean dosage of midazolam used. The correlation between level of presedation agitation and mean dosages of pentobarbital, overall adverse events, and hypoxia was not statistically significant. All airway adverse events resolved with airway alignment maneuvers (no ETT) and oxygen supplementation. Five children were admitted to the hospital overnight for observation, all of whom belonged to the control group. Two of them were admitted for non–Y-sedation–related reasons (one for arachnoid cyst fenestration and another for workup of seizures), and 3 were admitted secondary to sedation-related severe paradoxical reaction (Table 2). The study didn't find any difference in the depth of sedation between the 2 groups with sedatives used for PSA. This is an important take-home message when doing PSA in the emergency department.

E. C. Quintana, MD, MPH

Adherence to PALS Sepsis Guidelines and Hospital Length of Stay

Paul R, Neuman MI, Monuteaux MC, et al (Boston Children's Hosp, MA)
Pediatrics 130:e273-e280, 2012

Background and Objectives.—Few studies have evaluated sepsis guideline adherence in a tertiary pediatric emergency department setting. We sought to evaluate (1) adherence to 2006 Pediatric Advanced Life Support guidelines for severe sepsis and septic shock (SS), (2) barriers to adherence, and (3) hospital length of stay (LOS) contingent on guideline adherence.

Methods.—Prospective cohort study of children presenting to a large urban academic pediatric emergency department with SS. Adherence to

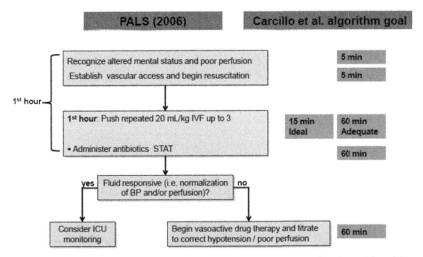

FIGURE 1.—Five time points evaluated for adherence from 2006 PALS algorithm. (Adapted from Carcillo JA, Fields AI; American College of Critical Care Medicine Task Force Committee Members. Clinical practice parameters for hemodynamic support of pediatric and neonatal patients in septic shock. *Crit Care Med.* 2002;30[6]:1370.)[6] *Editor's Note*: Please refer to original journal article for full references. (Reprinted from Paul R, Neuman MI, Monuteaux MC, et al. Adherence to PALS sepsis guidelines and hospital length of stay. *Pediatrics.* 2012;130:e273-e280, Copyright © [2012] by the American Academy of Pediatrics.)

TABLE 2.—Association of Fluid Adherence With LOS

	Fluid Adherence, $n = 46$, Mean No. Days[a]	Fluid Nonadherence, $n = 80$, Mean No. Days[a]	Decrease, %	P Value[b]
Hospital LOS	8	11.2	57	.039
ICU LOS	5.5	7.2	42	.024

[a]Unadjusted means.
[b]P value references "percent decrease in LOS" by using negative binomial regression, adjusting for PIM2 score at presentation and other comorbidities.

TABLE 3.—Association of Total Algorithm Adherence With LOS

	Algorithm Bundle Adherence, $n = 24$, Mean No. Days[a]	Algorithm Bundle Nonadherence, $n = 102$, Mean No. Days[a]	Decrease, %	P Value[b]
Hospital LOS	6.8	10.9	57	.009
ICU LOS	5.5	6.8	59	.035

[a]Unadjusted means.
[b]P value references "percent decrease in LOS" by using negative binomial regression, adjusting for PIM2 score at presentation and other comorbidities.

5 algorithmic time-specific goals was reviewed: early recognition of SS, obtaining vascular access, administering intravenous fluids, delivery of vasopressors for fluid refractory shock, and antibiotic administration. Adherence to each time-defined goal and adherence to all 5 components as a bundle were reviewed. A detailed electronic medical record analysis evaluated adherence barriers. The association between guideline adherence and hospital LOS was evaluated by using multivariate negative binomial regression.

Results.—A total of 126 patients had severe sepsis (14%) or septic shock (86%). The median age was 9 years (interquartile range, 3—16). There was a 37% and 35% adherence rate to fluid and inotrope guidelines, respectively. Nineteen percent adhered to the 5-component bundle. Patients who received 60 mL/kg of intravenous fluids within 60 minutes had a 57% shorter hospital LOS ($P = .039$) than children who did not. Complete bundle adherence resulted in a 57% shorter hospital LOS ($P = .009$).

Conclusions.—Overall adherence to Pediatric Advanced Life Support sepsis guidelines was low; however, when patients were managed within the guideline's recommendations, patients had significantly shorter duration of hospitalization (Fig 1, Tables 2 and 3).

▶ Severe sepsis and septic shock (SS) in children have a high morbidity and mortality, especially in those with chronic illnesses. Based on the proposed algorithm by Carcillo et al through the American College of Critical Care Medicine practice parameter, Pediatric Advanced Life Support (PALS) ideally recommends 60 mL/kg of intravenous fluids (IVFs) within 15 minutes of meeting the definition of SS, although administration within 60 minutes has been suggested as adequate resuscitation. Timely recognition and vascular access within 5 minutes, antibiotic delivery within 60 minutes, and initiation of vasoactive agents at 60 minutes are recommended (Fig 1). This study enrolled consecutive patients presenting to a tertiary pediatric emergency department (volume 58 000) with SS between November 2009 and March 2011 to determine adherence to the 5 main components of the PALS algorithm (Fig 1). Ninety-nine patients (79%) were recognized within 5 minutes of meeting the SS criteria. Eighty-five patients (67%) had intravenous access within 5 minutes of definition. Patients who adhered to fluid guidelines and the algorithm bundle had a significantly shorter hospital and intensive care unit (ICU) length of stay (LOS) (Tables 2 and 3). Patients who received 60 mL/kg of IVFs within 60 minutes had a 57% shorter hospital LOS ($P = .039$) and a 42% shorter ICU LOS ($P = .024$) than children with inadequate fluid delivery (Table 2). These findings, in addition to improved patient care, may decrease hospitalization and likely have significant cost implications.

E. C. Quintana, MD, MPH

ED point-of-care ultrasound in the diagnosis of ankle fractures in children
Taggart I, Voskoboynik N, Shah S, et al (Hasbro Children's Hosp, Providence, RI; Harborview Med Ctr, Seattle, WA)
Am J Emerg Med 30:1328.e1-1328.e3, 2012

In pediatric ankle injury, radiography is the current standard used to differentiate fracture from ligamentous injury; however, the associated cost, increased time, and radiation exposure pose a significant downside to this imaging modality. Point-of-care ultrasound may be an attractive alternative in this setting, as illustrated by this patient case. A 14-year-old boy presented to the emergency department with a left ankle inversion injury sustained while playing soccer. An emergency physician performed ultrasound

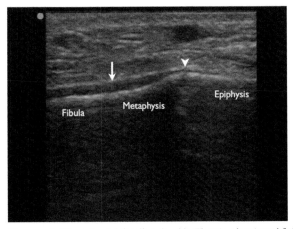

FIGURE 1.—Ultrasound of the patient's left (affected) ankle. There is subperiosteal fluid at the level of the metaphysis and distal fibula (arrow) and widening of the physis (arrowhead). (Reprinted from Taggart I, Voskoboynik N, Shah S, et al. ED point-of-care ultrasound in the diagnosis of ankle fractures in children. *Am J Emerg Med.* 2012;30:1328.e1-1328.e3, Copyright 2012, with permission from Elsevier.)

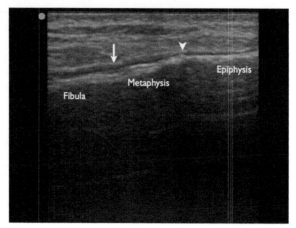

FIGURE 2.—Ultrasound of the patient's right (unaffected) ankle. There is normal subperiosteum (arrow) and no widening of the physis (arrowhead). (Reprinted from Taggart I, Voskoboynik N, Shah S, et al. ED point-of-care ultrasound in the diagnosis of ankle fractures in children. *Am J Emerg Med.* 2012;30:1328.e1-1328.e3, Copyright 2012, with permission from Elsevier.)

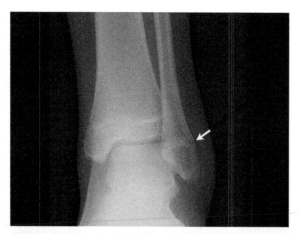

FIGURE 3.—Radiograph of the patient's left (affected) ankle. There is a slight widening of the distal fibular physis, suggestive of an SH I fracture (arrow). (Reprinted from Taggart I, Voskoboynik N, Shah S, et al. ED point-of-care ultrasound in the diagnosis of ankle fractures in children. *Am J Emerg Med.* 2012;30:1328.e1-1328.e3, Copyright 2012, with permission from Elsevier.)

examination that revealed findings consistent with a nondisplaced Salter-Harris I fracture of the distal fibula. The results of a formal radiograph confirmed this diagnosis. This case report presents the successful use of point-of-care ultrasound for detection of a Salter-Harris I ankle fracture, describes a stepwise approach for this new diagnostic technique in detail, and discusses its value in the setting of pediatric ankle injury (Figs 1-3).

▶ Ankle injuries are frequent in children, especially in the setting of sports-related trauma. This article presented a 14-year-old soccer player sustaining an inversion ankle injury that made a "pop" sound. A point-of-care ultrasound ankle examination using a 13-6 MHz linear array transducer at the point of maximal tenderness. Sonographic images of the injured left ankle revealed subperiosteal fluid at the level of the metaphysis and distal fibula and widening of the physis (Fig 1) as compared with the uninjured right ankle (Fig 2). X-rays (Fig 3) showed a slight widening of the distal fibular physis with adjacent soft tissue swelling, consistent with the diagnosis of Salter Harris I fracture. This introduces a potential alternative to x-rays, thus reducing radiation exposure.

E. C. Quintana, MD, MPH

Sonographic Diagnosis of Metaphyseal Forearm Fractures in Children: A Safe and Applicable Alternative to Standard X-Rays

Eckert K, Ackermann O, Schweiger B, et al (Elisabeth Hosp Essen, Germany; Klinikum Duisburg, Germany; Univ of Duisburg-Essen, Germany)
Pediatr Emerg Care 28:851-854, 2012

Objective.—Metaphyseal forearm fractures are very common in childhood. Radiography of the wrist is the standard diagnostic procedure. The aim of our study was to evaluate and confirm the safety and applicability of the ultrasound diagnostic procedure in comparison to x-ray diagnosis.

Methods.—We investigated 76 patients aged between 1 and 14 years. After clinical assessment, patients with suspected forearm fractures first underwent ultrasound examination of the metaphyseal forearm followed by standard 2-view radiographs of the wrist. Ultrasound and radiographic findings were then compared, and sensitivity and specificity for ultrasound were calculated

Results.—Of 76 patients, we found 42 patients with 52 metaphyseal forearm fractures by x-rays. By ultrasound, we also diagnosed 52 fractures. All

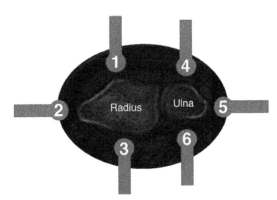

FIGURE 1.—Transducer positions on the distal forearm. (Reprinted from Eckert K, Ackermann O, Schweiger B, et al. Sonographic diagnosis of metaphyseal forearm fractures in children: a safe and applicable alternative to standard x-rays. *Pediatr Emerg Care.* 2012;28:851-854, with permission from Lippincott Williams & Wilkins.)

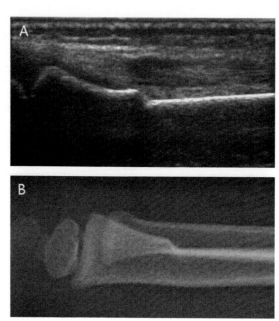

FIGURE 2.—Bulging fracture of the radius; dorsal view by ultrasound (A) and lateral x-ray view of the wrist (B). (Reprinted from Eckert K, Ackermann O, Schweiger B, et al. Sonographic diagnosis of metaphyseal forearm fractures in children: a safe and applicable alternative to standard x-rays. *Pediatr Emerg Care*. 2012;28:851-854, with permission from Lippincott Williams & Wilkins.)

patients with no fractures were correctly diagnosed as well. Referring to x-ray, we calculated for ultrasound a sensitivity of 96.1% and a specificity of 97%. Comparing axis deviation of displaced fractures, we found a mean difference of 2.1 degrees between sonographic and x-ray values.

Conclusions.—We confirm that ultrasound is an applicable and safe alternative tool to x-rays in nondisplaced or excluded metaphyseal forearm fractures in children (Figs 1-3).

▶ This study evaluated the use of ultrasound scan in diagnosis of forearm fractures as a potential alternative to x-rays. The ultrasound examination took about 3 to 4 minutes (Fig 1) and was safe and harmless without considerable strain or stress for the children. By ultrasound scan, 52 fractures were found, and all patients without a fracture were correctly diagnosed. All isolated radius and ulna fractures were detected by ultrasound scan, except for 1, when compared with x-rays (Figs 2 and 3). Eighty-two percent of ulna fractures were diagnosed by ultrasound scan versus x-rays. Of note, 2 concomitant ulna fractures that were diagnosed by x-rays were not seen sonographically; moreover, 2 concomitant ulna fractures were seen by ultrasound that were not confirmed by radiographs. The ultrasound scan method has a sensitivity of 96.1% and specificity of 97% with a positive predictive value of 94.3% and negative predictive value of 97.9%. This method warrants further studies as an alternative to x-rays.

E. C. Quintana, MD, MPH

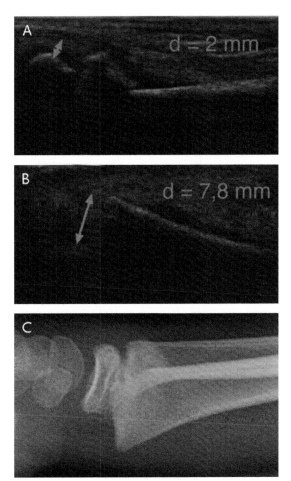

FIGURE 3.—Aitken-1 fracture of the distal radius; dorsal (A) and palmar (B) view by ultrasound and lateral x-ray view (C). (Reprinted from Eckert K, Ackermann O, Schweiger B, et al. Sonographic diagnosis of metaphyseal forearm fractures in children: a safe and applicable alternative to standard x-rays. *Pediatr Emerg Care*. 2012;28:851-854, with permission from Lippincott Williams & Wilkins.)

Randomized Trial Comparing Wound Packing to No Wound Packing Following Incision and Drainage of Superficial Skin Abscesses in the Pediatric Emergency Department

Kessler DO, Krantz A, Mojica M (Columbia Univ College of Physicians and Surgeons, NY)
Pediatr Emerg Care 28:514-517, 2012

Objective.—The objective of this study was to investigate the impact of wound packing versus no wound packing on short-term failure rates and long-term recurrences after incision and drainage (I&D) of a simple cutaneous abscess.

Methods.—In this randomized, single-blind, prospective study, subjects between the ages 1 and 25 years with skin abscesses needing an I&D were enrolled consecutively and randomized to be packed or not packed following the procedure. Treatment failure was assessed at a 48-hour follow-up visit by a masked observer who rated the need for a major intervention (repeat I&D or re-exploration) or minor intervention (antibiotics initiated or changed, need for packing, or repeat visit). Pain scores were assessed using color analog scales before and after the procedure and repeated at the 48-hour follow-up visit. Healing and abscess recurrence were assessed via telephone interview at 1 week and 1 month.

Results.—Fifty-seven subjects were enrolled over a 15-month period. Overall failure rates were similar between the groups, with 19 (70%) of 27 subjects in the packed group needing an intervention by 48 hours compared with 13 (59%) of 22 subjects in the nonpacked group who needed an intervention (difference, 11%; 95% confidence interval, −15% to 36%). Major and minor intervention rates were also similar. Pain scores did not significantly differ between groups.

Conclusions.—Wound packing does not appear to significantly impact the failure or recurrence rates after simple I&D. Larger studies are needed to better validate the equivalency of these 2 strategies. This trial was registered with the US National Institute of Health (clinicaltrials.gov identifier NCT00746109).

▶ The definition of standard management of skin and soft tissues, specifically abscesses, has been called into question recently—antibiotics or not, sterile procedure or not, etc. The authors of this randomized, single-blinded, prospective study assessed if the utilization of wound packing, in conjunction with incision and drainage, decreased the treatment failure rate. In pediatric patients, the recurrence rates were similar (19% in packing vs 13% in the no-packing group), but trended toward lower rates of recurrence in the no-packing group. These results suggest that packing could be eliminated when addressing cutaneous abscesses in pediatric patients. Without packing, a second procedure, ie, removal of the old packing and possible placement of new packing, could be avoided. Wound management, specifically warm soaks, may be facilitated because patients and their families would not be concerned about inadvertent removal of the packing. Adequate education about the potential for recurrence is probably of equal importance.

E. C. Bruno, MD

Topical anesthetic cream is associated with spontaneous cutaneous abscess drainage in children
Cassidy-Smith T, Mistry RD, Russo CJ, et al (UMDNJ-RWJMS at Camden; Children's Hosp of Philadelphia, PA; Al duPont Hosp for Children, Wilmington, DE)
Am J Emerg Med 30:104-109, 2012

Objective.—The objective of the study was to determine whether use of topical anesthetic cream increases spontaneous drainage of skin abscesses and reduces the need for procedural sedation.

Methods.—A retrospective multicenter cohort study from 3 academic pediatric emergency departments was conducted for randomly selected children with a cutaneous abscess in 2007. Children up to 18 years of age were eligible if they had a skin abscess at presentation. Demographics, abscess characteristics, and use of a topical analgesic were obtained from medical records.

Results.—Of 300 subjects, 58% were female and the median age was 7.8 years (interquartile range, 2-15 years). Mean abscess size was 3.5 ± 2.4 cm, most commonly located on the lower extremity (30%), buttocks (24%), and face (12%). A drainage procedure was required in 178 children, of whom 9 underwent drainage in the operating room. Of the remaining 169 children who underwent emergency department—based drainage, 110 (65%) had a topical anesthetic agent with an occlusive dressing placed on their abscess before drainage. Use of a topical anesthetic resulted in spontaneous abscess drainage in 26 patients, of whom 3 no longer required any further intervention. In the 166 patients who underwent additional manipulation, procedural sedation was required in 26 (24%) of those who had application of a topical anesthetic and in 24 (41%) of those who had no topical anesthetic (odds ratio, 0.45; 95% confidence interval, 0.23-0.89).

Conclusions.—Topical anesthetic cream application before drainage procedures promotes spontaneous drainage and decreases the need for procedural sedation for pediatric cutaneous abscess patients.

▶ Incision and drainage (I & D) of a simple cutaneous abscess is a common emergent procedure, but quickly becomes more complex with the patient is a child. Emergency physicians may be unable to rationalize the need for the procedure or alleviate the concerns about pain. Permitting I & D without the movement or screams, the procedural sedation carries its own set of limitations and complications. Elimination of the need for the procedure and subsequent procedural sedation may be a welcomed situation. The authors of this multicenter retrospective product assessed whether application of a topical anesthetic would obviate the need for procedural sedation. The anesthetic cream appears to promote spontaneous drainage, especially those abscesses that were ripe for rupture (pointing, less surrounding cellulitis). Balancing clinical improvement with efficiency is the priority. If the need for the procedure is eradicated, the length of stay may also be decreased. However, patients must have the topical anesthetic in place for 30 to 40 minutes to promote spontaneous drainage, and the pretreatment does not guarantee that I & D will not be necessary.

E. C. Bruno, MD

Dehydration Treatment Practices Among Pediatrics-Trained and Non–Pediatrics Trained Emergency Physicians
Nunez J, Liu DR, Nager AL (Univ of Southern California, Los Angeles, CA)
Pediatr Emerg Care 28:322-328, 2012

Objectives.—We sought to survey emergency physicians in the United States regarding the management of pediatric dehydration secondary to acute gastroenteritis. We hypothesized that responses from physicians with dedicated pediatric training (PT), that is, board certification in pediatrics or pediatric emergency medicine, would differ from responses of physicians with no dedicated pediatric training (non-PT).

Methods.—An anonymous survey was mailed to randomly selected members of the American College of Emergency Physicians and sent electronically to enrollees of Brown University pediatric emergency medicine listserv. The survey consisted of 17 multiple-choice questions based on a clinical scenario depicting a 2-year-old with acute gastroenteritis and moderate dehydration. Questions asked related to treatment preferences, practice setting, and training information.

Results.—One thousand sixty-nine surveys were received: 997 surveys were used for data analysis, including 269 PT physicians and 721 non-PT physicians. Seventy-nine percent of PT physicians correctly classified the scenario patient as moderately dehydrated versus 71% of non-PT physicians ($P = 0.063$). Among those who correctly classified the patient, 121 PT physicians (58%) and 350 non-PT physicians (68%) would initially hydrate the patient with intravenous fluids. Pediatrics-trained physicians were more likely to initially choose oral or nasogastric hydration compared with non-PT physicians ($P = 0.0127$). Pediatrics-trained physicians were less likely to perform laboratory testing compared with the non-PT group (n = 92, 45%, vs n = 337, 66%; $P < 0.0001$).

Conclusions.—Contrary to established recommendations for the management of moderately dehydrated children, significantly more PT physicians, compared with non-PT physicians, follow established guidelines.

▶ General emergency physicians (GEP) may be unnerved with the prospect of a pediatric patient with an inborn error of metabolism or a congenital heart defect, while pediatric emergency physicians (PEP) may be intimidated by an adult with a myocardial infarction or pulmonary embolism. Dehydration, however, falls in the purview of all emergency physicians (EP). The manner in which an EP treats the condition varies, based on experience, patient and family expectations, and available resources. To quantify this practice, the authors of this study surveyed both GEPs and PEPs to assess how each group tends to manage dehydration. The survey results found that PEPs were more likely to initiate oral or nasogastric rehydration and were less likely to order diagnostic blood tests compared with GEPs. These outcomes suggest that PEPs are more comfortable with a less-invasive approach to pediatric dehydration following the patient's clinical progress in the emergency department. Liberal when answering a survey, PEPs may act more conservatively when faced with the actual patient and her parents.

E. C. Bruno, MD

Induction Dose of Propofol for Pediatric Patients Undergoing Procedural Sedation in the Emergency Department

Jasiak KD, Phan H, Christich AC, et al (Univ of Arizona, Tucson; Univ of Michigan Health Systems, Ann Arbor; et al)
Pediatr Emerg Care 28:440-442, 2012

Objective.—This study aimed to determine if patient age is an independent predictor of the propofol dose required for the induction of sedation in pediatric patients for procedures performed in the emergency department (ED).

Methods.—This is a retrospective study conducted in an academic, tertiary ED between May 2005 and October 2009. Medical records of patients younger than 18 years who received propofol for procedural sedation were evaluated. Data collected included patient demographics, procedure type, propofol doses administered, time to sedation induction, pain scores before procedure, opioid administration, and adverse effects. Factors predictive of propofol induction dose were analyzed using linear regression analyses.

Results.—Eighty-eight patients were included in the final analyses. The mean age was 11 years (range, 1—17 years), and 75% were male. The mean induction dose required was 2.1 ± 1.3 mg/kg using a median of 3 boluses (interquartile range, 2—4). The mean time to induction was 3.9 ± 4.2 minutes. In the linear regression analyses ($R^2 = 0.07$), patient age was inversely predictive of the induction dose (in milligram per kilogram) of propofol (coefficient $= -0.074$; $P = 0.013$). Sex, race, procedure type, pain score before procedure, and opioid administration were not predictive of induction dose. Transient respiratory depression occurred in 13.6% and hypotension occurred in 8% of patients, without further complications.

Conclusions.—In pediatric patients undergoing procedural sedation in the ED, age is an independent predictor of the dose of propofol required for induction of sedation. Therefore, younger patients may require higher doses by body weight (in milligram per kilogram).

▶ Propofol, despite recent negative press, remains en vogue for utilization of rapid sequence induction as well as procedural sedation due to the rapid onset/rapid resolution profile of the medication. The dosing of the medication, initial and maintenance, is weight based, but the authors of this Chinese retrospective study found that a patient's age is an important predictor of dosing requirements. They discovered that younger (and predictably smaller) patients required higher per-kilogram dosing when compared with their older (and predictably larger) counterparts, although no explanation was presented. Presumably, body composition and paradoxical responses to sedation play a role in patient response and dosing requirements. The researchers also report wide ranges of dosing needs, and EPs must balance milligrams with somnolence. While propofol carries benefits, obstructionist behavior by pharmacy and therapeutics committees and the anesthesia stewards continues to limit more generalized use. The credentialing process for one medication, when alternatives remain, may be too arduous for EPs to pursue.

E. C. Bruno, MD

Intranasal Fentanyl and High-concentration Inhaled Nitrous Oxide for Procedural Sedation: A Prospective Observational Pilot Study of Adverse Events and Depth of Sedation

Seith RW, Theophilos T, Babl FE (Royal Children's Hosp, Parkville, Victoria, Australia)
Acad Emerg Med 19:31-36, 2012

Objectives.—Nitrous oxide (N_2O) is an attractive agent for pediatric procedural sedation and analgesia (PSA) with rapid onset and offset of sedation. However, it has limited analgesic efficacy. Intranasal fentanyl (INF) provides nonparenteral analgesia. There are currently no data on the combined use of N_2O and INF for PSA in children. The authors set out to prospectively assess the depth of sedation and incidence of adverse events when N_2O and INF are used in combination in pediatric patients.

Methods.—This was a prospective observational pilot study of combined N_2O and INF for PSA at a tertiary children's hospital emergency department (ED). INF was administered at a precalculated dose of 1.5 μg/kg for preascertained weight ranges. N_2O concentration, dose, timing of INF, adverse events, and sedation depth were recorded. Sedation depth was recorded using the University of Michigan Sedation Scale (UMSS).

Results.—A total of 41 patients, aged 1 to 14 years, received INF within 2 hours prior to N_2O. N_2O was administered at a maximal concentration of 70% in 40 patients, and at 50% in one patient. Most patients (80%) were minimally to moderately sedated (sedation score 1 or 2). Deep sedation (sedation score 3) was recorded in 14.6% of patients (95% confidence interval [CI] = 3.4% to 24.6%). No patients had serious adverse events; vomiting was recorded in 19.5% (95% CI = 7.4% to 31.6%). There were two patients (4.9%) who were deeply sedated and vomited during the procedure.

Conclusions.—There were no serious adverse events identified in this pilot study of combined N_2O and INF. However, there was an increased incidence of vomiting and deeper levels of sedation when compared to published data of single-agent use of N_2O, which could lead to more serious adverse events. Further investigation is needed to establish the analgesic efficacy of combining N_2O and INF and to clarify the safety profile before this combination can be recommended for PSA in children.

▶ In the quest for further reduction in pain and anxiety for pediatric patients in need of a painful procedure, the authors of this prospective observational series evaluated the safety and effectiveness of the combination of intranasal fentanyl (INF) and inhaled nitrous oxide (N_2O). The INF-N_2O duo is an attractive one because the patient does not require intravenous access and because of the short duration of action of the medications. The authors found that nearly 20% of the study's patients had adverse events, specifically vomiting. Vomiting in and of itself is not necessarily a reason to abort the practice, but likely necessitates further investigation into the process to search for a more secure protocol. The authors present a detailed study protocol excluding the rapidity of N_2O administration because this may be a contributing factor to the induction of vomiting. The treating emergency physician who decides to use the INF-N_2O combination must also be cognizant that the additive properties of the medications can approach general anesthesialike effects.

E. C. Bruno, MD

Pulmonary

Triage Nurse Initiation of Corticosteroids in Pediatric Asthma is Associated With Improved Emergency Department Efficiency
Zemek R, Plint A, Osmond MH, et al (Univ of Ottawa, Ontario, Canada; et al)
Pediatrics 129:671-680, 2012

Objective.—To assess the effectiveness of nurse-initiated administration of oral corticosteroids before physician assessment in moderate to severe acute asthma exacerbations in the pediatric ED.

Methods.—A time-series controlled trial evaluated nurse initiation of treatment with steroids before physician assessment in children with Pediatric Respiratory Assessment Measure score ≥4. One-to-one periods (physician-initiated and nurse-initiated) were analyzed from September 2009 through May 2010. In both phases, triage nurses initiated bronchodilator therapy before physician assessment, per Pediatric Respiratory Assessment Measure score. We reviewed charts of 644 consecutive children aged 2 to 17 years for the following outcomes: admission rate; times to clinical improvement, steroid receipt, mild status, and discharge; and rate of return ED visit and subsequent admission.

Results.—Nurse-initiated phase children improved earlier compared to physician-initiated phase (median difference: 24 minutes; 95% confidence interval [CI]: 1−50; $P = .04$). Admission was less likely if children received steroids at triage (odds ratio $= 0.56$; 95% CI: 0.36−0.87). Efficiency gains were made in time to steroid receipt (median difference: 44 minutes; 95% CI: 39−50; $P < .001$), time to mild status (median difference: 51 minutes; 95% CI: 17−84; $P = .04$), and time to discharge (median difference: 44

minutes; 95% CI: 17–68; $P = .02$). No differences were found in return visit rate or subsequent admission.

Conclusions.—Triage nurse initiation of oral corticosteroid before physician assessment was associated with reduced times to clinical improvement and discharge, and reduced admission rates in children presenting with moderate to severe acute asthma exacerbations.

▶ This before-and-after study from the Children's Hospital of Eastern Ontario demonstrates that a departmental procedure, or medical directive as they called it in this study, can be safely and effectively initiated and can result in improved medical care. These authors cut very nearly three-quarters of an hour off the time for children with moderate to severe asthma to improve to mild status and to get discharged just by having the triage nurse initiate oral dexamethasone therapy before physician evaluation. In a disease process such as asthma that is easy to identify and where there is a recognized best treatment approach, the development of departmental pathways can lead to improved turnaround times and to better medical care.

There are some limitations to studies of this type. Since it is not randomized but looks at treatment differences for 2 distinct time periods, the results can be skewed if there are confounding factors that change over the course of the study. In this analysis, the median emergency department (ED) length of stay was 1 hour longer during the second time period, the nurse-initiated phase, than in the prior physician-initiated phase. This information strengthens the result. Although the ED was more crowded and in general patients were waiting longer during the second time period, the asthma patients had a decline in their length of stay. Moreover, the results make sense because the time from administration of the medication until improvement was just over 3 hours in both groups, which is certainly in concert with the pharmacokinetics of oral steroids. We should all develop asthma pathways that let the triage nurse initiate bronchodilator therapy and administer oral corticosteroids prior to physician assessment.

E. A. Ramoska, MD, MPHE

Capnometry as a Predictor of Admission in Bronchiolitis
Lashkeri T, Howell JM, Place R (Inova Fairfax Hosp for Children, Falls Church, VA)
Pediatr Emerg Care 28:895-897, 2012

Objectives.—Bronchiolitis is a dynamic condition, and predicting clinical deterioration can be difficult. The objective of this study was to determine whether capnometry readings among bronchiolitic children admitted to the hospital are significantly different from those discharged from the emergency department.

Methods.—We prospectively studied a convenience sample of children younger than 24 months with clinical bronchiolitis. A single end-tidal CO_2 (ETCO2) reading was taken before treatment, and a clinical work of breathing score was assigned to each patient. Treating physicians and nurses

TABLE 1.—Capnometry Outcomes by Work of Breathing Categories

Work of Breathing Category	No. Patients	Mean Capnometry Reading (mm Hg)	95% CI (mm Hg)
Mild (scores of 1–4)	35	31.5	30–33
Moderate (scores of 5–8)	51	32.8	31–34
Severe (scores of 9–12)	19	33.6	30.7–36.5

were blinded to capnometry readings. The decision to admit was based on the judgment of the attending physician. Descriptive statistics and appropriate hypothesis testing were performed. A receiver operating characteristic curve was constructed for the association between admission and capnometry readings. The α was set at 0.05 for all comparisons.

Results.—One hundred five children with bronchiolitis were included for study. Capnometry readings for admitted (mean, 32.6 mm Hg; 95% confidence interval [CI], 30.3–34.9 mm Hg) and discharged (mean 31.4 mm Hg; 95% CI 29.8–33.0 mm Hg) bronchiolitic children were not significantly different. Capnometry readings for low (mean, 31.7 mm Hg; 95% CI, 29.5–33.8 mm Hg), intermediate (mean, 32.1 mm Hg; 95% CI, 30.1–34.1 mm Hg), and high (mean, 30.5 mm Hg; 95% CI, 19.3–41.7 mm Hg) work of breathing (score) ranges were not significantly different.

Conclusions.—Capnometry readings are not useful in predicting admission for children younger than 2 years with clinical bronchiolitis. There are no significant differences in capnometry readings among bronchiolitic children with low, medium, and high work of breathing scores (Table 1).

▶ Winter months will commonly bring 1 of the most prevalent viral diagnoses in the emergency department, bronchiolitis, that frequently leads to hospitalizations. This single-blinded prospective cohort study found that capnometry readings for admitted and discharged bronchiolitic children were not significantly different (32.6 vs 33.5, respectively) regardless of work of breathing category (Table 1). End-tidal carbon dioxide might be an easy, noninvasive, and objective way to determine ventilatory status and severity of illness in infants with bronchiolitis; however, single point measurements are not useful in determining admission/discharge disposition.

E. C. Quintana, MD, MPH

Complicated and Dislodged Airway Foreign Body in an Intubated Child: Case Report
Graw-Panzer KD, Wadowski SJ, Lee H (Children's Hosp at Downstate, Brooklyn, NY)
Pediatr Emerg Care 28:915-917, 2012

Objective.—We report a case of missed foreign body aspiration in a child presenting with status epilepticus. On admission, the patient was found to

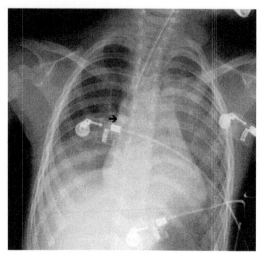

FIGURE 1.—Chest radiograph on admission with tip of the endotracheal tube at carina, right lower lobe. Consolidation with possible small pleural effusion and left lower and upper lobe patchy infiltrates. Round slightly radiopaque lesion overlying the head of the right seventh posterior rib (arrow). (Reprinted from Graw-Panzer KD, Wadowski SJ, Lee H. Complicated and dislodged airway foreign body in an intubated child: case report. *Pediatr Emerg Care.* 2012;28:915-917, with permission from Lippincott Williams & Wilkins.)

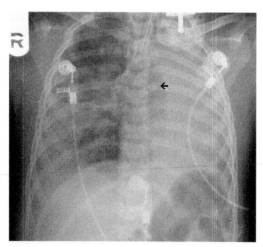

FIGURE 2.—Chest radiograph demonstrating tip of the endotracheal tube 5 mm above the carina, complete opacification of the left lung with silhouetting of the left hemidiaphragm and obscuration of the left costophrenic angle. Patchy infiltrates of right lung. Round slightly radiopaque lesion overlying the head of the left sixth posterior rib (arrow). (Reprinted from Graw-Panzer KD, Wadowski SJ, Lee H. Complicated and dislodged airway foreign body in an intubated child: case report. *Pediatr Emerg Care.* 2012;28:915-917, with permission from Lippincott Williams & Wilkins.)

have pneumonia, which progressed to respiratory failure and acute respiratory distress syndrome. While the patient was intubated and mechanically ventilated, the patient experienced acute respiratory deterioration.

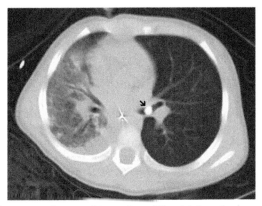

FIGURE 3.—Chest computed tomographic scan shows diffuse right lung alveolar opacities with air bronchogram and small right pleural effusion. There is a 6-mm focal hyperdensity within the left main bronchus (arrow). Hyperinflation of left lung with mediastinal shift to the right. (Reprinted from Graw-Panzer KD, Wadowski SJ, Lee H. Complicated and dislodged airway foreign body in an intubated child: case report. *Pediatr Emerg Care.* 2012;28:915-917, with permission from Lippincott Williams & Wilkins.)

Subsequently, it was determined that a previously undetected foreign body had dislodged from the right main to the left main bronchus and was the underlying cause for the child's illness.

Conclusions.—A combination of sudden change of physical and radiographic findings with unilateral lung hyperinflation is highly suspicious for an obstructing airway foreign body. This case demonstrates that foreign body aspiration can lead to significant morbidity. It should be in the differential diagnosis for any acute pulmonary process in an otherwise well child because there is no specific clinical or radiographic finding to rule it out (Figs 1-3).

▶ This case is of a 27-month-old, recently immigrated, African girl who was brought in by emergency medical services for self-limited generalized tonic-clonic seizure with a 2-day history of fever, worsening cough, and coryza. Her pre-illness and medical history were unremarkable. She was febrile, tachypneic, and tachycardic. Her pulse oximeter was 100% on a nonrebreather mask. Initially, she was postictal, but after a third seizure, she needed to be intubated for airway control after receiving lorazepam intravenously. Her laboratory levels were unremarkable with the exception of glucose 220 mg/dL, white blood cell count 31.5 K/KL, neutrophils 72%, bands 15%, lymphocytes 3%, monocytes 5%, eosinophils 1%, and atypical lymphocytes 2%. All cultures were negative and her chest x-ray (CXR) revealed right lower lobe consolidation with possible small pleural effusion and left upper and lower lobe patchy infiltrates (Fig 1). Her admission diagnoses to the pediatric intensive care unit were the diagnosis of complex febrile seizure secondary to fever from pneumonia, respiratory failure, and acute respiratory distress syndrome. On hospital day 4, she was switched to synchronized intermittent ventilation and decompensated her respiratory status after an episode of coughing. Manual bag-valve ventilation met increased airway resistance with diminished left lung field air entry. Repeat CXR, after endotracheal tube (ETT) replacement, showed left lung collapse with a good position of ETT and patchy infiltrates of the right lung (Fig 2). The lung reexpanded after nebulizer treatments and clindamycin adjuvant antibiotic, for possible aspiration pneumonia. Subsequently, she desaturated and began to wheeze again, with an exam showing monophonic central wheeze associated with decreased breath sounds on the left side. After pulmonary consultation, a chest computed tomography showed a 6-mm focal hyperdensity within the left main bronchus with distal hyperinflation likely consistent with a foreign body and diffuse interstitial and alveolar infiltrate with parapneumonic effusion on the right side (Fig 3). Of interest, her CXR had showed a round, slightly radiopaque lesion that had appeared in the right bronchus intermedius since admission. An orange, smooth, ovoid fragment of hard plastic measuring 6 mm in diameter was extracted out of the left main bronchus via rigid bronchoscopy. This is an atypical presentation for foreign body aspiration. Agitation of the patient and coughing could have led to foreign body dislodgment from the right into the left main bronchus. This is a reminder that sudden respiratory changes in lieu of a unilateral lung hyperinflation on CXR should heighten your suspicion for foreign body aspiration.

E. C. Quintana, MD, MPH

Fatal and Near-Fatal Asthma in Children: The Critical Care Perspective
Newth CJL, for the *Eunice Kennedy Shriver* National Institute of Child Health and Human Development Collaborative Pediatric Critical Care Research Network (Children's Hosp Los Angeles, CA; et al)
J Pediatr 161:214-221, 2012

Objective.—To characterize the clinical course, therapies, and outcomes of children with fatal and near-fatal asthma admitted to pediatric intensive care units (PICUs).

Study Design.—This was a retrospective chart abstraction across the 8 tertiary care PICUs of the Collaborative Pediatric Critical Care Research Network (CPCCRN). Inclusion criteria were children (aged 1-18 years) admitted between 2005 and 2009 (inclusive) for asthma who received ventilation (near-fatal) or died (fatal). Data collected included medications, ventilator strategies, concomitant therapies, demographic information, and risk variables.

Results.—Of the 261 eligible children, 33 (13%) had no previous history of asthma, 218 (84%) survived with no known complications, and 32 (12%) had complications. Eleven (4%) died, 10 of whom had experienced cardiac arrest before admission. Patients intubated outside the PICU had a shorter duration of ventilation (median, 25 hours vs 84 hours; $P < .001$). African-Americans were disproportionately represented among the intubated children and had a shorter duration of intubation. Barotrauma occurred in 15 children (6%) before admission. Pharmacologic therapy was highly variable, with similar outcomes.

Conclusion.—Of the children ventilated in the CPCCRN PICUs, 96% survived to hospital discharge. Most of the children who died experienced cardiac arrest before admission. Intubation outside the PICU was corre-lated with shorter duration of ventilation. Complications of barotrauma and neuromyopathy were uncommon. Practice patterns varied widely among the CPCCRN sites.

▶ This retrospective review of a pediatric critical care database evaluated the presentation, evaluation, management, and subsequent outcomes with severe asthma. This project represents the sickest of the sick, specifically those patients requiring intubation with mechanical ventilation or those patients who died. The extracted information demonstrated important findings related to intuba-tion and events that predicted death. The majority of patients (63%) had no prior admissions within 1 year of the presentation, showing that both acute and chronic asthma patients can require aggressive emergency medical care.

Regarding intubation, 69% of the included patients were intubated prior to arrival in the pediatric intensive care unit (PICU), though conventional teaching has been that intubation in asthma patients is a last resort. Of the 11 deaths, 10 patients were intubated, and 10 had a cardiopulmonary arrest prior to arrival in the PICU. The writers essentially stated that half of the fatalities were near death on arrival to the PICU, suggesting that patients should be moved to the PICU when they present with (or trend toward) severe symptoms.

The project is aptly titled. A clear bias is established in the discussion section, where the authors editorialize that patient outcomes would be better if PICU personnel were caring for these patients.

E. C. Bruno, MD

Effect of Honey on Nocturnal Cough and Sleep Quality: A Double-blind, Randomized, Placebo-Controlled Study
Cohen HA, Rozen J, Kristal H, et al (Pediatric Ambulatory Community Clinic, Petach Tikva, Israel; Tel Aviv Univ, Israel; et al)
Pediatrics 130:465-471, 2012

Objectives.—To compare the effects of a single nocturnal dose of 3 honey products (eucalyptus honey, citrus honey, or labiatae honey) to placebo (silan date extract) on nocturnal cough and difficulty sleeping associated with childhood upper respiratory tract infections (URIs).

Methods.—A survey was administered to parents on 2 consecutive days, first on the day of presentation, when no medication had been given the previous evening, and the following day, when the study preparation was given before bedtime, based on a double-blind randomization plan. Participants included 300 children aged 1 to 5 years with URIs, nocturnal cough, and illness duration of ≤7 days from 6 general pediatric commu-nity clinics. Eligible children received a single dose of 10 g of eucalyptus honey, citrus honey, labiatae honey, or placebo administered 30 minutes before bedtime. Main outcome measures were cough frequency, cough severity, bothersome nature of cough, and child and parent sleep quality.

Results.—In all 3 honey products and the placebo group, there was a significant improvement from the night before treatment to the night of treatment. However, the improvement was greater in the honey groups for all the main outcome measures.

Conclusions.—Parents rated the honey products higher than the silan date extract for symptomatic relief of their children's nocturnal cough and sleep difficulty due to URI. Honey may be a preferable treatment for cough and sleep difficulty associated with childhood URI.

▶ Emergency physicians (EP) are routinely faced with pediatric patients and their families who have complaints of persistent coughing related to upper respiratory infections (URIs). Frustration abounds when the coughing spells interrupt the sleep of the patient and the family. Over-the-counter cough formulations, though widely used, are likely ineffective for the suppression of cough and can be associated with adverse reactions. The authors of this study suggest a more natural agent: honey. Using a randomized, double-blind approach, the authors compared 3 different honey preparations with placebo. Data were obtained in a parent-completed questionnaire, and the results demonstrated that all 3 honey compounds were more effective than placebo in suppressing the patient's cough, which directly resulted in improved patient and parent sleep patterns. Advocating for honey as a cough suppressant sounds like grandmotherly advice, but it represents a safe, cheap, effective, and accessible treatment for URIs. EPs must emphasize avoidance in the younger (younger than 1 year old) patients.

E. C. Bruno, MD

Surgery

Trampoline Safety in Childhood and Adolescence
Council on Sports Medicine and Fitness
Pediatrics 130:774-779, 2012

Despite previous recommendations from the American Academy of Pediatrics discouraging home use of trampolines, recreational use of trampolines in the home setting continues to be a popular activity among children and adolescents. This policy statement is an update to previous statements, reflecting the current literature on prevalence, patterns, and mechanisms of trampoline-related injuries. Most trampoline injuries occur with multiple simultaneous users on the mat. Cervical spine injuries often occur with falls off the trampoline or with attempts at somersaults or flips. Studies on the efficacy of trampoline safety measures are reviewed, and although there is a paucity of data, current implementation of safety measures have not appeared to mitigate risk substantially. Therefore, the home use of trampolines is strongly discouraged. The role of trampoline as a competitive sport and in structured training settings is reviewed, and recommendations for enhancing safety in these environments are made.

▶ Although the prevalence of trampoline injuries is decreasing, concern persists regarding the severity of injuries sustained on the trampoline. Studies over the past decade in other countries revealed hospitalization rates between 3% and 14% vs 3% in the United States. It is concerning that although home trampoline use appears to be waning, commercial trampoline parks and other trampoline installations have been emerging over the past several years and that their safety has not been universally regulated. Several studies have revealed that approximately 75% of injuries occurred when multiple people were using the trampoline simultaneously and the smallest children were more likely to sustain injury relative to their heavier playmates. Current evidence suggests that the availability of enclosures/netting on the market has not significantly affected the proportions of injuries attributable to falls off the trampoline, and there does not appear to be an inverse correlation between presence of safety equipment and rates of injury. Children are often tempted to climb or grasp the netting, which may be an additional source of injury. Multiple studies reveal that approximately up to 50% of injuries occurred despite reported adult supervision. The most common trampoline-related injury is an ankle sprain. Although most trampoline injuries are sprains, strains, contusions, or other soft-tissue injury, younger children seem to be more prone to bony injury, especially upper extremity fracture after falling off the trampoline. Head and/or neck injuries accounted for up to 17% of all trampoline-related injuries, and 0.5% of all trampoline injuries resulted in permanent neurologic damage resulting from either hyperflexion or extension. There are several unique injuries associated with trampoline use: proximal tibial fractures (especially in children younger than 6 years old), sternal fracture or manubriosternal dislocation in children between 10 and 11 years old, vertebral artery dissections from abrupt cervical hyperextension and rotation, and atlantoaxial subluxation. Significant safety features in both home and professional locations are warranted to prevent significant injuries.

E. C. Quintana, MD, MPH

Are routine pelvic radiographs in major pediatric blunt trauma necessary?
Lagisetty J, Slovis T, Thomas R, et al (Memorial Hermann Med Ctr, Houston, TX; Wayne State Univ School of Medicine, Detroit, MI)
Pediatr Radiol 42:853-858, 2012

Background.—Screening pelvic radiographs to rule out pelvic fractures are routinely used for the initial evaluation of pediatric blunt trauma. Recently, the utility of routine pelvic radiographs in certain subsets of patients with blunt trauma has been questioned. There is a growing amount of evidence that shows the clinical exam is reliable enough to obviate the need for routine screening pelvic radiographs in children.

Objective.—To identify variables that help predict the presence or absence of pelvic fractures in pediatric blunt trauma.

Materials and Methods.—We conducted a retrospective study from January 2005 to January 2010 using the trauma registry at a level 1 pediatric trauma center. We analyzed all level 1 and level 2 trauma victims, evaluating history, exam and mechanism of injury for association with the presence or absence of a pelvic fracture.

Results.—Of 553 level 1 and 2 trauma patients who presented during the study period, 504 were included in the study. Most of these children, 486/504 (96.4%), showed no evidence of a pelvic fracture while 18/504 (3.6%) had a pelvic fracture. No factors were found to be predictive of a pelvic fracture. However, we developed a pelvic fracture screening tool that accurately rules out the presence of a pelvic fracture $P = 0.008$, NPV 99, sensitivity 96, 8.98 (1.52−52.8). This screening tool combines eight high-risk clinical findings (pelvic tenderness, laceration, ecchymosis, abrasion, GCS < 14, positive urinalysis, abdominal pain/tenderness, femur fracture) and five highrisk mechanisms of injury (unrestrained motor vehicle collision [MVC], MVC with ejection, MVC rollover, auto vs. pedestrian, auto vs. bicycle).

Conclusion.—Pelvic fractures in pediatric major blunt trauma can reliably be ruled out by using our pelvic trauma screening tool. Although no findings accurately identified the presence of a pelvic fracture, the screening tool accurately identified the absence of a fracture, suggesting that pelvic radiographs are not warranted in this subset of patients.

▶ Using screening pelvic x-rays to rule out pelvic fracture has been taught by the American College of Surgeons and the Advanced Trauma Life Support program for the initial evaluation of blunt abdominal trauma patients; however, the use of these x-rays in some subsets of pediatric blunt trauma patients has been questioned. This 5-year retrospective study found that 96.4% (486/504 patients) showed no evidence of a pelvic fracture, whereas 3.8% had an identifiable pelvic fracture. All were diagnosed in the initial emergency department evaluation, and didn't require any surgical intervention. Glasgow Coma Scale < 14 and pelvic tenderness were found to be significant predictors of a pelvic fracture; in contrast, concomitant femur fracture, other fractures, intra-abdominal injury, abdominal pain, head injury, or mechanism of injury weren't reliable predictors for a pelvic fracture. Prospective studies are warranted.

E. C. Quintana, MD, MPH

Spinal cord trauma in children under 10 years of age: clinical characteristics and prevention
de Amoreira Gepp R, Nadal LG (SARAH Network of Rehabilitation Hosps, Brasilia, Brazil)
Child's Nerv Syst 28:1919-1924, 2012

Purpose.—This study analyzed the clinical characteristics of spinal cord injury (SCI) in children 10 years of age and younger, forms of prevention, and ways to improve treatment.

Methods.—Ninety-three children were reviewed between 1996 and 2009. The variables studied were type, age, cause, neurological level, association between SCI and traumatic brain injury (TBI), arthrodesis surgery, time elapsed between trauma and diagnosis, and causes of death. The statistical evaluations were done using the chi-square and ANOVA scales, in the SPSS program version 11.0.

Results.—The most common cause was automobile crash accidents. Getting run over by a car was second (29.1%), followed by firearm injuries (11.8%). The thoracic spine was the most commonly impacted area. Evaluation showed that 83.9% had complete neurological injury. Associated TBI was present in 35.5% of the cases. Only 21.5% of the patients required arthrodesis of the spine. In 31.2% of the cases, myelopathy was not diagnosed at the time of the accident. There was no statistical correlation between TBI and a delayed diagnosis of SCI ($p = 0.231$). Five children (5.4%) died.

Conclusions.—The study showed that the cause of the trauma is associated to the child's age and that prevention is important. Trauma from automobile crash accidents was the main cause, and, in older children, firearm injuries are an important risk. Spinal cord injury was not always diagnosed in children at the time of accident. Educating family members and training emergency teams to adequately treat children with multiple traumas are measures that can help reduce the incidence of SCIs and neurological damage.

▶ Spinal cord injury (SCI) in children is considered a rare disease with serious consequences. In this study, 19 patients were between 0 and 2 years old at time of trauma, 34 were older than 2 and up to 5 years old, and 40 were between 5 and 10 years old; 58.1% of patients were male. The most common cause of the SCI was automobile accident (40.8%), followed by pedestrian strike (20.1%). Forty-two percent in the age group of up to 2 years old and 5-10 years old group had an SCI caused by automobile accidents, whereas 41% in the age group 2-5 years old was due to pedestrian strike. The thoracic spine was the vertebral segment most affected, at level T4 and T12. In the cervical spine region, the neurological level at C7 was the most common, with 7 cases (7.5%). The region of the medullary conus was affected by the L1 fracture in 8 cases (8.6%). Even though there was no statistical association on time for SCI diagnosis with incidental traumatic brain injuries (TBI) and patients' ages, the authors noted a trend of TBI delaying the SCI diagnosis. Throughout the long-term follow-up, 5 children died, representing 5.4% of the sample. The causes of death were complications from urological surgery, upper digestive tract hemorrhage, acute respiratory failure, septicemia with respiratory failure, and oncological disease not associated with the acquired SCI.

E. C. Quintana, MD, MPH

Race disparities in firearm injuries and outcomes among Tennessee children

Martin CA, Unni P, Landman MP, et al (Jr Children's Hosp at Vanderbilt Univ, Nashville, TN; et al)

J Pediatr Surg 47:1196-1202, 2012

Purpose.—The aim of this study was to identify race and socioeconomic factors associated with worse outcomes among Tennessee children who sustain firearm injuries.

Methods.—We queried our institutional pediatric trauma registry and the Davidson County Regional Medical Examiner database for children ages 15 years and younger who sustained firearm injuries between July 1998 and July 2010. Descriptive statistics and logistic regression modeling were used to analyze demographic data, circumstance of injury (unintentional or intentional), odds of death, and characteristics of zip codes (total population, race distribution, and median income) where injuries occurred.

Results.—One hundred eighty-eight children (median age, 13.2 years; range, 1.1-15.8 years) sustained a firearm injury and were either admitted to our institution or were referred directly to the medical examiner. More whites (n = 109, or 58%) sustained a firearm injury than blacks (n = 79, or 42%), but blacks were overrepresented 2.5-fold more compared with the general Tennessee population. Fifty-four children (29%) died, of whom 35 (65%) were black and 19 (35%) were white (*P* < .001). Ninety-three children sustained unintentional firearm injuries, and 84 were intentional (n = 67, assault; n = 17, suicide). When data were stratified by intent, 67% of blacks and 12% of whites were assaulted (*P* < .001). After controlling for age and intent, black children were 4 times more likely to die of firearm injuries than whites (*P* =.008; 95% confidence interval, 1.4-11.3).

Conclusion.—In a sample of firearm-injured Tennessee children, blacks were notably overrepresented and far more likely to die than whites. Using zip code data will help to establish firearm injury prevention programs specific to disparate populations and to reduce both violent and accidental childhood firearm injuries.

▶ The pediatric population has significant morbidity and mortality with firearm injuries. This cohort study (1998–2010) had a median age of 13.2 years (1.1–15.9 years); 155 children (82%) were boys. The racial distribution of the study population was 109 white (58%) and 79 black (42%) children. The annualized incidence of firearm injuries did not change significantly during the study period. Female sex was significantly associated with death compared with boys (*P* = .011). This study found that white children were more likely to sustain accidental or unintentional injuries, whereas black children were more likely to be victims of assault. The likely scenario of a firearm injury occurring in a white child playing with a parent's weapon who accidentally shoots himself or another sibling has been previously documented. Drawbacks of this study are the exclusion of children who were evaluated for minor firearm injuries in the emergency department, and geographic and regional cultural differences that can influence exposure to various weapons and to the type of firearm injury sustained. Nonetheless, these findings could be used to create injury prevention programs.

E. C. Quintana, MD, MPH

The acute compartment syndrome following fractures of the lower leg in children
Ferlic PW, Singer G, Kraus T, et al (Med Univ of Graz, Austria)
Injury 43:1743-1746, 2012

Introduction.—The acute compartment syndrome (ACS) of the lower leg is a rare but serious complication following either fractures or soft tissue injuries. An acute intervention consisting of fasciotomy is indicated as ACS may cause muscle and nerve damage. The aim of the present study was to evaluate the cause, the incidence, the time to fasciotomy and the outcome of ACS of the lower leg following fractures in a paediatric population.

Patients and Methods.—A retrospective analysis of all patients with ACS following a fracture of the lower leg treated from 1998 to 2010 was performed. The time from admission to occurrence of the ACS, the kind of fracture and surgical treatment was evaluated. Accident mechanisms were recorded.

Results.—A total of 1028 fractures of the lower leg were treated. 31 patients (3%) with a median age of 14.6 years (range 7.3—17.1 years) developed an ACS. In the group of patients younger than 12 years the incidence was even lower (1.3%). 81% of injuries leading to ACS were caused by high-energy trauma, with motorcycle accidents being the most common (45%). External fixation was used in 45%, including all open fractures. The diagnosis of an ACS was primarily based on clinical symptoms. In 23 cases an intracompartmental pressure of median 55 mmHg (range 40—100 mmHg) were measured. ACS was diagnosed after 19 h mean (range: 1.5—65 h). There was a tendency that the ACS occurred earlier after high-energy trauma than after low energy trauma (mean 16.9 vs. mean 28 h). No complications linked to the compartment syndrome were observed.

Discussion.—ACS can occur up to 65 h after an accident and therefore clinical monitoring is fundamental in order to be able to surgically intervene as soon as possible when needed. With early decompression complications can be prevented (Fig 1).

▶ This retrospective study found that acute compartment syndrome was a rare complication at a 3% incidence, lower in children younger than 12 years old. The most common injury mechanism was motorcycle accidents (45%), followed by sports injuries (skiing primarily) with fractures in the diaphyseal tibia/fibula (Fig 1). Acute compartment syndrome was diagnosed earlier after high-energy trauma (mean 17 hours) than after low-energy trauma (mean 28 hours), although it was not statistically significant ($P = .14$). An intracompartmental

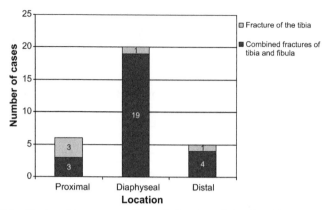

FIGURE 1.—Number of fractures according to the location and the affected bones. (Reprinted from Ferlic PW, Singer G, Kraus T, et al. The acute compartment syndrome following fractures of the lower leg in children. *Injury*. 2012;43:1743-1746, Copyright 2012, with permission from Elsevier.)

pressure measurement was performed in 23 cases for diagnosis, with a median measurement of 55 mm Hg, whereas there was a clinical diagnosis in 9 cases. There was a 19% complication rate that consisted of delayed bone healing, osteomyelitis, temporary peroneal nerve paresis, and decreased range of motion at the ankle. Ninety-four percent were asymptomatic at the last follow-up, with an excellent functional outcome.

E. C. Quintana, MD, MPH

Support for blood alcohol screening in pediatric trauma

Ley EJ, Singer MB, Short SS, et al (Cedars-Sinai Med Ctr, Los Angeles, CA)
Am J Surg 204:939–943, 2012

Background.—Alcohol intoxication in pediatric trauma is underappreciated. The aim of this study was to characterize alcohol screening rates in pediatric trauma.

Methods.—The Los Angeles County Trauma System Database was queried for all patients aged ≤ 18 years who required admission between 2003 and 2008. Patients were compared by age and gender.

Results.—A total of 18,598 patients met the inclusion criteria; 4,899 (26.3%) underwent blood alcohol screening, and 2,797 (57.1%) of those screened positive. Screening increased with age (3.3% for 0–9 years, 15.1% for 10–14 years, and 45.4% for 15–18 years; $P < .01$), as did alcohol intoxication (1.9% for 0–9 years, 5.8% 10–14 years, and 27.3% for 15–18 years; $P < .01$). Male gender predicted higher mortality in those aged 15 to 18 years (adjusted odds ratio, 1.7; $P < .01$), while alcohol intoxication did not (adjusted odds ratio, .97; $P = .84$).

TABLE 1.—Patient Demographics

Variable	All Patients (n = 18,598)	Age 0–9 Years (n = 5,612)	Age 10–14 Years (n = 3,518)	Age 15–18 Years (n = 9,068)	P
Age (y)	12.1 ± 5.6	4.5 ± 2.6	12.3 ± 1.4	16.8 ± 1.1	NA
Alcohol screened	26.3%	3.3%	15.1%	45.4%	<.01
Alcohol positive of total	15.0%	1.9%	5.8%	27.3%	<.01
Alcohol positive of those screened	57.1%	51.4%	38.4%	60.3%	<.01
Male	71.1%	63.4%	69.7%	76.3%	<.01
Admission SBP (mm Hg)	126.3 ± 19.6	117.8 ± 18.0	127.4 ± 17.0	131.1 ± 19.9	<.01
Admission SBP < 90 mm Hg	2.7%	4.5%	1.0%	2.2%	<.01
ISS	7.9 ± 8.4	7.0 ± 7.8	7.6 ± 7.9	8.6 ± 8.8	<.01
ISS ≥ 16	15.4%	12.3%	13.8%	17.9%	<.01
ISS ≥ 25	6.2%	5.0%	5.3%	7.4%	<.01
Admission GCS	14.2 ± 2.4	14.2 ± 2.3	14.2 ± 2.1	14.2 ± 2.5	<.01
Admission GCS ≤ 8	5.1%	5.1%	3.9%	5.6%	<.01
Head AIS	.58 ± 1.15	.7 ± 1.2	.6 ± 1.2	.5 ± 1.1	<.01
ICU admission	22.0%	20.3%	19.8%	24.0%	<.01
ICU LOS (d)	4.3 ± 7.8	3.8 ± 7.9	4.0 ± 7.5	4.7 ± 7.9	<.01
Hospital LOS (d)	3.4 ± 12.4	2.6 ± 6.7	3.3 ± 19.6	3.9 ± 11.1	<.01
Death	1.7%	1.3%	.9%	2.4%	<.01

Data are expressed as mean ± SD or as percentages.
LOS = length of stay; NA = not applicable.

TABLE 3.—Screened Patients: Alcohol Positive Versus Negative

Variable	Positive (n = 2,797)	Negative (n = 2,102)	P
Age (y)	16.2 ± 2.7	15.7 ± 2.9	<.01
Male	78.5%	72.7%	<.01
Admission SBP (mm Hg)	129.5 ± 20.4	133.5 ± 19.0	<.01
Admission SBP < 90 mm Hg	2.7%	1.3%	<.01
ISS	8.5 ± 8.4	10.1 ± 9.6	<.01
ISS ≥ 16	17.3%	23.6%	<.01
ISS ≥ 25	7.1%	9.5%	<.01
Admission GCS	13.9 ± 2.8	14.0 ± 2.7	.16
Admission GCS ≤ 8	7.2%	7.0%	.87
Head AIS	.6 ± 1.2	.9 ± 1.4	<.01
ICU admission	25.6%	28.6%	.02
ICU LOS (d)	4.2 ± 6.7	4.8 ± 9.1	.17
Hospital LOS (d)	3.8 ± 10.0	4.2 ± 8.5	.12
Death	2.2%	2.6%	.45

Data are expressed as mean ± SD or as percentages.
LOS = length of stay.

Conclusions.—Alcohol intoxication is common in adolescent trauma patients. Screening is encouraged for pediatric trauma patients aged ≥ 10 years who require admission (Tables 1 and 3).

▶ In the pediatric population, risky behaviors are associated with alcohol abuse/use. The authors hypothesized that alcohol screening is low in the pediatric population. Using the Los Angeles County Trauma System Database, 26.3% underwent blood alcohol screening and 15% (2797) tested positive. Rates of blood alcohol screening increased across age groups (3.3% vs 15.1% vs 45.4%, $P < .01$), as did rates of intoxication (1.9% vs 5.8% vs 27.3%, $P < .01$) (Table 1). The following demographic characteristics also increased with age, including the proportion of male patients (63.4% vs 69.7% vs 76.3%, $P < .01$), admission systolic blood pressure (117.8 vs 127.4 vs 131.1 mm Hg, $P < .01$), and Injury Severity Scale (ISS; 7.0 vs 7.6 vs 8.6, $P < .01$). Screened patients were older (16.0 vs 10.8 years, $P < .01$), were predominantly male (76.1% vs 69.3%, $P < .01$), had higher ISS (9.2 vs 7.4, $P < .01$), and had lower admission Glasgow Coma Scale scores (13.9 vs 14.4, $P < .01$) with more frequent intensive care unit admissions compared with those who were not screened (Table 3). Based on these findings, the authors suggest that routine screening for alcohol intoxication should be performed for all children aged ≥ 10 years who present for trauma evaluation.

E. C. Quintana, MD, MPH

Theoretical increase of thyroid cancer induction from cervical spine multidetector computed tomography in pediatric trauma patients
Muchow RD, Egan KR, Peppler WW, et al (Univ of Wisconsin—Madison)
J Trauma Acute Care Surg 72:403-409, 2012

Background.—The trend of increasing cervical spine multidirectional computed tomography (MDCT) imaging of pediatric trauma patients is characteristic of the overall dramatic increase in computed tomography utilization in the United States. The purpose of this study is to compare the amount of radiation a pediatric trauma patient absorbs to the thyroid from plain radiographs and MDCT of the cervical spine and to express risk by calculation of theoretical thyroid cancer induction.

Methods. A retrospective evaluation of pediatric trauma patients admitted from October 1, 2004, to October 31, 2009, was performed at an academic, Level I trauma center. Inclusion criteria were Level I/II trauma patients, cervical spine imaging performed at our institution, and age < 18 years. Absorbed thyroid radiation was calculated for patients receiving plain radiographs or MDCT. Thyroid cancer risk was calculated using the 2006 Biological Effects on Ionizing Radiation VII report.

Results.—Six hundred seventeen patients met inclusion criteria: 224 received cervical spine radiographs and 393 received cervical spine MDCT. The mean thyroid radiation absorbed from radiographs was 0.90 mGy for males and 0.96 mGy for females compared with 63.6 mGy (males) and 64.2 mGy (females) receiving MDCT ($p < 0.001$). The median excess relative risk of thyroid cancer induction from one cervical spine MDCT in males was 13.0% and females was 25.0%, compared with 0.24% (males) and 0.51% (females) for radiographs ($p < 0.001$).

Conclusions.—The significant difference in radiation that MDCT delivers to the pediatric trauma patient when compared with plain radiographs should temper routine use of computed tomography in pediatric cervical spine clearance algorithms (Tables 2 and 3).

▶ Pediatric cervical spine injuries are always concerning in blunt trauma, especially because of their devastating consequences if missed. Computed tomography (CT) use for pediatric cervical spine screening has increased nearly 4-fold because of easy access and sensitivity. In children, there is a concern for harmful effects of diagnostic radiation from cervical spine CT because of the age-related sensitivity of the thyroid to radiation, placing them at a higher risk over their life expectancy. In this theoretical study, the authors determine the risk factors for thyroid cancer with the use of diagnostic testing for cervical spine clearance. With x-rays, increased age was associated with significantly greater thyroid radiation absorption for both genders in the oldest age group (12–17 years) compared with the 2 younger groups (Table 2). For CT, the radiation dose received by the younger 2 age groups was significantly lower than the adolescent age groups but not significantly different between the youngest 2 age groups, males and females alike (Table 2). The overall median excess relative risk

TABLE 2.—Absorbed Radiation to the Thyroid in mGy for Males and Females From Plain Radiographs and CT Cervical Spine

	Plain Radiograph				CT			
	Male		Female		Male		Female	
Age Category	Number	mGy, Mean (SD)	Number	mGy, Mean (SD)	Number	mGy, Mean (SD)	Number	mGy, Mean (SD)
0–6	38	0.36 (0.16)	19	0.4 (0.25)	46	51.7 (24.3)	22	55.5 (21.0)
7–11	29	0.81 (0.33)	26	0.88 (0.28)	34	51.3 (18.79)	24	56.2 (16.8)
12–17	69	1.51 (0.61)*	43	1.59 (0.75)*	165	70.2 (20.1)*	102	68.3 (18.1)*
All	136	0.9 (0.69)	88	0.96 (0.73)	245	63.6 (21.6)	148	64.2 (19.2)

All absorbed thyroid radiation values (mGy) for CT were significantly greater ($p < 0.001$) than the respective plain radiograph values.
*Statistically significant difference in thyroid absorbed radiation between the 12- and 17-yr age group and the younger two age groups.

TABLE 3.—Excess Relative Risk of Thyroid Cancer Induction for CT Cervical Spine Versus Plain Radiographs

Age Category	Male Plain Radiograph	CT	P	Female Plain Radiograph	CT	p
0–6	0.16 (0.11–0.32)	21.5 (10.0–66.0)	<0.001	0.31 (0.02–0.48)	45.6 (17.0–116.0)	<0.001
7–11	0.22 (0.11–0.43)	13.5 (8.0–27.0)	<0.001	0.51 (0.27–0.77)	29.7 (15.0–55.0)	<0.001
12–17	0.29 (0.10–0.55)	12.0 (4.0–26.0)	<0.001	0.56 (0.18–1.32)	22.7 (8.0–42.0)	<0.001
All	0.24 (0.10–0.55)	13.0 (10.0–66.0)	<0.001	0.51 (0.02–1.32)	25.0 (8.0–116.0)	<0.001

Median values reported with the range in parentheses; p value indicates significance for age- and gender-matched groups comparing CT and plain radiographs.

for CT compared with plain radiographs was significantly higher 0.24% vs 13.0% for males and 0.51% vs 25.0% for females, for inducing thyroid cancer ($P < .001$). This was true across both genders and all age groups (Table 3). These findings warrant a judicious use of CT vs plain x-rays in the cervical evaluation.

E. C. Quintana, MD, MPH

Serum troponin-I as an indicator of clinically significant myocardial injury in paediatric trauma patients
Sangha GS, Pepelassis D, Buffo-Sequeira I, et al (Univ of Western Ontario, London, Canada; Univ of Manitoba, Winnipeg, Canada; et al)
Injury 43:2046-2050, 2012

Myocardial injury is a cause of mortality in paediatric trauma, but it is often difficult to diagnose. The objectives of this pilot study were to (1) determine the prevalence of elevated cardiac troponin I (TnI) in paediatric trauma patients and (2) to determine whether elevated TnI correlates with clinically significant myocardial injury, defined as abnormalities on echocardiogram (ECHO) and/or electrocardiograms (ECG). To this end, we investigated a convenient sample size of 59 paediatric trauma patients with an Injury Severity Score (ISS) > 12. TnI and creatine kinase-MB (CK-MB) were measured on admission, at then at regular intervals until TnI had normalized. Patients with elevated TnI levels had an ECHO performed within 24 h of admission and underwent daily ECGs until TnI normalized. Elevated serum TnI was found in $n = 16/59$ (27%; 95% CI: 18–40%) patients and was associated with elevated CK-MB in all cases. Abnormal ECHOs were seen in 4/16 patients with elevated TnI, but peak TnI values did not correlate with abnormalities on ECHO ($p = 0.23$). Only 1 patient had a clinically significant, albeit mild, decrease in cardiac function. All ECGs were normal. Patients with elevated TnI were more likely to be intubated ($p = 0.04$), to have higher Injury Severity Scores ($p = 0.02$), required more resuscitation fluid ($p = 0.001$), and to have thoracic injuries ($p < 0.001$). Our data indicates that the prevalence of elevated TnI in paediatric trauma patients is 27%; and whilst elevated TnI reflects overall trauma severity, it is frequently

TABLE 3.—Comparison of Paediatric Patients with Normal TnI versus Patients with Elevated TnI

Parameter	Normal TnI ($n = 43$)	Elevated TnI ($n = 16$)	p-Value
Age, yr	12.3 (SD = 4.5)	11.9 (SD = 4.8)	0.80
Weight, kg	53.4 (SD = 21.5)	50.8 (SD = 23.3)	0.68
Male:Female, n (%)	35:8 (81:19)	7:9 (44:56)	0.72
ISS	22.3 (SD = 7.1)	32.9 (SD = 16.2)	0.02
Episodes of hypotension[a]	0 (0, 0)	0 (0, 1.8)	0.15
Persistent tachycardia[a]	0 (0, 0)	0.5 (0, 1)	0.01
Total fluid, cc/kg[a]	81 (73, 111)	160 (105, 251)	0.001
Resuscitation fluid, cc/kg[a]	41 (20, 65)	110 (60, 180)	0.001
Inotropes used, n (%)	5 (12)	5 (31)	0.16
OR in first 24 h, n (%)	10 (23)	7 (44)	0.22
Intubated, n (%)	23(54)	14 (88)	0.04
Mechanism of injury, n (%)			
MVC	23 (54)	6 (38)	0.42
Ped vs MV	6 (14)	6 (38)	0.10
Fall	5 (12)	2 (13)	0.72
Toboggan vs tree	6 (14)	0 (0)	0.27
Bike vs MV	3 (7)	1 (6)	N/A
Assault	0 (0)	1 (6)	N/A
Associated injuries, n (%)			
Traumatic brain injury	26 (60)	10 (63)	0.87
Thoracic injury	16 (37)	15 (94)	<0.001
Abdominal injury	17 (40)	10 (63)	0.20
Orthopaedic injury	18 (42)	9 (56)	0.49
Facial injury	9 (21)	1 (6)	0.34
Spinal cord injury	1 (2)	1 (6)	N/A
Mortality	0 (0)	3 (19)	N/A

[a]In the first 24 h, reported as median (quartiles).

elevated without a clinically significance myocardial injury. Hence, large scale studies are required to determine if an elevated threshold TnI value can be identified to accurately diagnose severe myocardial injury in paediatric trauma (Table 3).

▶ The clinical significance of elevated troponin I (TnI) in the pediatric trauma population is unclear. Fifty-nine patients were enrolled in this pilot study. The most common mechanism of injury was a motor vehicle collision, with 49% traumatic brain injuries as the most common injury noted (61%). Ninety-four percent of the patients with elevated TnI levels had evidence of an associated pulmonary contusion. Twenty-seven percent of patients with blunt trauma had elevated TnI and creatine kinase MB. Pulmonary contusion was the most common thoracic injury. Twenty-five percent of these patients had abnormal echocardiograms with trivial pericardial effusions with normal ventricular function, 1 had mild septal wall hypokinesis with normal ventricular function, and 1 had low diastolic function and low-normal systolic function. A median value of 0.21 mg/L of TnI was found at 12 hours after admission. The group with elevated TnI levels had a larger proportion of intubated patients ($P = .04$), a higher mean Injury Severity Score ($P = .02$), more total fluid intake ($P = .001$), more resuscitation fluid ($P = .001$), and a larger proportion of patients with associated chest injuries ($P < .001$) (Table 3). All 3 patients who died in the study had elevated TnI levels. The

4 patients with abnormal echocardiograms had a TnI level of 0.37 mg/L; the peak level for the patient with mildly decreased function was 0.16 mg/L. These ranges could be considered as guidelines for further testing when evaluating blunt pediatric trauma.

E. C. Quintana, MD, MPH

The Predictive Value of a Normal Radiographic Anterior Fat Pad Sign Following Elbow Trauma in Children
Blumberg SM, Kunkov S, Crain EF, et al (Albert Einstein College of Medicine, Bronx, NY; Stony Brook Long Island Children's Hosp, NY)
Pediatr Emerg Care 27:596-600, 2011

Objective.—The purposes of this study were to describe the characteristics of a normal anterior fat pad (AFP) and to determine the association between a normal AFP and the absence of fracture.

Methods.—A prospective cohort of children aged 1 to 18 years with elbow trauma underwent radiographic examination. All patients received standard orthopedic management and follow-up 7 to 14 days after injury. A pediatric radiologist evaluated all radiographs for the presence or absence of fracture and documented whether the AFP was normal or abnormal on the lateral view. The radiologist also recorded specific measurements of the AFP including the apical angle, which is formed by the intersection of the humerus and the superior aspect of the AFP. The interpretation of the AFP on the initial lateral radiograph was compared with the final patient outcome (fracture/no fracture).

Results.—Two hundred thirty-one patients had elbow radiographs; 34 patients (15%) were lost to follow-up. A total of 56 fractures were identified: 49 (87%) on the initial radiograph and an additional 7 (13%) on follow-up radiographs. This latter group was defined as occult fractures. Among the 197 patients available for analysis, 113 (57%) had a normal AFP on the initial radiograph. Of these, 2 children had a final diagnosis of fracture. The sensitivity of a normal AFP was 96.4% (95% confidence interval, 86.6%−99.4%), and the negative predictive value was 98.2% (95% confidence interval, 93.1%−99.7%). There was a significant difference in mean AFP angle when the AFP was read as normal (14.7 [SD, 3.3] degrees) compared with when it was read as abnormal (27.0 [SD, 6.8] degrees) ($P < 0.01$).

Conclusions.—Our data suggest that a normal AFP is highly associated with absence of elbow fracture and that the determination of a normal AFP can be aided by measuring the apical angle of the AFP (Fig 1).

▶ Elbow trauma is a very common extremity injury in children. Posterior fat pad has been a better predictor of elbow fracture; however, some would state that an abnormal shape in an anterior fat pad is suggestive of fracture. The interpretation of the anterior fat pad as either abnormal or normal on initial x-ray was compared with final diagnosis of fracture or no fracture. Also specific measurements of

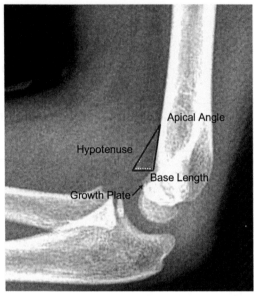

FIGURE 1.—The AFP triangle and its measurements. (1) Apical angle formed by the intersection of the anterior humerus and the proximal portion of the AFP; (2) base length, the distance from the anterior humerus to the most anterior and distal aspect of the AFP; (3) hypotenuse length, the distance from the proximal to the distal aspect of the AFP; and (4) length between the growth plate of the distal humerus and the base of the AFP. (Reprinted from Blumberg SM, Kunkov S, Crain EF, et al. The predictive value of a normal radiographic anterior fat pad sign following elbow trauma in children. *Pediatr Emerg Care.* 2011;27:596-600, with permission from Lippincott Williams & Wilkins.)

anterior fat pad (Fig 1) were compared when noted to be normal versus abnormal and compared with x-ray interpretation and final patient outcome. This study concluded that a normal anterior fat pad on an initial elbow x-ray was highly associated with the absence of elbow fracture in children. When compared with the posterior fat pad, the anterior fat pad had fewer false-negative cases and a higher sensitivity (96.4%) and negative predictive value (98%). Only the apical anterior fat pad was statistically significant with abnormal findings (measurement of more than 27 degrees). This simple guideline may be helpful in the management of elbow injuries.

E. C. Quintana, MD, MPH

Hidden attraction: a menacing meal of magnets and batteries
Brown JC, Murray KF, Javid PJ (Seattle Children's Hosp and Univ of Washington)
J Emerg Med 43:266-269, 2012

Background.—Magnet and button battery ingestions are increasingly common, and can result in significant morbidity. Timely identification of

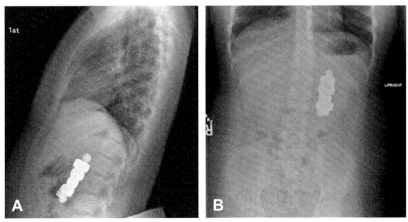

FIGURE 1.—Selected radiographs of the chest and abdomen, demonstrating a column of foreign bodies projecting over the stomach. (Reprinted from Brown JC, Murray KF, Javid PJ. Hidden attraction: a menacing meal of magnets and batteries. *J Emerg Med.* 2012;43:266-269, Copyright 2012, with permission from American Academy of Emergency Medicine.)

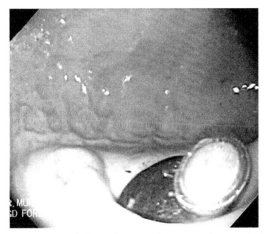

FIGURE 2.—Endoscopic image of a button battery and magnet in the stomach. An ulcer is visible to the right of these objects, on the greater curvature of the stomach. (Reprinted from Brown JC, Murray KF, Javid PJ. Hidden attraction: a menacing meal of magnets and batteries. *J Emerg Med.* 2012;43:266-269, Copyright 2012, with permission from American Academy of Emergency Medicine.)

hazardous foreign body ingestions can be difficult in non-verbal and non-disclosing children.

Objectives.—We aim to present a case that demonstrates some of the challenges around identifying and correctly locating magnets and batteries, and the importance of prompt identification and removal.

Case Report.—We describe an older child with the covert ingestion of multiple magnets and batteries, with magnets that attracted across the stomach and a loop of jejunum. Mild symptoms and signs resulted in a delayed diagnosis and serious consequences. Radiographs suggested a gastric location of the foreign bodies.

Conclusion.—Health care workers should consider the possibility of battery or magnet ingestions in children with vomiting and abdominal pain, even when well-appearing. Like esophageal batteries, multiple gastrointestinal magnets and combined magnet-battery ingestions can cause significant morbidity, and prompt identification is important. Providers should ask verbal children for ingestion histories, and consider radiographs when symptoms are atypical or persistent. Like esophageal batteries, gastrointestinal magnet-battery ingestions should be removed promptly to prevent complications. Caregivers should supervise or limit the use of toys that include magnets and batteries (Figs 1 and 2).

▶ Magnets are increasingly common as desktop and electronic toys for children and adults, and their ingestions are increasingly common and can be difficult to identify. This case study presented an 8-year-old female with abdominal pain and nonbilious, postprandial vomiting. On examination, she had mild nonlocalized abdominal tenderness without peritoneal signs and normal bowel sounds. Chest and abdominal radiographs revealed 7 metallic objects in a stack projecting over her stomach and were interpreted as likely gastric in location (Fig 1A, B). Two foreign bodies were found stuck together in the stomach: a button battery and a magnet (Fig 2) and were removed via esophagogastroduodenoscopy. At immediate laparotomy, the remaining 3 magnets and 2 batteries were found in a loop of jejunum approximately 10–15 cm from the ligament of Treitz with an associate full-thickness ulcer that required 10 cm of small bowel resection. On outpatient follow-up 2 weeks later, she had recovered full gastric function and was tolerating a regular diet and gaining weight. A psychiatric evaluation revealed that the patient was developmentally normal with mild academic difficulties. She reported that she didn't want to admit to the ingestion as she feared that her mother would get angry. The take-home lesson is that x-rays can show magnets in close proximity to each other and apparently touching when they are actually separated by bowel loops. Symptoms and signs may initially be mild, but further investigation is warranted to prevent pressure necrosis or full-thickness ulcers.

E. C. Quintana, MD, MPH

Diagnosis and treatment of tracheobronchial foreign bodies in 1024 children
Gang W, Zhengxia P, Hongbo L, et al (Children's Hosp of Chongqing Med Univ, China)
J Pediatr Surg 47:2004-2010, 2012

Objective.—This study sought to summarize the experience of diagnosis and treatment of tracheobronchial foreign bodies in children to effectively reduce complications and mortality.

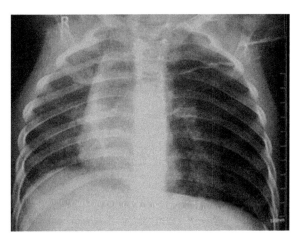

FIGURE 3.— Inspiratory and expiratory chest radiographs show obstructive emphysema and mediastinal flutter in the left lung. (Reprinted from Gang W, Zhengxia P, Hongbo L, et al. Diagnosis and treatment of tracheobronchial foreign bodies in 1024 children. *J Pediatr Surg*. 2012;47:2004-2010, with permission from Elsevier.)

Methods.—The medical records of 1024 pediatric patients admitted to our hospital from January 1997 to September 2011 and diagnosed with clinically suspected tracheobronchial foreign body aspiration were retrospectively analyzed.

Results.—Of the 1024 children patients, 674 were boys (65.8%) and 350 girls (34.2%). Two died of respiratory and circulatory failure (foreign bodies detected upon bronchoscopy but not retrieved) before surgery, 65 patients underwent direct bronchoscopic removal of foreign bodies due to their critical status, and 957 received chest radiographs and chest fluoroscopy or multidetector spiral computed tomographic scans (941 positive). Foreign bodies were expectorated before surgery in 3 cases. There were 953 cases of bronchoscopically proven airway foreign body aspiration, with a diagnostic accuracy of 94.5%. Ninety-eight foreign bodies were lodged in the main bronchus and/or bilateral bronchi, 506 in the right main bronchus, and 349 in the left main bronchus. Atelectasis was noted in 42 patients, including 11 with pulmonary consolidation, whose lungs were re-expanded by endobronchial lavage and sputum aspiration. In 3 patients with bronchiectasis, conservative treatment following foreign body removal was followed by no improvement, and pulmonary lobectomy was performed. Foreign bodies were successfully extracted at the first bronchoscopic attempt in 948 cases, accounting for 99.7% of the total. However, 3 patients had to undergo another bronchoscopy to remove the foreign bodies. The most common types of foreign bodies were peanuts, melon seeds, and beans.

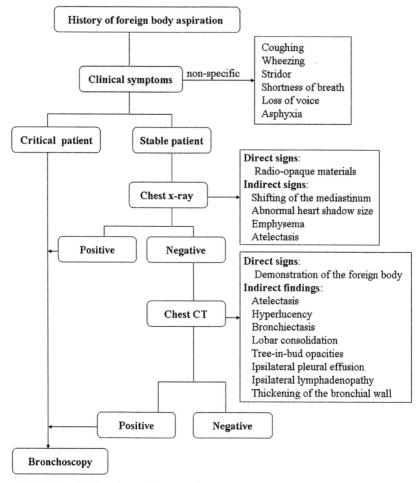

FIGURE 5.—The flow chart of diagnosis of tracheobronchial foreign body aspiration in children. (Reprinted from Gang W, Zhengxia P, Hongbo L, et al. Diagnosis and treatment of tracheobronchial foreign bodies in 1024 children. *J Pediatr Surg.* 2012;47:2004-2010, with permission from Elsevier.)

Conclusions.—Timely accurate diagnosis and treatment of tracheobronchial foreign bodies in children can avoid delay in treatment and effectively reduce complications and mortality (Figs 3 and 5).

▶ Tracheobronchial foreign body aspiration (FBA) in children can commonly present in the emergency department. This is a retrospective study of 1024 children with FBA. A clear history of foreign body aspiration was noted in 756 children (73.8%), whereas the other 268 cases did not (26.2%). One hundred and ninety-seven cases (20.1%) were misdiagnosed as pneumonia, tracheobronchitis, laryngitis, or asthma, with the duration of misdiagnosis lasting from 3 days to 2 years. Of the misdiagnosed cases, 65 (29.7%) were misdiagnosed for more than 6 months. All patients presented with paroxysmal cough and unilateral or bilateral decreased breath sounds on auscultation of the chest; wheezing or rales could be heard in 858 cases (83.8%); other respiratory symptoms were noted in 786 cases (76.8%); and 41 cases (4%) presented only with cough. There were 46 children who had "false-positive" chest radiographs and 9 had a "false-positive" multidetector spiral computed tomography (CT), but bronchoscopy failed to reveal any foreign body except for abundant viscous secretions. Foreign body removal was successful in most cases. Based on this study, the authors suggest criteria for diagnosis of tracheobronchial FBA (Fig 5). First, there is a history of clear or suspected FBA. In the current series, 73.8% of the children had a clear history of FBA. Second, paroxysmal cough, "roaring" unilateral or bilateral reduced breath sounds on auscultation, stridor, or wheezing are present; 83.8% patients in this study manifested such symptoms. Third, severe cases show dyspnea, inspiratory 3 depression sign, or cyanosis. Fourth, mediactinal shift abnormal heart shadow size, emphysema, or atelectasis is noted on chest radiographs (Fig 3). Their recommendations also include—for those children without a clear history of FBA or with negative chest radiographs and CT tests but present with notable respiratory symptoms—that tracheobronchoscopy should be performed, particularly for those who are treated for tracheobronchitis or pneumonia but show a recurrent course. Although a reasonable approach, the article didn't validate the algorithm presented. Another issue not addressed is the reduction of radiation exposure by using chest x-ray and subsequent CT of the chest in children.

E. C. Quintana, MD, MPH

C-Reactive Protein and Procalcitonin Are Predictors of the Severity of Acute Appendicitis in Children

Gavela T, Cabeza B, Serrano A, et al (Universidad Autónoma de Madrid, Madrid, Spain)
Pediatr Emerg Care 28:416-419, 2012

Objective.—The aim of this study was to evaluate the use of procalcitonin (PCT) and C-reactive protein (CRP) on admission as predictors of the severity of appendicitis in children.

Methods.—We prospectively studied 111 consecutive patients admitted with a diagnosis of acute appendicitis between July 2009 and February 2010 and recorded the following variables: age, sex, time since diagnosis, laboratory data, complications (abscess, intestinal obstruction), presence of hemodynamic instability, mortality, length of stay, and need for admission to the pediatric intensive care unit. Patients were divided into 2 groups according to the diagnosis confirmed during surgery (group 1, appendicitis; group 2, localized or generalized peritonitis).

Results.—Group 1 comprised 69 patients, and group 2 comprised 42 patients. Procalcitonin and CRP values were significantly lower in group 1 than in group 2 (0.15 vs 4.95 ng/mL [$P < 0.001$] and 3 vs 14.3 mg/dL [$P < 0.001$]). For a diagnosis of peritonitis, a PCT cutoff of 0.18 ng/mL gave a sensitivity of 97%, specificity of 80%, positive predictive value of 72%, and negative predictive value of 89.3%. The equivalent values for a CRP cutoff of 3 mg/dL were 95%, 74%, 68%, and 96.2%. Complications and the need for admission to the pediatric intensive care unit were more common in patients with peritonitis.

Conclusions.—On admission, CRP and PCT predict the outcome of pediatric patients with appendicitis. Children with CRP greater than 3 mg/dL and/or PCT greater than 0.18 ng/mL have a greater risk of complications; thus, intervention should be early, and patients should be monitored closely.

▶ Appendicitis remains the most common surgical emergency in pediatric patients and leads the differential diagnosis list of emergency physicians (EPs) treating pediatric patients with abdominal pain. Yet the diagnosis is elusive at times, and the inherent challenges of pediatric patients endure. The authors of this article suggest that C-reactive protein (CRP) and procalcitonin (PCT) can predicted acute appendicitis in the pediatric population. They found that increased PCT (> 0.18 ng/mL) and CRP (> 3 mg/dL) values predicted acute appendicitis with peritonitis.

Unfortunately, this article is wrought with limitations in terms of applicability to the general pediatric population. The majority (85%) of included patients had abdominal ultrasonography performed to make the appendicitis diagnoses, yet this radiographic modality is not universally available in emergency departments. While CRP levels are more readily available, obtaining a timely and clinically relevant PCT would be arduous.

EPs already struggle to get the surgeon to evaluate a patient with presumed appendicitis, and these additional laboratory tests generate further questions for the surgeon, such as "What is the white count?"

E. C. Bruno, MD

11 Emergency Medical Service Systems

General Issues

Global rating scale for the assessment of paramedic clinical competence

Tavares W, Boet S, Iheriault R, et al (Centennial College Paramedic Program, Toronto, Ontario, Canada; Ottawa Hosp, Ontario, Canada; Georgian College Paramedic Program, Barrie, Ontario, Canada; et al)
Prehosp Emerg Care 17:57-67, 2012

Objective.—The aim of this study was to develop and critically appraise a global rating scale (GRS) for the assessment of individual paramedic clinical competence at the entry-to-practice level.

Methods.—The development phase of this study involved task analysis by experts, contributions from a focus group, and a modified Delphi process using a national expert panel to establish evidence of content validity. The critical appraisal phase had two raters apply the GRS, developed in the first phase, to a series of sample performances from three groups: novice paramedic students (group 1), paramedic students at the entry-to-practice level (group 2), and experienced paramedics (group 3). Using data from this process, we examined the tool's reliability within each group and tested the discriminative validity hypothesis that higher scores would be associated with higher levels of training and experience.

Results.—The development phase resulted in a seven-dimension, seven-point adjectival GRS. The two independent blinded raters scored 81 recorded sample performances ($n = 25$ in group 1, $n = 33$ in group 2, $n = 23$ in group 3) using the GRS. For groups 1, 2, and 3, respectively, inter-rater reliability reached 0.75, 0.88, and 0.94. Intrarater reliability reached 0.94 and the internal consistency ranged from 0.53 to 0.89. Rater differences contributed 0–5.7% of the total variance. The GRS scores assigned to each group increased with level of experience, both using the overall rating (means = 2.3, 4.1, 5.0; $p < 0.001$) and considering each dimension separately. Applying a modified borderline group method, 54.9% of group 1, 13.4% of group 2, and 2.9% of group 3 were below the cut score.

Conclusion.—The results of this study provide evidence that the scores generated using this scale can be valid for the purpose of making decisions regarding paramedic clinical competence.

▶ Evaluating the effect of any educational activity is a complex process. Simple testing involves retrieving information that has been presented in a didactic session (ie, testing memory of and retention of information). At the next level, use and integration of this information is usually assessed by initiating or exposing students to "problem-solving" where the information they have is used to arrive at a solution to the challenge encountered; usually a word-type problem or scenario. When it comes to motor skills and complex decision making, the use of simulations or well planned scenarios with clear educational objectives and critical actions is usually the mode of evaluation used. Observation, video recording, and checklists are often also used as evaluation tools.

The training and evaluation of paramedics involves not only determining the efficacy of the educational process, but a process or tool also must be in place to provide evidence of competency in the skills taught and thorough familiarity with the didactic medical information provided during the training process. Failure to achieve competency prevents certification of an individual as capable of independent practice in the prehospital arena.

This study undertook the task to describe implementing an objective global rating scale that can be used to assess the clinical competency of medics in training. I find this to be a potentially very useful evaluation tool that should be considered by emergency medical educators.

B. M. Minczak, MS, MD, PhD

Comparison of emergency medical services systems across Pan-Asian countries: a Web-based survey
Shin SD, Hock Ong ME, Tanaka H, et al (Seoul Natl Univ College of Medicine, Chongno-Gu, Republic of Korea; Singapore General Hosp; Kokushikan Univ Graduate School of Sport System, Tokyo, Japan; et al)
Prehosp Emerg Care 16:477-496, 2012

Background.—There are great variations in out-of-hospital cardiac arrest (OHCA) survival outcomes among different countries and different emergency medical services (EMS) systems. The impact of different systems and their contribution to enhanced survival are poorly understood. This paper compares the EMS systems of several Asian sites making up the Pan-Asian Resuscitation Outcomes Study (PAROS) network. Some preliminary cardiac arrest outcomes are also reported.

Methods.—This is a cross-sectional descriptive survey study addressing population demographics, service levels, provider characteristics, system operations, budget and finance, medical direction (leadership), and oversight.

Results.—Most of the systems are single-tiered. Fire-based EMS systems are predominant. Bangkok and Kuala Lumpur have hospital-based systems. Service level is relatively low, from basic to intermediate in most of the communities. Korea, Japan, Singapore, and Bangkok have intermediate emergency medical technician (EMT) service levels, while Taiwan and Dubai have paramedic service levels. Medical direction and oversight have not been systemically established, except in some communities. Systems are mostly dependent on public funding. We found variations in available resources in terms of ambulances and providers. The number of ambulances is 0.3 to 3.2 per 100,000 population, and most ambulances are basic life support (BLS) vehicles. The number of human resources ranges from 4.0 per 100,000 population in Singapore to 55.7 per 100,000 population in Taipei. Average response times vary between 5.1 minutes (Tainan) and 22.5 minutes (Kuala Lumpur).

Conclusion.—We found substantial variation in 11 communities across the PAROS EMS systems. This study will provide the foundation for understanding subsequent studies arising from the PAROS effort.

▶ In an attempt to improve resuscitation outcomes from out-of-hospital cardiac arrest in Pan-Asian countries, there needs to be an effective review of outcomes data. However, the data generated are dependent on the services provided.

To appropriately analyze the information and arrive at the appropriate conclusions, the structure and function of the emergency medical system (EMS) must be known. Not only is the structure of this system important, but it is imperative that the scope of services and the delivery characteristics of these EMS systems be known.

This study undertook the task of comparing 11 EMS systems of 7 Pan-Asian countries. The study described the demographics of the population, what type of care/service is provided, how the system operates, the budgets, and how medical direction and oversight is provided.

Pan-Asian EMS systems are single-tiered, fire based entities. Service and level of care are not at a high level, and medical oversight is suboptimal.

The study described these systems and found much variability. To better understand the data, standardization must be introduced via future protocols, or the analysis of the current data must be appropriately processed to mitigate bias. One last concern that needs to be addressed is that the data are generated from an online survey that causes significant variability in the actual data. A more objective tool needs to be devised and validated in future studies.

B. M. Minczak, MS, MD, PhD

HEMS in Slovenia: One Country, Four Models, Different Quality Outcomes
Klemenc-Ketis Z, Tomazin I, Kersnik J (Univ of Maribor, Velenje, Slovenia; Univ of Ljubljana, Slovenia)
Air Med J 31:298-304, 2012

Objective.—The objective of this study was to determine the quality of patient care using quality indicators in 4 different Slovenian helicopter emergency medical service (HEMS) models.

Methods.—This was a cross-sectional study of all 4 HEMS in Slovenia. We collected data on quality for the period from July 2003 to August 2008, in a sample of all eligible patients that were managed by HEMS during the study period (N = 833). We obtained the following data on emergency operations: the time and organizational features of the operation; the description of the patients' condition; and the on-site diagnostic and treatment procedures. We used the following as quality indicators: the number of resuscitated patients that were intubated; the number of patients with a Glasgow Coma Scale (GCS) score of ≤ 8 that were intubated; the number of patients with acute coronary syndrome that received treatment with morphine, oxygen, nitroglycerine, and aspirin (MONA); the number of patients with a National Advisory Committee on Aeronautics (NACA) scale score of ≥ 4 with an intravenous line; the number of patients with a NACA score of ≥ 5 that were given oxygen; and the number of patients with a NACA score of ≥ 4 that were given appropriate analgesic treatment.

Results.—Across all HEMS bases, 36 (87.8%) resuscitated patients were intubated; 122 (81.9%) patients with GCS ≤ 8 were intubated; 149 (89.2%) patients with ACS were given MONA treatment; 52 (92.9%) patients with a NACA score of ≥ 4 were given an intravenous line; 254 (92.7%) patients with a NACA score of ≥ 5 were given oxygen; and 18 (32.7%) trauma patients with a NACA score of ≥ 4 were given intravenous analgesics. The quality of patient management in HEMS in Slovenia is affected by the callout procedure, the presence or absence of a fixed rope, the type of helicopter operator, and the provider of the doctor in the helicopter team.

Conclusions.—The data from our study indicates that the quality of patient management in HEMS in Slovenia is high. It also seems that organizational factors play a role in the quality management of patients in HEMS as well, but their effect remains unclear and needs further evaluation.

▶ The authors of this article attempt to objectively describe the quality of helicopter emergency medical services (HEMS) in Slovenia. When assessing the quality of HEMS, one must consider that EMS services often vary from region to region. In addition, these systems vary in configuration of crews (nurses, medics, doctors), type of equipment available (ie, the airframe or type of helicopter), and the structure of the aeromedical service company. The financial status of the organization and the specific protocols in place for the prehospital care of these patients are also factors in describing the quality of the HEMS service.

An additional issue that can affect the quality of HEMS operations is the terrain in which the rescue crews operate, whether it is mountainous areas, water rescue, or flat plains. Certain interventions may not be feasible under the conditions in which the patients are encountered.

These authors use the severity of illness or the patient's condition as described by various scores, such as the Glasgow Coma Score (GCS) and the National Advisory Committee on Aeronautics (NACA) score, to make decisions regarding the appropriateness and quality of care depending on the treatment that these patients received. Intubation success, resuscitation outcomes, and the utilization of intravenous therapy are also used as metrics to describe the quality of HEMS services in Slovenia. These authors also address administration of morphine, oxygen nitroglycerine, and aspirin to patients as indicators of care for patients with acute coronary syndromes.

The data, as collected in this article, suggest that the quality of care rendered by these services is quite good. However, quality indicators, such as timelines to care and timely disposition of a patient with severe injuries to a trauma center, transport of a patient complaining of chest pain to a facility capable of intervening and providing cardiac catheterization, or the delivery of a stroke patient to facilities capable of appropriately administering thrombolytics are not described. Furthermore, an assessment of the final outcomes for the patients of these time-sensitive interventions is not addressed. Also, the nature of the HEMS responses is not specifically described nor are they correlated to the final outcomes for the patients.

This study provides a favorable description of HEMS in Slovenia; however, I would also be interested in learning about the timeliness of the interventions that these services provide and the impact on the survival and final discharge diagnoses of the patients that they treat and transport.

B. M. Minczak, MS, MD, PhD

The core content of emergency medical services medicine
The EMS Examination Task Force, American Board of Emergency Medicine (American Board of Emergency Medicine, East Lansing, MI)
Prehosp Emerg Care 16:309-322, 2012

On September 23, 2010, the American Board of Medical Specialties (ABMS) approved emergency medical services (EMS) as a subspecialty of emergency medicine. As a result, the American Board of Emergency Medicine (ABEM) is planning to award the first certificates in EMS medicine in the fall of 2013. The purpose of subspecialty certification in EMS, as defined by ABEM, is to standardize physician training and qualifications for EMS practice, to improve patient safety and enhance the quality of emergency medical care provided to patients in the prehospital environment, and to facilitate integration of prehospital patient treatment into the continuum of patient care. In February 2011, ABEM established the EMS Examination Task Force to develop the Core Content of EMS Medicine (Core Content) that would be used to define the subspecialty and from which questions would be written for the examinations, to develop a blueprint for the examinations, and to develop a bank of test questions for use on the examinations. The Core Content defines the training parameters, resources, and knowledge of the treatment of prehospital patients necessary to practice EMS medicine. Additionally, it is intended to inform fellowship directors and candidates for certification of the full range of content that might appear on the examinations. This article describes the development of the Core Content and presents the Core Content in its entirety.

▶ Currently, many emergency medicine (EM) residency directors, EM chairs, future emergency medical services (EMS) fellowship directors, and EM residents interested in pursuing a fellowship and eventual certification in EMS are looking for direction and guidance regarding the requirements that will be set forth for the successful completion of an EMS fellowship.

In September 2010, the American Board of Medical Specialties approved EMS as a subspecialty of emergency medicine. An examination and subsequent issuing of certificates in EMS medicine was planned for Fall 2012. To this end, leaders in EM are working on developing academic and didactic experiences for future residents and fellows. Also, those physicians active in EM are being queried in an attempt to develop an appropriate pathway for certifying those already active in EMS medicine and for those physicians and residents who are pioneering the current advances in EM who did not undergo formal fellowship training. Many residencies are applying for accreditation as EMS fellowships and will need a set of curriculum guidelines in order to successfully apply and become accredited as EMS fellowship sites.

This Special Contribution was drafted as a result of the efforts of the EMS Examination Task Force working with the American Board of Emergency Medicine and the Accreditation Council for Graduate Medical Education. This core content is meant to be a dynamic document that will keep pace with future advances in EMS medicine and incorporate the latest material pertinent to providing an appropriate educational and practical experience to physicians in fellowship training.

Regarding the specific components of this publication, it addresses the various aspects of the clinical aspects of EMS medicine (ie, assessment, treatment, and procedural aspects of prehospital medicine; medical oversight principles; and quality management and research in EMS medicine and special operations). The individual subheadings are significantly detailed and will be a great help to fellowship directors preparing schedules and allocating resources for the fellows' training and they will be useful to EM residency directors interested in enhancing the EM residency EMS experience.

This document needs to be disseminated among EM leaders interested in developing and running an EMS medicine fellowship and it should also be reviewed by EM residency directors interested in enhancing the EMS curriculum of their current residency.

B. M. Minczak, MS, MD, PhD

Disparities in Trauma Center Access of Older Injured Motor Vehicular Crash Occupants

Ryb GE, Dischinger PC (Univ of Maryland, Baltimore)
J Trauma 71:742-747, 2011

Background.—To evaluate whether older injured motor vehicular crash (MVC) occupants' access to trauma centers (TC) reflects the lower threshold suggested in triaging recommendations.

Methods.—Adult front seat occupants of MVCs transported to a hospital from 1999 through 2006 included in the National Automotive Sampling System (NASS) were studied. Cases were classified by their age in years (≤60 years or >60 years). Younger and older injured MVC occupants were compared in relation to their likelihood of being transported to a TC. Multiple logistic regression models were built to adjust for confounders.

Results.—A total of 35,830 cases representing 7,894,940 cases after weighting were analyzed. Older occupants were less likely to be transported to a TC than younger ones (47% vs. 55%, $p < 0.0001$). Older individuals were more likely to be restrained, passengers, and seated on the impacted side of lateral crashes. Injury severity was higher among the older group (mean Injury Severity Score, 4.1 vs. 3.1; $p < 0.0001$) and so was the resulting mortality (1.7% vs. 0.6%, $p < 0.0001$). Multiple logistic regression models after adjusting for confounders (i.e., other triage criteria) revealed a lower likelihood of TC transport (odds ratio, 0.75 [0.57–0.98]) for the older group.

Conclusion.—In contrast to the American College of Surgeons triaging recommendations, injured MVC occupants older than 60 years are less likely to be transported to a TC than their younger counterparts. Further studies should establish whether the lower access to TC experienced by the older population is a function of geographical factors, emergency medical services unconscious bias, or other factors.

▶ This article presents another view of the apparent age-related bias in patient transport to trauma centers after injuries. Age has been included as a factor in consideration for need to transport patients to a trauma center since 1986, but what is the actual practice?

The authors analyzed a sample representing a nationwide picture of patients after motor vehicle crashes. The National Automotive Sampling System (NASS) data (collected by trained abstractors in response to police-reported accidents) were used to describe what was known about the accident, as well as patient and injury characteristics, to seek factors that might influence the decision by prehospital providers on whether a patient should be transported to a trauma center (level 1 or 2) or to a lower level of care.

In essence, the authors are stating that prehospital providers are not using age-related factors appropriately when it comes to deciding who should be transported to a trauma center. First and foremost, they are ignoring the "if a patient is over 55 years of age" criterion for trauma center transport set by the American College of Surgeons' Committee on Trauma. It could be that they think that trauma care is not needed or is not valuable for these older patients. But neither of these ideas are part of prehospital provider training. So the decision process is being modified by some preexisting "knowledge."

Are there any limitations to their work? Sure there are. This dataset did not include any vital signs, so it could be argued that it is not possible to describe completely the image that prehospital providers would see at the scene. The authors are able to make some assumptions about how these missing data would affect their results, further strengthening their suggestion that bias is significant. Another deficit is that there is no information available to determine if geographic factors might explain the difference in rates of transport to trauma centers. (The sampling and weighting done in the NASS is performed to create a nationwide picture of what happens in accidents.) Suppose that most motor vehicle accidents occur near home and that there are significantly greater numbers of elderly people living in regions where trauma centers are not accessible. This would reduce the disparity found by the authors.

Is there an age bias carryover once the patients reach the hospital? I think we should be alert to the possibility. After all, it might be that prehospital providers are bending clinical guidelines just like we might.

N. B. Handly, MD, MSc, MS

Safety and Resource Utilization

A pilot study of emergency medical technicians' field assessment of intoxicated patients' need for ED care

Cornwall AH, Zaller N, Warren O, et al (The Miriam Hosp, Providence, RI; Rhode Island Hosp, Providence; et al)
Am J Emerg Med 30:1224-1228, 2012

Objective.—Alcohol–intoxicated individuals account for a significant proportion of emergency department care and may be eligible for care at alternative sobering facilities. This pilot study sought to examine intermediate-level emergency medical technician (EMT) ability to identify intoxicated individuals who may be eligible for diversion to an alternative sobering facility.

Methods.—Intermediate-level EMTs in an urban fire department completed patient assessment surveys for individual intoxicated patients between May and August 2010. Corresponding patient medical records were retrospectively reviewed for diagnosis, disposition, and blood alcohol content. Statistical analysis was conducted to determine correlates of survey response, diagnosis, and disposition; and survey sensitivity and specificity were calculated.

Results.—One hundred ninety-seven patient transports and medical records were analyzed. Emergency medical technicians indicated 139 patients (71%) needed hospital-based care, and 155 patients (79%) had a primary ethanol diagnosis. Fourteen patients (7%) were admitted to the hospital, and EMTs identified 93% of admitted patients as requiring hospital-based care. Overall sensitivity and specificity of the survey were

93% (95% confidence interval, 66.1-99.8) and 40% (95% confidence interval, 33.3-47.9), respectively.

Conclusion.—Intermediate-level EMTs may be able to play an important role in facilitating triage of intoxicated patients to alternate sobering facilities.

▶ What to do with people who are intoxicated in public is a question for which US society still has not found an adequate answer. Historically, society has used the "drunk tank," where police take inebriated individuals to the local jail and let them sober up overnight. (They may or may not be charged with a crime.) Occasionally, one of them would be ill or injured or even die in police custody. This led to the police bringing drunken individuals to the emergency department (ED) for medical clearance before taking them to jail or even just to sober up. All emergency physicians see intoxicated patients to varying degrees. On a weekend night, especially if there is a local event in the area, the ED can fill up with patients whose only medical issue is intoxication. Some localities have created sobering facilities to help decrease the crowding of the ED.

This preliminary investigation from Rhode Island examined whether intermediate-level emergency medical technicians could assess intoxicated patients and determine whether they required medical care or just needed sobering. This is a situation where you would want a high sensitivity so that patients with medical conditions or trauma are not missed. The overall sensitivity is reported as 93%, but could be as low as 66%. These are not good numbers, but then again this is a pilot study. There are quite a few limitations with these data; most important, the authors only looked at the diagnosis, disposition, and blood alcohol content of the participants. They did not perform a medical record review. Therefore, they may have overlooked whether patients had critical medical interventions in the ED but were eventually discharged. Moreover, physicians may not have listed every medical condition encountered as a diagnosis. This is an intriguing concept that needs to be further explored with more research before it can be implemented.

E. A. Ramoska, MD, MPHE

Can nebulized naloxone be used safely and effectively by emergency medical services for suspected opioid overdose?
Weber JM, Tataris KL, Hoffman JD, et al (Cook County Hosp, Chicago, IL; Chicago Fire Dept, IL)
Prehosp Emerg Care 16:289-292, 2012

Background.—Emergency medical services (EMS) traditionally administer naloxone using a needle. Needleless naloxone may be easier when intravenous (IV) access is difficult and may decrease occupational blood-borne exposure in this high-risk population. Several studies have examined intranasal naloxone, but nebulized naloxone as an alternative needleless route has not been examined in the prehospital setting.

Objective.—We sought to determine whether nebulized naloxone can be used safely and effectively by prehospital providers for patients with suspected opioid overdose.

Methods.—We performed a retrospective analysis of all consecutive cases administered nebulized naloxone from January 1 to June 30, 2010, by the Chicago Fire Department. All clinical data were entered in real time into a structured EMS database and data abstraction was performed in a systematic manner. Included were cases of suspected opioid overdose, altered mental status, and respiratory depression; excluded were cases where nebulized naloxone was given for opioid-triggered asthma and cases with incomplete outcome data. The primary outcome was patient response to nebulized naloxone. Secondary outcomes included need for rescue naloxone (IV or intramuscular), need for assisted ventilation, and adverse antidote events. Kappa interrater reliability was calculated and study data were analyzed using descriptive statistics.

Results.—Out of 129 cases, 105 met the inclusion criteria. Of these, 23 (22%) had complete response, 62 (59%) had partial response, and 20 (19%) had no response. Eleven cases (10%) received rescue naloxone, no case required assisted ventilation, and no adverse events occurred. The kappa score was 0.993.

Conclusion.—Nebulized naloxone is a safe and effective needleless alternative for prehospital treatment of suspected opioid overdose in patients with spontaneous respirations.

▶ Deaths from unintentional drug overdoses have been on the rise for several decades, and they are now the second-leading cause of accidental death in the United States. Most of this increase is because of the rising number of opioid (synthetic narcotic) overdoses. Emergency medical services (EMS) personnel commonly administer naloxone for suspected overdose with these agents by a variety of routes. This retrospective analysis from Cook County Hospital and the Chicago Fire Department demonstrates that EMS personnel can safely nebulize naloxone and that this method of delivery appears to be effective in reversing opioid toxicity.

This manner of administration is important since these patients are often at high risk for blood-borne infections, such as hepatitis B and C and human immunodeficiency virus, and needle sticks and blood exposure are significant occupational hazards for EMS workers. Moreover, it has been suggested, although not proven, that nebulized naloxone administration can more gently awaken a patient than intravenous bolus administration, thus averting sudden patient agitation and florid withdrawal symptoms. Whether this is true is not established by this analysis.

The major limitation of a study like this is that it has no comparison or control group of any sort. The message is, "We do it. We like it. You should try it, too." Perhaps as a next step a comparison of intravenous versus nebulized naloxone will be conducted. In the meantime, advising your medics that this may be an alternate route of naloxone administration seems a reasonable approach.

E. A. Ramoska, MD, MPHE

Intravenous Access During Out-of-Hospital Emergency Care of Noninjured Patients: A Population-Based Outcome Study

Seymour CW, Cooke CR, Hebert PL, et al (Univ of Washington, Seattle; Univ of Michigan, Ann Arbor)

Ann Emerg Med 59:296-303, 2012

Study Objective.—Advanced, out-of-hospital procedures such as intravenous access are commonly performed by emergency medical services (EMS) personnel, yet little evidence supports their use among noninjured patients. We evaluate the association between out-of-hospital, intravenous access and mortality among noninjured, non—cardiac arrest patients.

Methods.—We analyzed a population-based cohort of adult (aged ≥18 years) noninjured, non cardiac arrest patients transported by 4 advanced life support agencies to one of 16 hospitals from January 1, 2002, until December 31, 2006. We linked eligible EMS records to hospital administrative data and used multivariable logistic regression to determine the risk-adjusted association between out-of-hospital intravenous access and hospital mortality. We also tested whether this association differed by patient acuity by using a previously published, out-of-hospital triage score.

Results.—Among 56,332 eligible patients, half (N = 28,078; 50%) received out-of-hospital intravenous access from EMS personnel. Overall hospital mortality for patients who did and did not receive intravenous access was 3%. However, in multivariable analyses, the placement of out-of-hospital, intravenous access was associated with an overall reduction in odds of hospital mortality (odds ratio = 0.68; 95% confidence interval [CI] 0.56 to 0.81). The beneficial association of intravenous access appeared to depend on patient acuity (P = .13 for interaction). For example, the odds ratio of mortality associated with intravenous access was 1.38 (95% CI 0.28 to 7.0) among patients with lowest acuity (score = 0). In contrast, the odds ratio of mortality associated with intravenous access was 0.38 (95% CI 0.17 to 0.9) among patients with highest acuity (score ≥ 6).

Conclusion.—In this population-based cohort, out-of-hospital efforts to establish intravenous access were associated with a reduction in hospital mortality among noninjured, non—cardiac arrest patients with the highest acuity. Reasons why this occurred (cause and effect) could not be determined in this model.

▶ The controversy about whether to load and go or stay and play has waged for some time in the emergency medical services (EMS) literature, mainly with regard to trauma patients. This retrospective cohort study from King County EMS in Washington showed that intravenous (IV) access was associated with lower odds of mortality in the subgroup of seriously ill patients. There was no mortality difference overall between those patients who had an IV line placed and those who did not. Two-thirds of the patients who did not have an IV line placed had an EMS severity code of nonurgent, whereas more than four-fifths of those who had an IV line had an EMS severity code as either urgent or life threatening. This analysis did not look at whether the IV lines were used to administer medication or fluids, only that they were placed. On-scene time was increased by 5 minutes in patients who received IV access.

Prior research has found that only 17% to 39% of out-of-hospital IV lines placed in nontrauma patients are actually used to administer fluids or medications. This study suggests that IV access is warranted in the sickest patients because they may incur a survival advantage. The benefit of having a field IV line placed in most noninjured patients remains unknown.

E. A. Ramoska, MD, MPHE

Life Flight Network
Borland E (Life Flight Network in Aurora, OR)
Air Med J 31:216-217, 2012

Background.—Life Flight Network (LFN) is a not-for-profit air medical program serving the Pacific Northwest and Intermountain West areas of the United States. Begun in 1978, it is the largest emergency air medical service provider in Oregon, Idaho, and Washington and operates 12 medical helicopters, five fixed-wing aircraft, and four ground ambulances at 13 bases. LFT is accredited by the Commission on Accreditation of Medical Transport Systems and has safely transported more than 65 000 patients in its 34 years of operation. Its mission, scope of care, and future plans were outlined.

Mission.—Among the guiding principles of the company are establishing bases where they are best able to serve patients who need critical care air ambulance services. They strive to provide the highest level of critical care transport, to understand customers' needs, to proactively respond to changing environments, and to keep customers informed. Their flight crews, clinical educators, and customer service managers provide various educational and informational outreach programs for medical professionals, law enforcement personnel, and the public. Various free seminars and state and regional conference sponsorships also help to ensure that patients and communities are adequately served.

Scope of Care.—The flight nurse/flight paramedic team of LFN merges the expertise and knowledge of hospital critical care with prehospital emergency and transport environments. LFN transport crews must demonstrate a minimum of 5 years of experience, which ensures medical excellence and safety. Teams have the medical resources, training, and experience to manage pediatric and adult patients who suffer from conditions related to situations such as trauma, neurology, obstetrics, cardiac (ST elevation myocardial infarction [STEMI]), vascular, pulmonary, and sepsis. As a result, they have received numerous honors for their excellence and their business success.

Future Plans.—To provide the most modern, safest, and best equipped fleet of EMS aircraft in their area, LFN has contracted to acquire 15 AgustaWestland AW119 Ke helicopters, which will permit faster response times, flexibility in medical cabin configuration, and full-body access.

Cockpits will be outfitted with Garmin G-1000H controls with synthetic vision. IFN is also expanding to include four new state-of-the-art Pilatus PC-12 NG fixed-wing aircraft that will provide an electric lift rated for up to 650 pounds, larger interior space, and the most advanced avionics package. Their communications center is being expanded to incorporate technology and process improvements that will provide better detail and quality of information to EMS and hospital customers.

▶ This brief article describes the history, educational programs, and community services that Life Flight Network (LFN) provides in the Pacific Northwest and Intermountain West. The author also describes the configuration of the flights crews and their qualifications. From this description, the reader can glean that this company may be able to provide useful educational opportunities and has the capability to provide some unique training experiences for medical personnel

The author describes the goals the company is ascribing to attain with future equipment and training programs.

In addition, the author provides a listing of the accomplishments of the company and that it operates as a not-for-profit organization that started out as Emanuel Life Flight in 1978.

This description can serve as a template for the development of and/or the restructuring of current air medical transport companies.

B. M. Minczak, MS, MD, PhD

Effects of physician-based emergency medical service dispatch in severe traumatic brain injury on prehospital run time
Franschman G, Verburg N, Brens-Heldens V, et al (VU Univ Med Ctr, Amsterdam, The Netherlands; Radboud Univ Nijmegen Med Ctr, The Netherlands; et al)
Injury 43:1838-1842, 2012

Introduction.—Prehospital care by physician-based helicopter emergency medical services (P-HEMS) may prolong total prehospital run time. This has raised an issue of debate about the benefits of these services in traumatic brain injury (TBI). We therefore investigated the effects of P-HEMS dispatch on prehospital run time and outcome in severe TBI.

Methods.—Prehospital run times of 497 patients with severe TBI who were solely treated by a paramedic EMS ($n = 125$) or an EMS/P-HEMS combination ($n = 372$) were retrospectively analyzed. Other study parameters included the injury severity score (ISS), Glasgow Coma Scale (GCS), prehospital endotracheal intubation and predicted and observed outcome rates.

Results.—Patients who received P-HEMS care were younger and had higher ISS values than solely EMS-treated patients (10%; $P = 0.04$). The overall prehospital run time was 74 ± 54 min, with similar out-of-hospital times for EMS and P-HEMS treated patients. Prehospital endotracheal intubation was more frequently performed in the P-HEMS group (88%) than in the EMS group (35%; $P < 0.001$). The prehospital run time for intubated patients was similar for P-HEMS (66 (51—80) min) and EMS-treated patients (59 (41—88) min). Unexpectedly, mortality probability scores and observed outcome scores were less favourable for EMS-treated patients when compared to patients treated by P-HEMS.

Conclusion.—P-HEMS dispatch does not increase prehospital run times in severe TBI, while it assures prehospital intubation of TBI patients by a well-trained physician. Our data however suggest that a subgroup of the most severely injured patients received prehospital care by an EMS, while international guidelines recommend advanced life support by a physician-based EMS in these cases.

▶ Prehospital medicine has developed over the past few decades into a specialty that has a specific body of knowledge and skills. First responders, emergency medical technicians, and paramedics provide emergency medical services routinely. The skills and knowledge that they have brings life-saving techniques to the scene of a medical emergency. These services save time and provide timely treatment that is invaluable to time-sensitive injuries. Having a physician on scene may bring additional skills, some of which may impede expedient initiation of transport to the hospital and not bring any additional benefit to the patient's final outcome. This study examines this issue.

This publication demonstrated that having a physician on scene may enhance certain treatments such as endotracheal intubation or rhythm recognition and provide the opportunity for establishing quick diagnoses; however, it does not necessarily increase scene time or cause significant transport delays. The physicians responding to these emergencies need to have the situational awareness needed to be able to provide a meaningful presence at the prehospital scene.

This study suggests that physicians involved in prehospital emergency medical services should have exposure to appropriate training that will facilitate and enhance the value of their presence in the field.

B. M. Minczak, MS, MD, PhD

Medical preparation for the 2008 Republican National Convention: A practical guide
Dries DJ, Frascone RJ, Hick JL, et al (HealthPartners Med Group, Bloomington, MN; Univ of Minnesota, Minneapolis; et al)
J Trauma Acute Care Surg 73:1614-1623, 2012

Background.—Events identified as National Special Security Events (NSSEs) include the Olympics, major political conventions, presidential inaugurations, and special large multinational meetings. The operational security plan for these events is under the direction of the US Secret Service (USSS), the Federal Bureau of Investigation (FBI) handles crisis response, and the Federal Emergency Management Agency (FEMA) is responsible for crisis or consequence management. Planners must also prepare for low-probability, high-impact incidents such as nuclear, biologic, and chemical attacks or explosions. In addition, medical emergencies and general medical care must be included in the planning. Minneapolis-n-St Paul, Minnesota, served as the site for the Republican National Convention (RNC) in 2008. The plans for medical care provision formed to manage all the foreseeable scenarios were outlined, supplying a needed resource for future NSSE planners. Analysis of effective past responses identified four factors that contribute to the best outcomes: systems, space, staffing, and supplies.

Systems.—Planning began about 2 years before the RNC and involved multiple subcommittees and a single steering committee. The Emergency Medical Services (EMSs) of the St Paul area participate in multiagency coordination exercises and responses that focus on cross-jurisdictional care delivery. Medical resource control centers (MRCCs) are based at Level I trauma centers and provide redundant medical direction should one center become overloaded or unable to respond. Coordinated responses begin with EMS and ambulance function and progress to hospital coordination. The subcommittees were co-chaired by USSS personnel and included hospital representatives, EMS, public health officials, and police and fire departments. They met regularly, and all resource allocations were reviewed by the USSS.

Space.—Six months before the convention, a hospital planning group was formed to address issues related to fire, life safety, and hazardous materials and facilitate city-specific planning. Hospital capacities were identified, and surge capacity planning done for each facility. Multiple resources were deployed within the convention center itself.

Staffing.—Local medical resources were supplemented by numerous federal assets, including four joint hazard assessment teams and four joint hazard explosive response teams. Thirteen Mobile Field Forces teams were responsible for managing riots or security threats and included 80 or more police officers and two tactical paramedics. Federal assets provided resources to address the potential need for rapid mass decontamination of 25,000 to 40,000 persons after a chemical incident. The US Marine Corps Chemical Biologic Incident Response Force (CBIRF) team covered the restricted vehicle area and provided facilities for decontaminating 490 victims per hour. Two separate 10-person disaster medical assistance teams (DMATs) aided the CBIRF teams, with an additional small CBIRF-DMAT contingent stationed at the jail facility. Hospitals scheduled all surgical services with immediate responsibility for managing injured patients, emergency department, and critical care teams for on-call duty, with vacations for attending trauma surgeons and emergency department physicians canceled. A staffed treatment area provided high-volume, low-acuity patient care. DMATs and decontamination personnel were also stationed at hospitals closest to the convention center and at downtown hospital locations to facilitate triage for multiple casualty incidents. "Street medics" who accompany protest groups to care for them were perhaps the busiest of the medical groups. They had a facility in a church basement where they provided first aid, psychological support, massage, and nontraditional therapies.

At the convention venue itself, medical resources were available to handle needs ranging from cardiac arrests to distribution of over-the-counter medications. A health care center (HCC) was permanently located on the main floor of the convention center and included two beds, a restroom, basic monitoring equipment, and medical supplies. Because this HCC was too small to address the anticipated medical needs, an additional space was commandeered contiguous to the permanent location, offering four additional beds and serving as the main treatment area. Full advanced cardiac life support (ACLS) capability, sophisticated airway management, and other services were available, making this essentially a small emergency department. A Pyxis machine was used to enhance pharmaceutical dispensing. Two registered nurses, one midlevel provider, and one staff physician served in the HCC from noon to midnight, with overlap for double coverage during the peak hours of 2 to 10 PM. This facility was supplemented by nine roaming two-person paramedic teams who were in constant radio communication with the HCC. An all-terrain, multiwheeled vehicle was used to transport stable patients from the HCC to a fully staffed ambulance outside the security perimeter fence. The plan was for unstable patients to be placed immediately in an ambulance and transferred directly to the Level-1 hospital for care, but this situation never presented itself.

Supplies.—Among the federal assets provided were 400 impact ventilators, nerve agent antidote kits, and chemical, nuclear, and biologic response materials. Chemical response "packs" were distributed to seven local hospitals and six EMS agencies. The Strategic National Stockpile (SNS) is a repository of antibiotics, chemical antidotes, antitoxins, life-support medications, intravenous administration equipment, airway maintenance supplies, and medical-surgical items. Rapid delivery of the closest SNS push packs was assured. In addition, a 250-bed mobile hospital that could add additional modules in 250-bed increments was put on-call for the event.

Conclusions.—Web-based systems, conference calls, and daily incident action plans were used to achieve excellent information exchange among EMS, hospital, and public safety personnel. Flexible use of DMATs facilitated active patient care and could have been critical if a mass casualty or mass contamination incident had occurred. The RNC was treated as a full-scale functional exercise with exercise grant funding, which permitted data feedback useful for refining the operations of the system. Although protestor groups were poorly monitored by design, coordination with their care providers would support early recognition of communicable or food-based illnesses. Improvements suggested by this experience include the inclusion of a medical subcommittee directed by federal and local medical personnel; specific health appropriations in NSSE funding; flexibility in patient egress routing; greater priority given to accurate credentialing of EMS, medical, and fire personnel; and the incorporation of street medics or alternative health care facilities into the conventional health care system.

▶ Any mass gathering such as a major political convention has the potential for things to go wrong. Some of the problems or events are inevitable, whereas others can be anticipated. A political convention, the Olympics, a presidential inauguration, or a meeting with dignitaries from various nations is classified as National Special Security Event. Presidential Directive 62 designates that the United States Secret Service (USSS) must design and implement an operational security plan.

Because these events involve individuals who are under the protection of the USSS, planning for such an event becomes more complicated. The possibility of violence from terrorists or political activists becomes a factor in the planning of these types of events, which can bring about the potential involvement by the Federal Bureau of Investigation or the Federal Emergency Management Agency.

Possible events that may occur are categorized into high-probability low-impact events, such as a foodborne outbreak, a weather-related problem, or an unexpected uprising from political activists, to low-probability high-impact events such as an explosion, dissemination of a biological agent, drinking water contamination, or an aircraft crash.

To plan such an event, the various agencies and systems must assess the needs, assess the current resources, plan solutions to the anticipated problems, and initiate interagency communication.

The planning must involve the systems, the space/location, both inside and outside the actual convention floor of the event, the staff, and the supplies available. The medical needs must be anticipated, and the appropriate response vehicles and equipment must be available to provide access and treatment to all participants. Supply lists must be prepared and potential unexpected challenges must be anticipated and the appropriate mitigations planned.

This special report addresses many of these issues and can serve as a template for the planning of future events by various organizations.

B. M. Minczak, MS, MD, PhD

The methodology of the Australian Prehospital Outcomes Study of Longitudinal Epidemiology (APOStLE) Project
Cone DC, Irvine KA, Middleton PM (Yale Univ School of Medicine, New Haven, CT; Cancer Inst NSW, Eveleigh, Australia; Univ of Sydney, Australia)
Prehosp Emerg Care 16:505-512, 2012

This paper describes the methodology of a large emergency medical services (EMS) data linkage research project currently under way in the statewide EMS system of New South Wales, Australia. The paper is intended to provide the reader with an understanding of how linkage techniques can be used to facilitate EMS research. This project, the Australian Prehospital Outcomes Study of Longitudinal Epidemiology (APOStLE) Project, links data from six statewide sources (computer-assisted dispatch, EMS patient health care reports, emergency department data, inpatient data, and two death registries) to enable researchers to examine the patient's entire journey through the health care system, from the emergency 0-0-0 call to the emergency department and inpatient setting, through to discharge or death, for approximately 2.6 million patients transported by the Ambulance Service of New South Wales to emergency departments between June 2006 and

July 2009. Manual, deterministic, and probabilistic data linkages are described, and potential applications of linked data in EMS research are outlined.

▶ To conduct a meaningful research study, the investigator(s) must have a well-thought-out experimental design or plan and have access to reliable data. If the study is going to be a longitudinal type of study, then the complete timeline of pertinent data points must be available, that is, from dispatch to disposition.

Doing research relevant to emergency medical services (EMS) is often difficult for multiple reasons. Once the experimental protocols have been approved, and internal review board approval is obtained, then the research team faces new challenges. First, there must be a means of obtaining consent, where applicable, from the patients to get access to their medical records and demographic information. Gaining access to all pertinent medical records without compromising the privacy of patients can be an issue. Being able to access paper records and various electronic databases, some of which are not easily accessed or able to be interfaced with, the methodology of the given experimenters is still an issue today, even as various EMS systems are transitioning to the electronic medical record (EMR). Furthermore, these issues can become confounders for the interpretation of the data and they can even cause selection bias, depending on how the data were captured. Therefore, it would be a great benefit to have a means of accessing multiple databases without the problems associated with interfacing various electronic medical records (EMR).

This study describes how linkage techniques can be used to provide a useful, simple interface among six databases: computer-aided dispatch, EMS data from the prehospital interaction, emergency department records, inpatient charts, and death registries. These techniques provide a continuum of data from the initial call to the final disposition of the patient. Because of encryption and data manipulation capabilities, patient confidentiality can be protected. The availability of these data facilitates the assessment of previous performance outcomes to various problems and can serve as a database for the formulation of predictive correlations, which could help in the development of future protocols. Also, these methods increase the number of subjects and data points that are available because of the easier access, and this can lead to better sensitivity and specificity of the study, provided the design and sampling are appropriately scripted into the project. I strongly suggest that individuals interested in EMS research take a look at this article and consider some of the proposed options in the design of their projects.

B. M. Minczak, MS, MD, PhD

Three insulation methods to minimize intravenous fluid administration set heat loss

Piek R, Stein C (Univ of Johannesburg, Doornfontein, South Africa)

Prehosp Emerg Care 17:68-72, 2013

Objective.—To assess the effect of three methods for insulating an intravenous (IV) fluid administration set on the temperature of warmed fluid delivered rapidly in a cold environment.

Methods.—The three chosen techniques for insulation of the IV fluid administration set involved enclosing the tubing of the set in 1) a cotton conforming bandage, 2) a reflective emergency blanket, and 3) a combination of technique 2 followed by technique 1. Intravenous fluid warmed to 44°C was infused through a 20-drop/mL 180-cm-long fluid administration set in a controlled environmental temperature of 5°C. Temperatures in the IV fluid bag, the distal end of the fluid administration set, and the environment were continuously measured with resistance thermosensors. Twenty repetitions were performed in four conditions, namely, a control condition (with no insulation) and the three different insulation methods described above. One-way analysis of variance was used to assess the mean difference in temperature between the IV fluid bag and the distal fluid administration set under the four conditions.

Results.—In the control condition, a mean of 5.28°C was lost between the IV fluid bag and the distal end of the fluid administration set. There was a significant difference found between the four conditions ($p < 0.001$). A mean of 3.53°C was lost between the IV fluid bag and the distal end of the fluid administration set for both the bandage and reflective emergency blanket, and a mean of 3.06°C was lost when the two methods were combined.

Conclusion.—Using inexpensive and readily available materials to insulate a fluid administration set can result in a reduction of heat loss in rapidly infused, warmed IV fluid in a cold environment.

▶ Hypothermia can be a great adjunct in the treatment of a patient in cardiac arrest, but when it comes to the treatment of a trauma patient, it can cause problems. When a trauma patient is being resuscitated, the likelihood of the patient receiving intravenous (IV) fluids is high. These fluids, even at room temperature, can ultimately contribute to a drop in the core body temperature of the patient if a significant volume of fluid is given. To prevent this from being an issue, warmed fluids can be administered to the patient. To accomplish this in the prehospital setting, the fluid must be appropriately warmed and safely stored. However, when it is time to administer the fluids, because the solution runs through IV tubing that is at a lower temperature than the solution, the fluid will be cooled via conduction of heat through the tubing, and the tubing will be cooled via convection and radiation to the atmosphere. This study offers a simple, affordable solution: Insulate the tubing with the most effective insulator. A future study to determine the effects of this method versus others on the core body temperature would help reinforce this method.

B. M. Minczak, MS, MD, PhD

The 60-Day Temperature-Dependent Degradation of Midazolam and Lorazepam in the Prehospital Environment

McMullan JT, on behalf of the Neurological Emergencies Treatment Trials investigators (Univ of Cincinnati, OH; et al)
Prehosp Emerg Care 17:1-7, 2012

Background.—The choice of the optimal benzodiazepine to treat prehospital status epilepticus is unclear. Lorazepam is preferred in the emergency department, but concerns about nonrefrigerated storage limits emergency medical services (EMS) use. Midazolam is increasingly popular, but its heat stability is undocumented.

Objective.—This study evaluated temperature-dependent degradation of lorazepam and midazolam after 60 days in the EMS environment.

Methods.—Lorazepam or midazolam samples were collected prior to ($n = 139$) or after ($n = 229$) 60 days of EMS deployment during spring-summer months in 14 metropolitan areas across the United States. Medications were stored in study boxes that logged temperature every minute and were stored in EMS units per local agency policy. Mean kinetic temperature (MKT) exposure was derived for each sample. Drug concentrations were determined in a central laboratory by high-performance liquid chromatography. Concentration as a function of MKT was analyzed by linear regression.

Results.—Prior to deployment, measured concentrations of both benzodiazepines were 1.0 relative to labeled concentration. After 60 days, midazolam showed no degradation (mean relative concentration 1.00, 95% confidence interval [CI] 1.00–1.00) and was stable across temperature exposures (adjusted R^2 −0.008). Lorazepam experienced little degradation (mean relative concentration 0.99, 95% CI 0.98–0.99), but degradation was correlated to increasing MKT (adjusted R^2 0.278). The difference between the temperature dependence of degradation of midazolam and lorazepam was statistically significant ($T = -5.172$, $p < 0.001$).

Conclusions.—Lorazepam experiences small but statistically significant temperature-dependent degradation after 60 days in the EMS environment. Additional study is needed to evaluate whether clinically significant deterioration occurs after 60 days. Midazolam shows no degradation over this duration, even in high-heat conditions.

▶ Emergency medical services (EMS) personnel carry significant varieties of medication in order to treat a plethora of conditions in the prehospital setting.

The list of medications carried may vary depending on the type of service and the crew configuration of the service. Most of the medications EMS carry are usually in liquid form; therefore, these chemicals are susceptible to chemical degradation. Chemical degradation can occur because of time elapsed from preparation of the solution, temperature variation, or agitation from vibration in either the ambulance or aircraft. As a result, these medications may become ineffective because of changes in chemical composition, concentration, or pH, or from contamination of the packaging. The medication may also precipitate out of solution, causing the medication to become ineffective.

This study attempts to quantify the effects of temperature on 2 benzodiazepines over a 2-month period. The clinical relevance of these findings needs to be evaluated further.

However, these findings suggest that EMS systems should keep a close watch on the inventory and shelf life of the medications they use to prevent the use of expired medications. Furthermore, if there are various extraneous circumstances the medications should be rotated, especially if there has been a significant variation in temperature, either hot or cold. Medication solutions should be physically checked and if found to be discolored, cloudy, or in any way look compromised, these medications should be discarded and replaced with fresh solutions. More studies regarding the degree of degradation should be contemplated; studies to determine if the degradation has a significant effect on the therapeutic value of the medication should be planned. Furthermore, communication with the manufacturer/drug company regarding medication stability should be a priority in the periodic surveillance of EMS operations and supplies, especially medications in solution.

B. M. Minczak, MS, MD, PhD

Successful Administration of Intranasal Glucagon in the Out-of-Hospital Environment

Sibley T, Jacobsen R, Salomone J (Truman Med Ctr, Kansas City, MO)
Prehosp Emerg Care 17:98-102, 2012

We present a case of successful prehospital treatment of hypoglycemia with intranasal (IN) glucagon. Episodes of hypoglycemia can be of varying severity and often requires quick reversal to prevent alteration in mental status or hypoglycemic coma. Glucagon has been shown to be as effective as glucose for the treatment of hypoglycemia. The inability to obtain intravenous (IV) access often impairs delivery of this peptide and is therefore frequently given via the intramuscular (IM) route. Intranasal administration of glucagon has been shown to be as effective as the IV route and may be used for rapid correction of hypoglycemic episodes where IV access is difficult or unavailable and IM administration is undesirable. We describe the first documentation in the peer-reviewed literature of the successful treatment and reversal of an insulin-induced hypoglycemic episode with IN glucagon in the prehospital setting. We also present a review of the literature regarding this novel medication administration route.

▶ The title of this publication does not do justice to the content. There are several messages that can be derived from this publication.

Using a case report, the article basically describes how a hypoglycemic patient with no vascular access was successfully treated with 1 mg of intranasal (IN) glucagon. It also elaborates on how effective this treatment modality is in comparison with intramuscular (IM) administration of varying doses of glucagon and oral (PO) glucose (using 2 mg of IN glucagon).

In addition to providing a useful in-depth discussion of this safe, practical, potentially very useful, noninvasive treatment modality for hypoglycemia, the authors provide a thought-provoking, comprehensive discussion of this alternative route of medication administration that can be extrapolated and applied to the administration of other medications in various urgent medical situations (such as the administration of naloxone to a patient who is an intravenous drug user with bad veins in respiratory suppression from an apparent opiate overdose, or for the sedation of an agitated patient with IN midazolam of an agitated patient in whom vascular access is not easily obtained).

When a patient has a time-sensitive, potentially life-threatening issue that needs immediate treatment and gaining vascular access is a problem, the nasal mucosa serves as an excellent portal for administering medication to a patient without requiring sterile preparation or the use of sharp needles. This in turn decreases the potential risk of exposure to potential blood-borne pathogens via needlesticks. In addition, as the medication is absorbed from the nasal mucosa, first-pass metabolism on the drug is mitigated and delivery of the drug into the bloodstream is faster than the intramuscular route. Furthermore, performing this procedure takes less time and does not require extensive training. Thus medical directors of emergency medical services (EMS) should consider reviewing the current prehospital protocols and possibly contemplate adding this modality to the medics' scope of practice. This technique could even possibly be performed by emergency medical technicians in basic emergency medical services, when confronted with a patient who is presumptively hypoglycemic. I strongly believe that EMS medical directors should take a closer look at this and related literature and give the possibilities some thought.

Just as an aside, training of first responders and family members of diabetic patients on how to perform this technique should also be considered because administration of medication when patients become unresponsive from hypoglycemia could prove to be a lifesaving intervention and/or decrease the potential unnecessary morbidity.

B. M. Minczak, MS, MD, PhD

Lithium Battery Fires: Implications for Air Medical Transport
Thomas F, Mills G, Howe R, et al (Intermountain Life Flight, Salt Lake City, UT; Intermountain Med Ctr, Salt Lake City, UT)
Air Med J 31:242-248, 2012

Lithium-ion batteries provide more power and longer life to electronic medical devices, with the benefits of reduced size and weight. It is no wonder medical device manufacturers are designing these batteries into their products. Lithium batteries are found in cell phones, electronic tablets, computers, and portable medical devices such as ventilators, intravenous pumps, pacemakers, incubators, and ventricular assist devices. Yet, if improperly handled, lithium batteries can pose a serious fire threat to air medical transport personnel. Specifically, this article discusses how lithium-ion batteries work, the fire danger associated with them, preventive measures to reduce the likelihood of a lithium battery fire, and emergency procedures that should be performed in that event.

▶ Medical devices in use today by emergency medical services (EMS) personnel require batteries designed to store a vast amount of electrical power and to be small in size and light in weight. This makes the devices that they are used in more portable and easier to work with in the prehospital setting. In addition, the batteries used in this equipment need to be resistant to various circumstances that can be encountered in the prehospital environment, such as extreme variations in temperature, moisture, vibration, and physical forces that can cause damage to the structure of the battery.

Many of the batteries are specially designed to interact with the equipment they are used in so that there is an appropriate rate of discharge and a failsafe in place to prevent overcharging and damage to the battery. The type of battery that appears to best meet these specifications is the lithium-ion battery. This battery type can be found in many medical devices used both outside and inside the hospital. Numerous ventilators, intravenous pumps, pacemakers, pediatric incubators, and left ventricular devices have the lithium-ion battery inside for either primary power or as backup power sources. However, it is imperative that the medical personnel using the equipment with these types of batteries be totally familiar with how to store backup batteries, be aware of how they should be installed in the device being used, and know how to charge these batteries appropriately. Failure to do so has led to tragic outcomes such as having the batteries overheat, ignite, and burst into flames and even explode, causing injuries to EMS personnel and patients.

This article presents a case report in which a mishap occurred secondary to a lithium-ion battery malfunction during a helicopter transport in progress. Fortunately, the incident occurred while the patient and crew were still on the ground. An in-flight incident with a fatal outcome is also discussed in the article. Aside from describing these accidents, the article provides 12 tips on how to prevent mishaps with lithium batteries such as not mixing battery types in a single device, using the appropriate charging devices, and following proper procedures when charging these types of batteries. Also listed are tips on how to store spare batteries and how to properly dispose of them.

This article also provides a list of do's and don'ts in the event that a lithium battery fire should occur.

I find this article informative and full of information that every flight crew working in the helicopter EMS services should read. This article also has relevance for ground crews and in-patient staff who use lithium battery—powered equipment in a patient care environment.

B. M. Minczak, MS, MD, PhD

Major incident preparation for acute hospitals: Current state-of-the-art, training needs analysis, and the role of novel virtual worlds simulation technologies

Cohen DC, Sevdalis N, Patel V, et al (Imperial College London, UK; et al)
J Emerg Med 43:1029-1037, 2012

Background.—There is growing evidence that health systems in developed countries are poorly prepared to deal with major incidents.

Study Objectives.—This study aimed to determine the skills required for successful major incident response, the factors that contribute to a successful major incident exercise, and whether there is a role for using novel simulation training (virtual worlds) in preparing for major incidents.

Methods.—This was a qualitative semi-structured interview study. Fourteen health care staff with experience of major incident planning and training in the United Kingdom were recruited. Interviews were content-analyzed to identify emergent themes.

Results.—The aims and benefits of current exercises were categorized into three major themes: Organizational, Interpersonal, and Cognitive. Participants felt that the main objective of current exercises is to see how a major incident plan is implemented, rather than training individual staff. Communications was the most frequently commented-on area requiring improvement. Participants felt that lack of constructive feedback reduced the effectiveness of the exercises. All participants commented that virtual worlds technology could be successfully utilized for training. The creation of an immersive environment, increased training opportunity, and improved participant feedback were thought to be amongst the greatest benefits.

Conclusion.—There are clear deficiencies with current major incident preparation. Utilizing virtual worlds technology as an adjunct to existing exercises could improve training and response in the future.

▶ The past, both immediate and distant, is peppered with incidents that have at times overwhelmed routine service system arrangements. These events, often termed disasters, exhaust the resources available at the time the situation occurs. These incidents can be caused by weather, transportation accidents, earthquakes, or terrorist activities. The recovery to a normal state of operations can take days to weeks. To potentially prevent these problems from occurring, having a protocol or disaster plan in place is imperative. However, having the plan does not ensure that the situation will be dealt with successfully. This plan must be made known to the potential respondents and practiced to ensure compliance and efficiency in the execution of the plan. This requires participation in occasional exercises or drills.

However, these activities are usually geared toward evaluating and enhancing the performance of the participants/respondents to the disaster or major incident. This study attempts to test the plan itself for its practicality and applicability to a disaster. The authors also tried to assess the approach to training the respondents for the incident response and to determine how use of virtual simulation can be used to accomplish this.

This study describes the aims and benefits of current exercises focusing on communication(s), organization, cognitive issues, and interpersonal interactions.

The methods used were prospective, qualitative semistructured interviews and the application of virtual world simulation. This process was intended to discover gaps in training, communication systems, patient flow, and familiarization of documentation under the organizational skills portion. The interpersonal skills session analyzed leadership/provision of command and multiteam interaction. The cognitive skills portion assessed situational awareness, decision making, and management capabilities of the participants and of the plan.

All of these challenges were posed to the test subjects with the help of using virtual worlds to enhance fidelity to the actual event. This method may prove to be better than tabletop exercises, drills, and even full-scale exercises because of immediate feedback and better definition of educational objectives. The simulations are predicable, reliable, and reproducible. Also, they are resource-sparing events, saving on the cost of conducting such a training event.

In addition, this approach may lead to more efficient, useful preparation of hospitals and supportive resources in anticipation of a major incident with mass casualties.

B. M. Minczak, MS, MD, PhD

Factors associated with ambulance use among patients with low-acuity conditions
Durant E, Fahimi J (Univ of California—Berkeley)
Prehosp Emerg Care 16:329-337, 2012

Background.—The use of ambulances for low-acuity medical complaints depletes emergency medical services (EMS) resources that could be used for higher-acuity conditions and contributes to emergency department (ED) overcrowding and ambulance diversion.

Objective.—We sought to understand the characteristics of patients who use ambulances for low-acuity conditions. We hypothesized that patients who arrive to the ED by ambulance for low-acuity conditions are more likely to be members of vulnerable populations.

Methods.—A secondary analysis was performed on the National Hospital Ambulatory Medical Care Survey (NHAMCS). We included only patients aged 18 years or older who were triaged to the "nonurgent" category upon presentation to the ED. To compare patients who arrived by ambulance with those who arrived by all other modes, multivariate logistic regression was performed using a generalized linear model, and adjusted relative risks (ARRs) were calculated.

Results.—A total of 16,109 records from 1997 to 2008 (excluding 2001—2002) were included in the analysis. Significantly higher rates of ambulance use for low-acuity conditions were associated with: 1) older age (ARR 1.30, 95% confidence interval CI: 1.18—1.43; per 10 years); 2) Medicare or Medicaid insurance (ARR 1.81, 95% CI: 1.36—2.41, and ARR 1.46, 95% CI: 1.12—1.91, respectively); 3) homelessness (ARR

3.30, 95% CI: 1.61−6.78); 4) arrival between 11 PM and 6:59 AM (ARR 1.80, 95% CI: 1.43−2.27); and 5) certain chief complaint categories: psychiatric (ARR 1.78, 95% CI: 1.03−3.07), toxicologic/poisoning (ARR 3.26, 95% CI: 1.85−5.76), and neurologic/psychological (ARR 1.71, 95% CI: 1.34−2.18). Patients who arrived by ambulance were more likely than nonambulance patients to receive laboratory diagnostic tests (ARR 3.50, 95% CI: 2.80−4.39), radiographic imaging (ARR 2.26, 95% CI: 1.91−2.68), and admission to the hospital (ARR 3.99, 95% CI: 3.03−5.27).

Conclusion.—Our study builds on a body of work highlighting the factors associated with ambulance transport to EDs, confirms that certain vulnerable populations disproportionately use ambulances, and may inform interventions aimed at increasing access to nonambulance transportation and urgent care for these patients.

▶ Many emergency departments (ED) experience overcrowding, which occurs for many reasons. Many patients presenting to the ED have no primary physician. Yet other patients who have no insurance come to the ED as a self-pay seeking care. Some of the patients perceive the ED as 24-hour access to care and use the ED on a convenience basis, coming when they have a spare moment for evaluation and treatment. Many patients have come to the ED and asked to be evaluated for a "second opinion" regarding their presumed medical condition. Parents of small children often are directed by their pediatrician to "go to the ED" if they are concerned. In addition, many physicians send their patient to the afterhours clinic for evaluation and treatment.

This publication addresses how many patients use emergency medical services (EMS) as a means of transport to the ED, even when their chief complaint is not a true emergency (ie, of low acuity). Most of these patients arrive via ambulance or EMS. An ambulance ride is usually a 911 call away. Although the cost of an ambulance trip is significantly greater than a cab or some other means of public transportation, many nonetheless call EMS with the hope of getting to the hospital sooner without a substantial wait for their ride. These patients then receive door-to-door service and the attention of the medics. Furthermore, there is the perception that if an ambulance brings the patient to the ED, they will be seen sooner, which is not always the case.

This study attempts to demonstrate who uses the EMS system inappropriately and provides data that could be used to help develop other means of transporting patients to either the hospital or some alternate health care delivery agency, such as a clinic or urgent care center. Furthermore, this study points to reasons that cause decreased patient satisfaction in patients who are experiencing long waits and delays in their care because of the volume of patients that ultimately must be triaged and processed. This causes delays in the evaluation and treatment of patients who do need the resources and services that the ED was designed to provide. Hospital administrators should review these data and incorporate the information into future policies and procedures for managing patient flow. Furthermore, thought should go into planning alternative means of providing the service to those patients who inappropriately use the EMS/ambulance system.

Many of these patients need mental health care, rehabilitation, or simply access to a primary care center with health care staff capable of providing the needed services.

B. M. Minczak, MS, MD, PhD

Ten-year trends in intoxications and requests for emergency ambulance service
Holzer BM, Minder CE, Schätti G, et al (Univ Hosp Zurich, Switzerland; et al)
Prehosp Emerg Care 16:497-504, 2012

Background.—Intoxication, whether from alcohol, drugs, or alcohol and drugs in combination, remains a challenging burden on emergency departments. The increasing alcohol consumption among adolescents and young adults, particularly heavy episodic drinking, and the resulting increase in the use of health care resources for alcohol intoxication has been a widely discussed topic.

Objective.—The aim of our study was to assess and characterize the use of emergency ambulance services that was required as a result of alcohol and drug intoxication in a major metropolitan area.

Methods.—We conducted a retrospective, longitudinal study over a 10-year period in the greater metropolitan area of Zurich, Switzerland. The study population included intoxicated patients assessed and initially treated by paramedics of the emergency ambulance service. Data were extracted from the ambulance service reports. The primary outcomes measured were trends over time in the numbers and types of intoxication and trends with respect to gender and age distributions of intoxicated patients.

Results.—An annual increase of about 5% in the number of intoxicated patients requiring emergency ambulance service was observed over the study period. Alcohol use was present in 73% of the cases. The highest number of cases was among patients 25—44 years of age. The greatest increase in the number of cases over time was among patients under 25 years of age. Women comprised 41% of the patients under 25 years of age but only about 35% of older patients. The number of severe injuries and suicide attempts was small, but the number of suicide attempts increased at a higher rate than the overall number of cases of intoxication. There was a significant increase (17.64% per year on average) in the incidence of aggressive behavior toward paramedics from intoxicated patients, although still small in numbers.

Conclusions.—Our findings suggest two main vulnerable groups: young persons under 25 years of age, with a particular focus on women, having the greatest increase over time, and middle-aged men, having the greatest proportion among all cases observed. Intervention efforts should include a high-risk approach to reduce alcohol-related problems.

▶ Abuse of alcohol is common in today's society. Substance abuse is also a common problem. Frequently, persons who abuse alcohol also abuse street drugs. This behavior often leads to these individuals behaving aberrantly, having suicidal tendencies, getting into motor vehicle accidents, and suffering various injuries. Sometimes this alcohol and substance abuse even leads to aggressive behavior toward others and even arrests.

Many times, these behaviors are recreational in nature. However, most of these people are addicted to alcohol or drugs. Those that suffer from addiction often have underlying psychiatric issues or are living under circumstances that could possibly be mitigated.

A significant number of intoxicated patients are brought to the emergency department (ED) for observation and treatment. The treatment is usually some combination of a physical examination, a blood glucose check, intravenous fluids, some vitamin supplements in the IV, possibly an alcohol level, and a urine drug screen. They may be placed on a cardiac monitor/pulse oximeter and observed until they are sober and can be safely discharged. During this ED experience, they are utilizing a hospital bed.

Current data indicate that EDs are experiencing increased patient volume, overcrowding, and long waits. Patients are frequently leaving without being seen. Patients who do not need to be evaluated and treated in the ED are contributing to this problem. As a result, bed availability is compromised.

The authors of this study attempted to describe how alcohol and substance abuse problems affect ambulance utilization today. The data were obtained by retrospectively reviewing prehospital emergency medical services (EMS) patient care charts of emergency medical units that were involved in responding to patients found to be intoxicated. However, many times EMS units are dispatched to calls such as unresponsive patient, sick unknown, passed out, syncope, fell out, or seizure. Even after EMS personnel arrive on scene and evaluate these patients, the cause of their mishap is not always obvious until they are further evaluated in the hospital. This may confound the data, potentially compromise the conclusions, and decrease the accuracy of the data.

The data obtained in this study did show that most of the patients brought to the ED under the influence of alcohol or drugs are young men less than 25 years of age. The number of patients in this state is increasing. In addition, there is an increase in the number of young women being brought to the ED intoxicated. The number of men that arrive to the ED drunk still exceeds that of women. Based on these findings, it can be concluded that the problem with alcohol abuse needs to be addressed.

This study shows that alcohol and substance abuse is adversely affecting EMS and EDs. The number of hospital beds is compromised and resources are unnecessarily consumed. If feedback from EMS to government agencies and social services were to be provided, this may lead to the preparation of a plausible solution to this problem. Doing so may ultimately help mitigate the issues concerning EMS utilization and enhance ED flow.

B. M. Minczak, MS, MD, PhD

Helicopter Emergency Medical Service in Tehran, Iran: A Descriptive Study

Hassani SA, Moharari RS, Sarvar M, et al (Tehran Univ of Med Sciences, Iran)
Air Med J 31:294-297, 2012

Objective.—The study provides descriptive information regarding missions performed by Tehran helicopter emergency medical services (HEMS) during a 1-year period.

Methods.—All patients transferred by Tehran HEMS between March 2006 and March 2007 were enrolled in this descriptive study. Based on HEMS records, information was gathered on flight time, the number of patients transferred in each flight, and mission outcomes.

Results.—During the 1-year study, a total of 353 patients were transported via 138 helicopter flights to 4 medical care centers in Tehran. The mean flight time, the time from the initial call until the patient was delivered to a medical facility, was 36.56 ± 18.44 minutes.

Conclusion.—Tehran HEMS is still far from attaining optimal values, particularly regarding flight time. More efforts are needed to improve the timing as a component of care and the quality of care provided by this system.

▶ Helicopter emergency medical service(s) (HEMS) is now a global industry. Many countries are now utilizing helicopters to provide timely prehospital care to patients with life-threatening injuries. Flight crews are dispatched to accident scenes to treat and fly patients to trauma centers and they also fly in to extract injured parties from challenging terrain. In addition, helicopters are used in interfacility transport of patients who have time-sensitive pathology, such as an evolving myocardial infarction or an ischemic stroke that may require thrombolytics.

Many helicopter services are now also doing what could be described as *specialized* transports of patients who are on intra-aortic balloon pumps, left ventricular assist devices, and other advanced cardiac care equipment. Some services do interfacility transports of pediatric patients in incubators, taking babies to children's hospitals.

These HEMs are structured to be available 24/7, have medical supervision by physicians experienced in the nuances of transport medicine, and have protocols in place to deal with a variety of issues that may occur in the prehospital or inter-facility transfer. The helicopters are well equipped and the pilots well trained with the capability of flying in variable conditions in which visibility may be suboptimal; that is, they can use visual flight rules, instrument flight rules, or night vision goggles to fly into a scene or land on a hospital rooftop after dark.

This publication describes HEMS in Tehran, Iran. This system appears to be growing and developing. Currently, the flights crew consists of a physician and either a nurse or an appropriately skilled medic. The helicopters in service can carry up to 4 patients, and the helicopter bases are located in reasonable proximity to the receiving hospitals. The staff works exclusively for the HEMs service. The cost to patients is not an issue because the services are supported by the government. However, the availability of the helicopter service is currently sunrise to sunset. The helicopter services each cover a vast amount of square miles, with just 9 HEMS operating. At the time of this publication, there are no specialized service capabilities available. Thus, the missions consist primarily of flights to motor vehicle and motorcycle crashes, postcardiac resuscitation flights, frostbite situations, higher elevations, intoxication situations, and gastrointestinal bleeds.

Despite much hard work and planning in the development of these services, the actual overall flight times seem to be high. This may be caused by increased scene times. To fulfill the major premise of utilizing HEMS to get patients to definitive care sooner, work needs to be done to decrease overall transport times and improve efficiency in these areas. This article demonstrated that there is an interest in looking at outcome measures and improving the service.

B. M. Minczak, MS, MD, PhD

Effects of an emergency medical services–based resource access program on frequent users of health services

Tadros AS, Castillo EM, Chan TC, et al (Univ of California, San Diego; et al)
Prehosp Emerg Care 16:541-547, 2012

Background.—A small group of adults disproportionately and ineffectively use acute services including emergency medical services (EMS) and emergency departments (EDs). The resulting episodic, uncoordinated care is of lower quality and higher cost and simultaneously consumes valuable public safety and acute care resources.

Objective.—To address this issue, we measured the impact of a pilot, EMS-based case management and referral intervention termed the San Diego Resource Access Program (RAP) to reduce EMS, ED, and inpatient (IP) visits.

Methods.—This was a historical cohort study of RAP records and billing data of EMS and one urban hospital for 51 individuals sequentially enrolled in the program. The study sample consisted of adults with ≥ 10 EMS transports within 12 months and others reported by prehospital personnel with significant recent increases in transports. Data were collected over a 31-month time period from December 2006 to June 2009. Data were collected for equal pre- and postenrollment time periods based on date of initial RAP contact, and comparisons were made using the Wilcoxon signed-rank test. Overall use for subjects is reported.

Results.—The majority of subjects were male (64.7%), homeless (58.8%), and 40 to 59 years of age (72.5%). Between the pre and post periods, EMS encounters declined 37.6% from 736 to 459 ($p = 0.001$), resulting in a 32.1% decrease in EMS charges from \$689,743 to \$468,394 ($p = 0.004$). The EMS task time and mileage decreased by 39.8% and 47.5%, respectively, accounting for 262 ($p = 0.008$) hours and 1,940 ($p = 0.006$) miles. The number of ED encounters at the one participating hospital declined 28.1% from 199 to 143, which correlated with a 12.7% decrease in charges from \$413,410 to \$360,779. The number of IP admissions declined by 9.1% from 33 to 30, corresponding to a 5.9% decrease in IP charges from \$687,306 to \$646,881. Hospital length of stay declined 27.9%, from 122 to 88 days. Across all services, total charges declined by $314,406.

Conclusions.—This pilot study demonstrated that an EMS-based case management and referral program was an effective means of decreasing EMS transports by frequent users, but had only a limited impact on use of hospital services.

▶ Many homeless, mentally ill, and alcoholic people wander the streets of our cities daily. In addition to having the aforementioned issues, many of these people have chronic medical conditions, inconsistent medical care, and no financial or emotional support. In an effort to survive, they go to various locations such as shelters, transit stations, or hotel lobbies, and when they are turned away or put out, they declare that they are having chest pain, initiate movements emulating a seizure, or complain of abdominal pain. Sometimes they drink to excess, use illicit street drugs, and collapse or lay down in a public place. Workers at these facilities or bystanders usually call 911, summoning emergency medical services (EMS) personnel or police, who transport these patients to a local hospital. These events recur frequently, leading to inappropriate use of EMS and loss of available, much-needed beds in the emergency department(s) (EDs). This, in turn, leads to overcrowding, compromised access, and delays in care for those patients experiencing a true medical emergency.

A potential solution to this problem of inappropriate use of EMS and ED resources is to have a resources access program in which the problems of these individuals can be analyzed and the real needs of the patient(s) met. For example, the patient who is homeless and winds up sleeping in ED beds as a myocardial rule out might be placed in an appropriate shelter or be directed to an appropriate housing facility. The patient who needs insulin to treat his diabetes may be referred to an outpatient medical facility where treatment and medication may be provided.

To do this, a database needs to be created and appropriately utilized. Based on the demographics recorded, appropriate services and interventions can be initiated in an attempt to mitigate the problems of these persons. This may decrease the frequency of inappropriate use of EMS. Subsequently, ED/hospital resources may be spared to some degree. Walk-in patients will still present, but with appropriate analysis and a broader implementation of this resource access system, even this problem may be reduced. This article addressed such an attempt.

B. M. Minczak, MS, MD, PhD

Inappropriate helicopter emergency medical services transports: results of a national cohort utilization review
Hafner JW, Downs M, Cox K, et al (Univ of Illinois College of Medicine at Peoria; et al)
Prehosp Emerg Care 16:434-442, 2012

Background.—Medical transport using helicopter emergency medical services (HEMS) has rapidly proliferated over the past decade. Because of issues of cost and safety, appropriate utilization is of increasing concern.

Objective.—This study sought to describe the medical appropriateness of HEMS transports, using established guidelines, in a large national patient cohort.

Methods.—A review was performed of all flights designated as inappropriate by a large national air medical company, Air Evac EMS Inc. (which operates Air Evac Lifeteam AEL), for the period from January 1, 2009, through December 31, 2009. Every flight was reviewed initially through a resource utilization process as well as a utilization review process. Medical appropriateness review criteria were derived from the *Medicare Benefit Policy Manual* and industry guidelines outlined by the Commission on Accreditation of Medical Transport Systems (CAMTS), Air Medical Physicians Association (AMPA) position papers, the Centers for Disease Control and Prevention (CDC) *Morbidity and Mortality Weekly Report* (MMWR) Guidelines for Field Triage, and published clinical peer-reviewed articles, as well as previous interactions with Medicare contractors and reimbursement appeal decisions. Higher scrutiny was given to flights of <30 or >100 miles. Records indicating a possible inappropriate flight (i.e., review criteria were not satisfied, but special circumstances existed) were further reviewed by a senior quality assurance/quality improvement (QA/QI) nurse and/or senior medical director and were categorized.

Results.—During the study period, 27,697 flights were completed and reviewed, with 582 (2.1%) flights identified for further review by a senior QA/QI nurse and/or senior medical director. Of those, 367 (1.3%) were determined to be medically inappropriate flights. Inappropriate flights were most often on-scene flights (59.9%), were most often for adult patients (92.9%; median age 56.9 years; 25–75% interquartile range 42–75 years), and most often represented medical diagnoses (57.8%).

Conclusions.—Based on established criteria, only 1.3% of total flights were determined to be inappropriate. This large national cohort demonstrated compliance with current industry standards.

▶ The use of medical helicopters in emergency medical services (HEMS) has increased dramatically in the past decade. The number of HEMS flights has increased, as have the costs and the accidents. Concern for maintaining the safety of flight operations and keeping the risk:benefit ratio of flying patients to medical facilities low versus using ground transport has prompted a review of previous flights and initiated a quest to establish standardized universal criteria that would deem dispatching and flying a patient appropriate. However, the mission to accomplish this is a difficult one because there are often many mitigating and confounding circumstances that arise concerning why a patient was flown from 1 facility to another. Some of the reasons for these HEMS flights are patient/family requests and interfacility transfers to centers with a higher level of care, especially if there is a time-sensitive issue that needs to be urgently addressed. Some patients are injured far away from home and request transfer to a facility proximal to their homes. When transfer via ground necessitates a long ride via ground ambulance, some patients and their families opt to use HEMS.

When HEMS is dispatched to the scene of a motor vehicle crash or a construction site where there may be life-threatening injuries sustained by the patient, often it is the ground crew that requests HEMS for expedient transfer of the patient to a trauma center or otherwise appropriate facility. Once the helicopter crew has arrived, the patient is usually transported. This fact alone confounds the interpretation of the results. The helicopter crew is responding to a scene as a result of a decision that was made by emergency medical services personnel at the scene. If there is concern that the victim(s) of the mishap may have significant injuries that might need a high level of evaluation and care, as can be provided at a trauma center, then the patient should be flown. If after evaluation the patient can be discharged, even the same day, then there is the confidence that an appropriate level of screening was done and the flight was appropriate.

This study attempted to ascertain if the flights made by a large national air medical company were appropriate. There are several levels of bias that can be noted in this publication. Some of the data selected and the criteria used to evaluate the appropriateness of the HEMS mission were tainted with selection bias and lack of validation of the criteria used in determining the appropriateness of the flight(s).

Overall, despite some of the issues, the study suggests that the majority of the flights were appropriate. Future surveillance and scrutiny of criteria for the appropriateness of patient transfers need to be a dynamic work in progress. Overall, HEMS serves a valuable useful purpose, especially in situations where there are high-acuity, time-sensitive injuries, or there is a need for expedient access to a higher level of care.

Also, HEMS is invaluable for difficult terrain rescues and these data need to be appropriately reviewed and factored into the final assessment of overall statistics describing the appropriateness of flights.

B. M. Minczak, MS, MD, PhD

Accuracy of prehospital diagnosis and triage of a Swiss helicopter emergency medical service
Hasler RM, Kehl C, Exadaktylos AK, et al (Univ Hosp Bern, Switzerland; et al)
J Trauma Acute Care Surg 73:709-715, 2012

Background.—Helicopter emergency medical services (HEMSs) have become a standard element of modern prehospital emergency medicine. This study determines the percentage of injured HEMS patients whose injuries were correctly recognized by HEMS physicians.

Methods.—A retrospective level III evidence prognostic study using data from the largest Swiss HEMS, REGA (*Rettungsflugwacht/Guarde Aérienne*), on adult patients with trauma transported to a Level I trauma center (January 2006—December 2007). National Advisory Committee on Aeronautics (NACA) scores and the Injury Severity Score (ISS) were assessed to identify severely injured patients. Injured body regions diagnosed by REGA physicians were compared with emergency department discharge diagnoses.

Results.—Four hundred thirty-three patients were analyzed. Median age was 42.1 years (interquartile range, 25.5—57.9). Three hundred twenty-three (74.6%) were men. Patients were severely injured, with an in-hospital NACA score of 4 or higher in 88.7% of patients and median ISS of 13. REGA physicians correctly recognized injuries to the head in 92.9%, to the femur in 90.5%, and to the tibia/fibula in 83.8% of patients. Injuries to these body regions were overdiagnosed in less than 30%. Abdominal injuries were missed in 56.1%, pelvic injuries in 51.8%, spinal injuries in 40.1%, and chest injuries in 31.2% of patients.

Conclusion.—This study shows that patients are adequately triaged by REGA physicians reflected by a NACA score 4 or higher in 88.7% of patients and a median ISS of 13. However, recognition of injured body regions seems to be challenging in the prehospital setting. Prospective studies on specific training of HEMS physicians for recognition of these injuries (e.g., portable ultrasonography, telemedicine) might help in the future.

Level of Evidence.—Prognostic study, level III.

▶ This study attempts to compare the accuracy of prehospital evaluations, diagnoses, and triage decisions made by helicopter emergency medical service (HEMS) personnel with the findings obtained at the receiving medical facilities.

The data presented in this retrospective cohort study must be interpreted within the appropriate context. The assessment and triage decisions made by HEMS crews are usually performed under challenging circumstances. On landing at the site of an accident or where the patient has had a mishap, the crew has to deal with multiple issues. There may be multiple barriers in the way of initiating patient assessment and the provision of care. The scene may be unsecure and fraught with potential hazards (eg, an unstable vehicle that may be an explosion hazard, a hostile crowd of bystanders may be present at the scene, a distraught family may be anxious and try to expedite the actions of the rescuers). If a ground crew is present and has initiated assessment and treatment of the patient, data from the initial injury may become unavailable as the ground crew stabilizes and, if needed, extricates or moves the patient from the initial injury site. Information about the mechanism of injury may be sparse due to either the lack of witnesses to the event or the patient/victim not being able to provide pertinent information regarding the nature of the problem. The chief complaint, history of present illness, mechanism of injury, current medications that may be a clue to occult pathology, such as an increased potential for a head bleed, and medication allergies may not be readily available on initial prehospital patient contact. The HEMS crew may have to surmise what and how the patient was injured based on a superficial visual assessment of the scene.

Regarding the patient, a physical evaluation of the victim is not as complete due to the limitations in exposing the patient appropriately and maintaining an appropriate environment for a thorough examination of the patient. Therefore, some obvious injuries such as those to the head and extremities may be more easily detected and treated, whereas injuries to the torso, which may affect the cervical spine, chest, abdomen, and pelvis, may be hidden by clothing and not be perceived on initial contact. Furthermore, internal injuries may be subtle and declare themselves some time after the injury has occurred, when the patient is in the hospital.

HEMS crews usually do not have all of the equipment readily available that is necessary to conduct a comprehensive evaluation of the patient. They are usually limited to physical assessment skills and portable monitoring equipment. In addition, the helicopter crew configuration is usually 3 people: an EMS physician, a HEMS paramedic, and the pilot. Evaluation and treatment of a patient during flight is complicated by noise, vibration, and at times compromised illumination.

In contrast, once the patient is at the trauma center, the patient evaluation begins in a controlled, well-lit, temperature-controlled environment. The evaluation is conducted by the emergency medicine and trauma teams, which usually includes an emergency physician, a trauma surgeon, emergency department and surgical nurses, respiratory therapy, and anesthesia. Advanced monitoring and imaging equipment is available for enhancing the evaluation of the patient's injurie as are supportive services (ie, radiology for x-rays, computed tomography scans, magnetic resonance imaging, and ultrasonography and laboratory services). As the patient is evaluated and treated, surgical consultation with the capability to perform surgical exploration of the inured organs is usually available. Often family and friends may subsequently arrive at the hospital and provide pertinent medical history that was not initially available to the prehospital rescue team.

In light of these issues, it is not unreasonable to conclude that there may be significant differences in the initial prehospital diagnostic findings and the final emergency department discharge diagnoses.

This study reports that the majority of evaluations and diagnoses by HEMS personnel are comparable to the findings presented in the emergency department discharge diagnoses. However, some of the injuries to the torso that involve the spine, chest, abdomen, and pelvis that are not initially detected may potentially be mitigated by the provision of timely feedback regarding additional findings from the receiving trauma center to the HEMS crews. This may increase the index of suspicion for the injury when the HEMS team responds to a similar call in the future. Initiation of this process could be designed to provide education for both the prehospital and trauma center staff and even serve as a potential source of continuing education opportunities. Nonetheless, it appears that the HEMS crews are doing a pretty good job overall.

B. M. Minczak, MS, MD, PhD

The impact of distance on triage to trauma center care in an urban trauma system
Doumouras AG, Haas B, Gomez D, et al (Univ of Toronto, Ontario, Canada; et al)
Prehosp Emerg Care 16:456-462, 2012

Background.—Urban trauma systems are characterized by high population density, availability of trauma centers, and acceptable road transport times (within 30 minutes). In such systems, patients meeting field trauma triage (FTT) criteria should be transported directly to a trauma center, bypassing closer nontrauma centers.

Objective.—We evaluated emergency medical services (EMS) triage practices to identify opportunities for improving care delivery.

Objective.—Specifically, we evaluated the effect of the additional distance to a trauma center, compared with a closer non—trauma center, on the noncompliance with trauma destination criteria by EMS personnel in an urban environment.

Methods.—This was a retrospective cohort study of adults having at least one physiologic derangement and meeting Toronto EMS field trauma triage criteria from 2005 to 2010. Road travel distances between the site of injury, the closest non—trauma center, and the closest trauma center were estimated using geographic information systems. For patients who were transported to non—trauma centers, we estimated "differential distance": the additional travel distance required to transport directly to a trauma center. Logistic regression was used to analyze the effect of differential distance on triage decisions, adjusting for other patient characteristics.

Results.—Inclusion criteria identified 898 patients; 53 were transported directly to a trauma center. Falls, female gender, and age greater than 65 years were associated with transport to non—trauma centers. Differential distances greater than 1 mile were associated with a decreased likelihood of triage to a trauma center.

Conclusion.—Differential distance between the closest non—trauma center and the closest trauma center was associated with lower compliance with triage protocols, even in an urban setting where trauma centers can be accessed within approximately 30 minutes. Our findings suggest that there are opportunities for reducing the gap between ideal and actual application of field trauma triage guidelines through a process of education and feedback.

▶ On arrival at the scene of an accident that has caused trauma to the victim(s), the emergency medical services (EMS) personnel are confronted with many decisions: assessing the scene and determining the mechanism of injury, the number of victims, the need to call additional units or a helicopter, and which treatment to initiate, etc.

After the assessment(s) are completed, the victims are stabilized and prepared for transport. At this time, a decision has to be made regarding the destination hospital. Protocols, policies, and checklists are usually in place to facilitate this decision-making process and they are used by the crews either directly or are incorporated as needed into the decision-making process based on crew experience and level of training. These protocols include anatomic, physiologic, and demographic data that help characterize the patients' injuries. Data such as age and gender are also included in the triage process regarding appropriate destination hospital(s) for the patient. When it comes to helicopter EMS, weather conditions, setting up a landing zone rendezvous point, and flight distances and times enter into the decision-making process.

In this study, the authors point out how the decision-making process of EMS can be affected by yet another factor, something they termed "differential distance." Differential distance is defined as the additional distance the team must travel with the patient from a nearby hospital to deliver the patient to an actual trauma center. To accomplish this, the authors conducted a retrospective review of a cohort of patients, looking at their injuries and where the patients were taken. The data analysis demonstrated that medics decided to take patients to the closest hospital if the differential distance exceeded 1 mile. In addition, patients who fell, were females, and/or were older than 65 years of age were also taken to the nearest hospitals instead of the trauma center, which was more than 1 mile or so away. The exact reasons for this decision are not delineated in the study. Of note, travel to an appropriate trauma center in this urban model under study did not exceed 30 minutes. Therefore, in this particular urban setting, the decision to go to a trauma center should not have been affected by relative distance or speculated travel time. If this study were to be conducted in a rural area where geographical constraints caused travel times to be excessive, the decision to proceed to the nearest medical facility might be appropriate. However the data in this study indicate that the medics gave more consideration to the differential distance than they did to the specifications in the field trauma criteria. To mitigate this, a consensus of opinion suggests that if the destination hospitals provide timely feedback and education to the EMS personnel and there is open dialogue for quality assurance purposes, this might lead to the development of a database, analysis of operational trends, and potentially a revision in triage protocols, policies, and procedures. Subsequently, patients that are severely injured will appropriately go to trauma centers, whereas those patients with minor injuries will go to the appropriate nontrauma centers.

In the experience of this editor, I have encountered situations in which medics have taken patients to the nearest hospital because the medics perceived the patient to be "unstable" for transport to a more distant facility. On conducting a retrospective review of the case, it was found that the patient would have probably benefited from direct transport to a specialized facility that was just a few miles farther, translating into several more minutes of travel time. By transporting the patient to the nearest facility, there were more delays in initiating appropriate diagnostics and treatments because of the lack of available services. Therefore, I believe that this study brings to light an important issue that needs prompt attention of medical directors and EMS supervisors.

B. M. Minczak, MS, MD, PhD

Effect of gender on prehospital refusal of medical aid
Waldron R, Finalle C, Tsang J, et al (New York Hosp Queens, Flushing; Feinstein Inst for Med Res, Manhasset, NY)
J Emerg Med 43:283-290, 2012

Background.—"Refusal of medical aid" (RMA) is the term commonly used by emergency medical technicians (EMTs) when someone calls 911 for care (usually the patient or a family member) but, after the initial encounter with the EMTs, the patient refuses emergency medical services transport to the hospital. Some intervention may have been performed, such as taking vital signs or an electrocardiogram, before the RMA.

Although there have been multiple studies of the characteristics and outcomes of patients who RMA, little analysis has been done of the role of EMTs in these cases.

Objective.—To analyze the association between EMT gender and the patient's decision to refuse medical aid in the prehospital setting.

Methods.—The study was performed using data from one hospital-based ambulance service in an urban setting that participates in the 911 system. This was a case control study that examined the data from consecutive patients who refused medical aid for a 1-year period compared to a control group of non-RMA patients.

Results.—There was a significantly higher representation of all-male EMT teams in the RMA group ($p < 0.0001$). Using propensity score-matching methodology to control for other factors, all-male EMT teams were 4.75 times more likely to generate an RMA as compared to all-female and mixed-gender EMT teams (95% confidence interval 1.63–13.96, $p = 0.0046$).

Conclusion.—We found that the gender of the EMTs was one of the most important factors associated with RMA, with a much higher frequency of RMAs occurring when both members of the team were male.

▶ Sure, there are limitations to this study based on its retrospective nature, so at best we can say this is a hypothesis discovery effort and not a determination of cause and effect. However, the authors' study offers an interesting peek into prehospital and clinical culture.

Let's evolve a model for what might be going on between a patient and the prehospital crew (PHC). Perhaps the simplest model might be one in which some patients have the plan to not go to the hospital even before the call to 911 is initiated. Some factor about the patient not involving any interaction with the PHC might be discovered that predicts refusal of further medical care (such as age, gender, or time of day). However, the authors used propensity scoring to remove the effects of these commonly observable factors from likely contributing to the difference of refusing or accepting transport.

A more complicated model of decision making by the patient would include a number of other covariates that described the interaction of the patient with the PHC. Some of these covariates considered in this study included how many hours the PHC had been on duty or whether the PHC contacted emergency physicians about the possible refusal. Yet these variables also were eliminated from comparison by propensity scoring method. Note that there are a great number of other interaction variables possible but these were not recorded. Did the PHC smile or shake hands with the patient? Did the PHC exhibit a disdain for the patient by facial expression or tone of voice?

What can be applied from this study to the problem of patients leaving without being seen? It is likely that there are a number of interactions that may operate similarly in both settings.

N. B. Handly, MD, MSc, MS

Cardiovascular

Termination of resuscitation for adult traumatic cardiopulmonary arrest
The National Association of EMS Physicians and American College of Surgeons Committee on Trauma (Johns Hopkins Univ Dept of Emergency Medicine, Towson, MD)
Prehosp Emerg Care 16:571, 2012

The National Association of EMS Physicians (NAEMSP) and the American College of Surgeons Committee on Trauma (ACS-COT) believe that emergency medical services (EMS) systems should have protocols that allow EMS providers to terminate resuscitative efforts for certain adult patients in traumatic cardiopulmonary arrest. This document is the official position of the NAEMSP and ACS COT.

▶ This publication is a position paper from the National Association of Emergency Medical Services (EMS) Physicians and the American College of Surgeons—Committee on Trauma that addresses the prehospital termination of resuscitation for patients who have succumbed to a traumatic cardiac arrest.

EMS personnel occasionally encounter situations in which a patient is found to be in cardiac arrest after a trauma. After the EMS crew initiates and conducts resuscitation for a significant period (15 minutes), if there is no return of spontaneous circulation, they often transport the patient to the hospital with red lights and siren, risking an accident and potential injury to the crew and others encountered enroute, such as other motorists or pedestrians.

This document describes 8 points that should be considered and applied toward the decision of making a field pronouncement or termination of the resuscitation. These points are basically that on scene time should be limited, especially in patients who are suffering correctable blood loss; protocols should be made available to allow termination of the resuscitation if the outcome appears to be futile; and some process should be in place to deal with the deceased patient and the potentially grieving family. In addition, the document calls for mandatory direct medical oversight when making the decision to stop treatment interventions.

However, the decision to terminate the resuscitation should include an evaluation of any potential confounding/mitigating circumstance that could affect the futility of the resuscitation, such as hypothermia or code status of the patient. More research and discussion are needed to determine the appropriateness of the 15-minute interval of the resuscitation before termination.

B. M. Minczak, MS, MD, PhD

Non-Urgent Commercial Air Travel After Acute Myocardial Infarction: A Review of the Literature and Commentary on the Recommendations

Wang W, Brady WJ, O'Connor RE, et al (Univ of Virginia in Charlottesville; et al)
Air Med J 31:231-237, 2012

Background.—With more people traveling by air abroad, the risk of experiencing an acute coronary syndrome (AMS), including acute myocardial infarction (AMI), has increased. ACS is the leading cause of death during vacation travel. Thus air medical repatriation of patients who have been hospitalized for cardiac reasons abroad has become a concern. Early repatriation can save patients money and psychological stress but may also risk straining the already compromised cardiovascular system. The physiologic effects of flying, current recommendations and the evidence supporting them, and suggestions for better patient management were discussed.

Effects of Flying.—Factors occurring before, during, and after flying play a role in patient safety for those who have suffered an ACS. Before flying, heightened airport security measures, flight delays, and overexertion can create anxiety and physical strain that aggravate cardiac ischemia through the release of catecholamines. During the flight, prolonged immobility, dehydration, and changes in circadian rhythm can lead to fatigue and insomnia and increase the risk of deep vein thrombosis and pulmonary emboli. Hypoxia and anxiety are the main problems directly related to myocardial compromise. In addition, patients' medical status and treatment regimens can influence safe travel. Patients with uncomplicated myocardial infarctions and successful reperfusion tend to fare well even with hypoxia and anxiety, whereas those with irreversible heart injury suffer decreased pumping function and a higher risk for complications.

Current Guidelines and Evidence.—The myocardial infarction-n-related air travel guidelines available are not evidence based and vary widely. For uncomplicated AMI, guidelines suggest postponing air travel for anywhere from 7 to 10 days up to 2 to 8 weeks. Patients at medium risk for repeat ACS are advised to delay flying for 10 days, with further recommendations based on coronary medical history and type of treatment administered. Invasive therapy such as percutaneous coronary intervention (PCI) are associated with better outcomes, so flight delays are shorter than for patients whose therapy is less successful in lowering complication risks. For patients with complicated AMI, which includes ongoing and/or recurrent ischemia, compromising dysrhythmia, and pump failure, guidelines suggest delays of 2 to 6 weeks, or "until the condition stabilizes." Few data support these recommendations. Although PCI is mentioned in several guidelines, it is largely unavailable in many areas of the world, so few data indicate the safety of air travel after revascularization. Some expert groups indicate a delay of just 5 days is safe. After coronary artery bypass graft (CABG), patients are advised to wait 10 to 14 days before traveling for uncomplicated cases, and to based their delay on physician opinion for more involved cases.

Recommendations and Conclusions.—The existing database on the safety of commercial air flight after AMI is limited to just five studies performed over the course of 30 years without no recent reviews. Few data look specifically at post-flight adverse events related to air travel. Many measures are based on theoretical analysis of what happens during flight and how it might affect patients. Often recommendations require risk stratification, which can be impossible. A two-step perspective is suggested, focusing on, the type of AMI (uncomplicated or complicated) and the nature of the initial therapy (reperfusion, fibrinolysis, or CABG versus minimal or noninvasive measures.

▶ The potential for developing heart disease increases if a person has or is exposed to various risk factors such as hypertension, cigarette smoking, and high cholesterol. In addition, if someone is diabetic, has a sedentary lifestyle, is obese, or has a family history of cardiac disease, the person is at greater risk for experiencing an acute coronary syndrome (ACS) and/or a myocardial infarction (MI)

Many people have these risk factors and travel daily. When these people travel by airplane, a mode of transportation regarded as safer than travel by automobile by some actuaries, they are exposing themselves to additional risk factors that can put stress on the cardiovascular and pulmonary systems. If these people are going to be passengers on an aircraft, they may experience stress resulting from anxiety of waiting in long lines, going through airport security, crowding on the aircraft, and noise during flight. This anxiety can lead to increased catecholamine levels in the blood, which can cause an increase in heart rate, cardiac work, and blood pressure. Furthermore, once on board, the passengers usually sit in small confined seats for a significant interval, risking the development of a deep venous thrombus or a pulmonary embolism. Once the aircraft levels off at its assigned cruising altitude, the actual barometric pressure in the passenger compartment is lower than on the ground, setting the stage for hypobaric hypoxia. The changes in humidity can lead to dehydration and volume contraction, also increasing the stress on the cardiovascular system. All of these factors increase the potential for problems in a relatively healthy patient, let alone a patient with an undiagnosed cardiopulmonary condition. What if a passenger travels far away from home or to another country and experiences an ACS or an MI?

Many people are traveling abroad today for business and pleasure. Statistics demonstrate that MI is the leading cause of mortality when people are away from home on vacation. If they survive the MI or ACS, they want to return home. Knowing what pathophysiological risks are part of air travel, the question arises as to when they can safely fly back home. Numerous recommendations are available. This article provides a discussion on the physiology of air travel and addresses how to determine when it is safe to fly and after what type of cardiac event.

B. M. Minczak, MS, MD, PhD

EMS Medical Direction and Prehospital Practices for Acute Cardiovascular Events

Greer S, Williams I, Valderrama AL, et al (Ctrs for Disease Control and Prevention, Atlanta, GA; et al)
Prehosp Emerg Care 17:38-45, 2013

Objective.—The purpose of this analysis was to determine whether there is an association between type of emergency medical services (EMS) medical direction and local EMS agency practices and characteristics specifically related to emergency response for acute cardiovascular events.

Methods.—We surveyed 1,292 EMS agencies in nine states. For each cardiovascular prehospital procedure or practice, we compared the proportion of agencies that employed paid (full- or part-time) medical directors with the proportion of agencies that employed volunteer medical directors. We also compared the proportion of EMS agencies who reported direct interaction between emergency medical technicians (EMTs) and their medical director within the previous four weeks with the proportion of agencies who reported no direct interaction. Chi-square tests were used to assess statistical differences in proportion of agencies with a specific procedure by medical director employment status and medical director interaction. We repeated these comparisons using t-tests to evaluate mean differences in call volume.

Results.—The EMS agencies with prehospital cardiovascular response policies were more likely to report employment of a paid medical director and less likely to report employment of a volunteer medical director. Similarly, agencies with prehospital cardiovascular response practices were more likely to report recent medical director interaction and less likely to report absence of recent medical director interaction. Mean call volumes for chest pain, cardiac arrest, and stroke were higher among agencies having paid medical directors (compared with agencies having volunteer medical directors) and agencies having recent medical director interaction (compared with agencies not having recent medical director interaction).

Conclusions.—Our study demonstrated that EMS agencies with a paid medical director and agencies with medical director interaction with EMTs in the previous four weeks were more likely to have prehospital cardiovascular procedures in place. Given the strong relationship that both employment status and direct interaction have with the presence of these practices, agencies with limited resources to provide a paid medical director or a medical director that can be actively involved with EMTs should be supported through partnerships and other interventions to ensure that they receive the necessary levels of medical director oversight.

▶ This article makes me think of several old sayings. The first is, "While the cat's away the mice will play."

It is rather well established that people often behave differently when they are watched, that is, the Hawthorne effect. The bottom line of this work is that if there is medical supervision and direction provided to emergency medical technicians

(EMTs) on a regular basis, they perform better on the job and patient outcomes most likely are better.

To elaborate, with consistent medical supervision, there is an opportunity to do retrospective debriefings and chart reviews. Some of the metrics that can be assessed to ensure quality are choice of destination hospitals, stroke assessments, response times to chest pain calls, and compliance with advanced life support guidelines. This can provide prompt personal feedback to the EMTs and initiate timely input so that their performance is enhanced. The lessons learned from the data examined in the debriefings can serve as an educational experience for the staff. This can facilitate maintenance of certification requirements for the EMTs. Furthermore, if there are system problems, policies and procedures can be reviewed and, if needed, protocols can be revised.

In addition to the quality improvement that can be achieved, the medical supervisor/director can provide education on new methods, treatments, medications, and procedures that may be applied to patients by the EMTs.

This, in turn, will broaden the service line of the particular emergency medical service (EMS) and possibly increase utilization of this particular system if word gets out that they are good at what they do! On the other hand, if an EMS service has infrequent interaction with the medical director, the EMTs do not always successfully maintain their skills, certifications lapse, protocols are often violated without consequence, and the quality of patient care suffers. The EMTs are unaware of innovations and the organizational morale can deteriorate.

The other issue is how do you ensure that the medical directors comply with these obligations? If the medical director has a contract and is financially compensated for his or her work, there seems to be a more consistent degree of commitment to providing medical direction. However, if the medical director is a volunteer, then the medical supervision is often only provided infrequently on an as-needed basis or not at all. This makes me think of the saying: "Out of sight, out of mind." This article reviews the issues mentioned above in more detail.

B. M. Minczak, MS, MD, PhD

Treatment and Imaging

Occult traumatic loculated tension pneumothorax—a sonographic diagnostic dilemma
Burns BJ, Aguirrebarrena G (Greater Sydney Area HEMS, Bankstown, Australia)
Prehosp Emerg Care 17:92-94, 2013

This case outlines a rarely seen disease in prehospital emergency care—namely, a traumatic loculated tension pneumothorax. Prehospital thoracic ultrasound as part of a standard extended focused assessment with sonography in trauma (EFAST) algorithm failed to diagnose this life-threatening injury. We have subsequently added scanning the lateral chest wall in the fifth intercostal space to the algorithm.

▶ The premise behind emergency medical services (EMS) is to bring rapid assessment and care to patients injured or suffering consequences of time-sensitive, pathophysiological processes. Currently, advanced life support units usually carry defibrillators/pacemakers/monitors, various intravenous fluids, and medications. Now with the advances in microelectronics, medical equipment has become smaller, lighter, and more portable. This has made it possible to bring yet another piece of equipment to the prehospital arena, the portable ultrasound.

Use of ultrasound in the prehospital setting is currently being investigated. Potential applications include the use of ultrasound for optimizing intravenous access, determining the presence or absence of cardiac activity during cardiac arrest, looking for the presence of free fluid in the abdomen, detecting a pneumothorax, or evaluating a gravid uterus.

In this case report, ultrasonographic diagnosis of a pneumothorax was attempted. Because the pneumothorax was a loculated tension pneumothorax, the operators failed to detect the presence of this abnormality.

Use of ultrasound can facilitate certain procedures such as vascular access, but use of this modality can also prevent the performance of an unnecessary procedure such as decompression of a suspected tension pneumothorax based on clinical assessment, when in reality there is no pneumothorax present. For this to happen, the ultrasonographer must be able to accurately detect the presence or absence of a pneumothorax. This case demonstrates that there are potential confounders in the data collected that can lead to misdiagnoses or missed diagnoses.

I find this report intellectually stimulating and thought provoking. To enhance the utility and accuracy of this modality, more work needs to be conducted in order to establish appropriate procedures and techniques that will increase the sensitivity and specificity of this technique, especially in the prehospital setting.

B. M. Minczak, MS, MD, PhD

12 Toxicology

A Case of Histamine Fish Poisoning in a Young Atopic Woman
Wilson BJ, Musto RJ, Ghali WA (Univ of Calgary, Alberta, Canada; Alberta Health Services, Calgary, Canada)
J Gen Intern Med 27:878-881, 2012

Histamine fish poisoning, also known as scombroid poisoning, is a histamine toxicity syndrome that results from eating specific types of spoiled fish. Although typically a benign syndrome, characterized by self-limited flushing, headache, and gastrointestinal symptoms, we describe a case unique in its severity and as a precipitant of an asthma exacerbation.

A 25-year-old woman presented to the emergency department (ED) with one hour of tongue and face swelling, an erythematous pruritic rash, and dyspnea with wheezing after consuming a tuna sandwich. She developed abdominal pain, diarrhea and hypotension in the ED requiring admission to the hospital. A diagnosis of histamine fish poisoning was made and the patient was treated supportively and discharged within 24 hours, but was readmitted within 3 hours due to an asthma exacerbation. Her course was complicated by recurrent admissions for asthma exacerbations.

▶ Scombroid is the other name for histamine fish poisoning. For a fish to cause this, it must be rich in the amino acid histidine, colonizing gram-negative enteric bacteria must contain histidine decarboxylase to convert histidine into histamine, and the fish must have been left in a warm environment long enough, exposed to relatively warm temperatures to permit bacterial replication and histidine metabolism. The authors note that freshly caught fish typically have tissue histamine levels less than 1 mg/100 g, and 20 mg/100 g is roughly the level necessary to cause disease. Usually we think twice about making this diagnosis when the patient has consumed canned tuna, because that industry has much more rigorous control than the fresh fish industry, but it is still quite possible.

R. J. Hamilton, MD

Long-term neurotoxic effects of dimethylamine borane intoxication

Liu C-H, Wang H-M, Lin K-J, et al (Chang Gung Memorial Hosp and Univ College of Medicine, Taipei, Taiwan; Chang Gung Memorial Hosp, Linkou, Taiwan; et al)
J Neurol Sci 319:147-151, 2012

Objectives.—To investigate the long-term neurotoxic effects in a patient with acute dimethylamine borane (DMAB) intoxication.

Patients.—A 38-year-old man, working in a semiconductor factory, with acute DMAB intoxication presented with confusion, and drowsiness, followed by cognitive impairments and motor-predominant axonal polyneuropathy.

Investigations.—We performed serial neurobehavioral assessments and functional neuroimaging studies, including brain ^{99m}Tc-TRODAT single photon emission computed tomography (SPECT) and brain positron emission tomography (PET) scan to monitor the long-term central nervous system (CNS) effects of DMAB intoxication.

Results.—Neurobehavioral tests revealed a persistent impairment in episodic memory of visual retention semantic category retrieval and working memory of digit span (backward). Brain ^{99m}Tc-TRODAT SPECT scan showed a lower radioactivity uptake in the left striatum and F-18 FDG PET scan revealed a relatively decreased cerebral metabolism at the anterior cingulate gyrus and both frontal regions. Follow-up neurobehavioral tests showed that the cognitive improvements were mainly documented in intelligence, attention function, conceptual shift, perceptual motor speed, verbal learning and working memory but were limited in visual memory and executive functions.

Conclusion.—Patients with acute DMAB intoxication may have a long-lasting CNS toxicity on the cognitive dysfunction, parkinsonism, and an impaired metabolic activity of the brain. Clinical improvements may sustain during the long-term follow-up period.

▶ Dimethylamine borane is corrosive to the skin and mucosa on exposure, and is an irritant to the throat, causing epigastralgia, vomiting, diarrhea, and pulmonary edema. In addition, it can cause damage to the peripheral nerves and central nervous system. It is reported to cause acute cerebellar edema and a delayed axonal degeneration in the peripheral nerves.

R. J. Hamilton, MD

Use of haloperidol in PCP-intoxicated individuals

Macneal JJ, Cone DC, Sinha V, et al (Mercy Health System, Janesville, WI; Yale Univ School of Medicine, New Haven, CT; Yale-New Haven Hosp, Janesville, WI)
Clin Toxicol 50:851-853, 2012

Context.—Emergency medical workers often experience violence while performing their job functions. Phencyclidine (PCP)-intoxicated patients are often violent and difficult to control physically. A chemical restraint is frequently needed to assist in protecting both patients and staff from agitated persons.

Objective.—This study evaluated haloperidol as a chemical restraint in PCP-intoxicated patients.

Methods.—This is a retrospective case series of all PCP-positive patients who received haloperidol for behavioral control from April 2008 to April 2011 at a single large (944 bed), urban, tertiary-care hospital. All patients receiving haloperidol and having a toxicology screen positive for PCP were identified using an electronic medical record. Identified cases were then manually reviewed by investigators for adverse events.

Results.—Subjects included 59 adult patients who were acutely agitated requiring chemical restraint or sedation with haloperidol, and who tested positive for PCP. There were 20 females and 39 males, ranging in age from 19 to 54 years. Patients received haloperidol via the PO, IM, or IV routes in doses ranging from 1 to 10 mg. There were two adverse events (mild hypoxia and mild hypotension) found during chart review; neither were serious nor required change in patient disposition.

Conclusions.—In this study, haloperidol does not seem to cause harm when used in the management of PCP-intoxicated patients. Caution must always be exercised in the use of chemical restraint; further prospective study is warranted.

▶ I have never had an adverse event related to the use of Haldol in the agitated overdose patient who has taken phencyclidine. Yet the literature has plenty of case reports that would give clinicians pause. I agree with the author's conclusion that standard does of Haldol appear to be a safe choice. However, I would suggest avoiding excessive doses (> 5 mg). Instead, add a benzodiazepine.

R. J. Hamilton, MD

Severe Colchicine Intoxication in a Renal Transplant Recipient on Cyclosporine

Garrouste C, Philipponnet C, Kaysi S, et al (Univ Hosp, Clermont-Ferrand, France; et al)
Transplant Proc 44:2851-2852, 2012

Using colchicine to treat an acute gout crisis in an organ transplant recipient (TR) on cyclosporine (CsA) may result in life-threatening intoxication. We report the case of a 59-year-old kidney transplant recipient on CsA who was treated with colchicine for acute gout crisis. Seven days later, he developed rhabdomyolysis with progressive quadriparesis, hematologic toxicity and acute renal failure. CsA inhibits P-glycoprotein resulting in decreased hepatic metabolism and renal excretion of colchicine. Colchicine and CsA withdrawal as well as appropriate supportive treatments were effective to manage all of these complications.

▶ This was an unfortunate outcome from a series of drug interactions that could not have been predicted with certainty, but nonetheless could have been avoided. A single dose or 2 of colchicine for the acute crisis would have been more than enough given that drug's narrow therapeutic to toxic window.

R. J. Hamilton, MD

A rare cause of poisoning in childhood: yellow phosphorus
Taskesen M, Adguzel S (Dicle Univ Faculty of Medicine, Diyarbakir, Turkey)
J Emerg Med 43:270-272, 2012

Background.—Yellow phosphorus poisoning is rare, but when it occurs, it may result in pathological changes in almost all organs of the body, especially the liver, heart, kidney, spleen, and brain, and it has a significant mortality rate.

Objectives.—This report presents two cases of poisoning by yellow phosphorus in children. Yellow phosphorus ingestion rarely has been reported among the pediatric population.

> *Case Report.*—This report presents two cases of yellow phosphorus poisoning in children. The patients were admitted with upper abdominal pain, vomiting, lethargy, and respiratory distress. Laboratory testing revealed hepatotoxicity and coagulation disorder. Yellow phosphorus poisoning was treated with conservative therapy in both patients, and one patient died.

Conclusion.—Yellow phosphorus poisoning is a rare clinical entity and should be considered a dangerous toxic ingestion in children.

▶ Yellow phosphorus ingestion has a high mortality. I would have been interested in finding out how these 2 children were able to come in contact with this explosive material. One of the principles of toxicology is that it is better to prevent a lethal poisoning than treat it—and there should be some public health lesson available here.

R. J. Hamilton, MD

A Review of Disaster-Related Carbon Monoxide Poisoning: Surveillance, Epidemiology, and Opportunities for Prevention

Iqbal S, Clower JH, Hernandez SA, et al (Ctrs for Disease Control and Prevention, Atlanta, GA)
Am J Public Health 102:1957-1963, 2012

Objectives.—We conducted a systematic literature review to better understand aspects of disaster-related carbon monoxide (CO) poisoning surveillance and determine potentially effective prevention strategies.

Methods.—This review included information from 28 journal articles on disaster-related CO poisoning cases occurring between 1991 and 2009 in the United States.

Results.—We identified 362 incidents and 1888 disaster-related CO poisoning cases, including 75 fatalities. Fatalities occurred primarily among persons who were aged 18 years or older (88%) and male (79%). Hispanics and Asians accounted for 20% and 14% of fatal cases and 21% and 7% of nonfatal cases, respectively. Generators were the primary exposure source for 83% of fatal and 54% of nonfatal cases; 67% of these fatal cases were caused by indoor generator placement. Charcoal grills were a major source of exposure during winter storms. Most fatalities (94%) occurred at home. Nearly 89% of fatal and 53% of nonfatal cases occurred within 3 days of disaster onset.

Conclusions.—Public health prevention efforts could benefit from emphasizing predisaster risk communication and tailoring interventions for racial, ethnic, and linguistic minorities. These findings highlight the need for surveillance and CO related information as components of disaster preparedness, response, and prevention.

▶ I saw a lot of public health announcements about the safe use of generators and gas grills in the days that followed Superstorm Sandy this past fall, and I am not sure if any of them were on Spanish or Asian language—based media. A good public health project would be to increase awareness of carbon monoxide toxicity in those communities.

R. J. Hamilton, MD

A rare cause of atrial fibrillation: mad honey intoxication

Bayram NA, Keles T, Durmaz T, et al (Ataturk Education and Res Hosp, Bilkent, Ankara, Turkey)
J Emerg Med 43:e389-e391, 2012

Background.—Mad honey intoxication occurs after ingestion of honey containing grayanotoxin.

Case Report.—We report the case of a 36-year-old man who ingested mad honey and developed atrial fibrillation.

Discussion.—Mad honey intoxication is often characterized by symptoms such as hypotension, bradycardia, and syncope. Patients may also experience gastrointestinal, neurologic, and cardiovascular symptoms due to intoxication. Cardiac rhythm abnormalities, including sinus bradycardia, atrioventricular blocks, and nodal rhythms, also may be observed. To our knowledge, this is the first case report of a 36-year old man developing atrial fibrillation with a slow ventricular response after mad honey ingestion.

▶ Mad honey intoxication used to be low on the working list of differential diagnoses for patients with digoxin overdoses. However, digoxin use and overdose have become quite rare! This is a nice review of the toxicity of the cardiac glycoside grayanotoxin but also a reminder of how unusual this problem has become.

R. J. Hamilton, MD

Aminorex poisoning in cocaine abusers

Karch SB, Mari F, Bartolini V, et al (Consultant Pathologist/Toxicologist, Berkeley, CA; Univ of Florence, Italy)
Int J Cardiol 158:344-346, 2012

Levamisole is found in more than 80% of illicit cocaine seized within United States borders. Percentages are somewhat lower in Europe. In 2009, controlled in vivo studies demonstrated that horses metabolize levamisole to aminorex. Earlier this year our laboratory demonstrated that the same conversion occurs in man. Levamisole itself causes aplastic anemia and numerous reports have begun to appear in the literature, but the conversion of levamisole to aminorex is of much more concern. Aminorex ingestion was responsible for a five-year epidemic (1967–1972) of idiopathic pulmonary hypertension (IPH) confined to Switzerland, Austria, and Germany, the only countries where aminorex had been marketed as an anorectic. The incidence of IPH reverted to normal levels as soon as aminorex was withdrawn. In most cases onset of symptoms in IPH began after six to nine months of aminorex use, with average dosage ranges of 10 to 40 mg per day. The outcome was almost uniformly fatal. The conversion rate of levamisole to aminorex has not been established, but given the high daily intake of cocaine by many abusers, it seems likely that many of them will have ingested enough contaminated cocaine to ultimately cause IPH. Until the disease is well established, the symptoms of IPH are vague, and existing drug registries specifically exclude drug abusers, making it difficult to track these cases. This review is intended to draw attention to what may be a slowly emerging new epidemic.

▶ This is an excellent article for toxicologists because they will be consulted regarding many patients who use cocaine. Watching for the clinical trends might help further the concept that aminorex is what is causing the problem—not just the cocaine.

R. J. Hamilton, MD

Anaphylaxis at image-guided epidural pain block secondary to corticosteroid compound
Moran DE, Moynagh MR, Alzanki M, et al (Cappagh Natl Orthopaedic Hosp, Finglas Dublin, Ireland)
Skelet Radiol 41:1317-1318, 2012

Anaphylaxis during image-guided interventional procedures is a rare but potentially fatal event. Anaphylaxis to iodinated contrast is an established and well-recognized adverse effect. However, anaphylaxis to some of the other frequently administered medications given during interventional procedures, such as corticosteroids, is not common knowledge. During caudal epidural injection, iodinated contrast is used to confirm needle placement in the epidural space at the level of the sacral hiatus. A combination of corticosteroid, local anesthetic, and saline is subsequently injected. We describe a very rare case of anaphylaxis to a component of the steroid medication instilled in the caudal epidural space.

▶ Further abstracting from the article:
Tests for methylprednisolone, iohexol, bupivacaine, and latex were negative. On review of the summary of product characteristics of Depo-Medrone, it was found to contain polyethylene glycol 3350 (also known as macrogol 3350). Skin-prick testing to Depo-Medrone and Movicol (a laxative that also contains macrogol 3350, [Norgine Ltd, Uxbridge, UK]) was strongly positive. The patient's episode of anaphylaxis was due to polyethylene glycol or macrogol allergy. This is the second article this year that implicates macrogol in a depo steroid preparation as a trigger for anaphylaxis. Good tidbit to keep in mind.

R. J. Hamilton, MD

Rapid and Complete Bioavailability of Antidotes for Organophosphorus Nerve Agent and Cyanide Poisoning in Minipigs After Intraosseous Administration
Murray DB, Eddleston M, Thomas S, et al (Royal Infirmary of Edinburgh, UK; Univ of Newcastle, UK; et al)
Ann Emerg Med 60:424-430, 2012

Study objective.—Management of chemical weapon casualties includes the timely administration of antidotes without contamination of rescuers. Personal protective equipment makes intravenous access difficult but does not prevent intraosseous drug administration. We therefore measured the systemic bioavailability of antidotes for organophosphorus nerve agent and cyanide poisoning when administered by the intraosseous, intravenous, and intramuscular routes in a small study of Göttingen minipigs.

Methods.—Animals were randomly allocated to sequentially receive atropine (0.12 mg/kg by rapid injection), pralidoxime (25 mg/kg by injection during 2 minutes), and hydroxocobalamin (75 mg/kg during 10 minutes) by the intravenous or intraosseous route, or atropine and pralidoxime by the intramuscular route. Plasma concentrations were measured for 6 hours to characterize the antidote concentration-time profiles for each route.

Results.—Maximum plasma concentrations of atropine and pralidoxime occurred within 2 minutes when administered by the intraosseous route compared with 8 minutes by the intramuscular route. Maximum plasma hydroxocobalamin concentration occurred at the end of the infusion when administered by the intraosseous route. The mean area under the concentration-time curve by the intraosseous route was similar to the intravenous route for all 3 drugs and similar to the intramuscular route for atropine and pralidoxime.

Conclusion.—This study showed rapid and substantial antidote bioavailability after intraosseous administration that appeared similar to that of the intravenous route. The intraosseous route of antidote administration should be considered when intravenous access is difficult.

▶ This is a very nice study that clearly demonstrates a role for intraosseous administration for these antidotes.

R. J. Hamilton, MD

Gastro-intestinal poisoning due to consumption of daffodils mistaken for vegetables at commercial markets, Bristol, United Kingdom
Matulkova P, Gobin M, Evans M, et al (Health Protection Agency South West, Temple Quay, Bristol, UK; et al)
Clin Toxicol 50:788-790, 2012

Introduction.—In February 2012, we investigated a cluster of people who presented at a local emergency department with sudden onset of vomiting after mistaken consumption of daffodils.

Methods.—We interviewed patients to collect information on daffodil purchase and consumption. With Local Authority we investigated points of sale to understand the source of confusion.

Results.—We identified 11 patients (median age: 23 years, range 5—60 years, eight females) among Bristol (UK) residents of Chinese origin. The most commonly reported symptoms were vomiting (n = 11) and nausea (n = 9) that developed within 12 h of daffodil consumption. There were no hospitalisations or deaths. Patients were clustered in two family dinners and one party. Bunches of pre-bloom daffodil stalks were purchased in two stores of one supermarket chain, which displayed daffodils next to vegetables, not marked as non-edible. Patients cooked and consumed daffodils mistaking them for Chinese chives/onions.

Discussion.—Gastro-intestinal poisoning should be considered in differential diagnoses of gastroenteritis. Multi-cultural societies are at risk of confusion between non-edible and edible plants. Supermarket presentation of daffodils may have contributed to mistaken consumption. We recommended explicit labelling and positioning of daffodils, away from produce. The supermarket chain introduced graphic 'non-edible' labels. No further patients were reported following action.

▶ Further proof that poison prevention is the cornerstone of toxicologic safety—merely placing the daffodil bulbs in such a manner as to suggest they were bunches of chives resulted in the sickening of 11 patients. Lesson RE-learned!

R. J. Hamilton, MD

Maternal exposure to moderate ambient carbon monoxide is associated with decreased risk of preeclampsia
Zhai D, Guo Y, Smith G, et al (Central South Univ, Changsha, Hunan, People's Republic of China; Univ of Ottawa Faculty of Medicine, Ontario, Canada; Queen's Univ, Kingston, Ontario, Canada)
Am J Obstet Gynecol 207:57.e1-57.e9, 2012

Objective.—Carbon monoxide (CO) in cigarette smoke may be the mechanism by which tobacco use during pregnancy decreases the risk of the development of preeclampsia. We attempted to test this hypothesis by examining the effect of maternal exposure to ambient CO on preeclampsia.

Study Design.—Births that occurred between 2004 and 2009 in the Canadian province of Ontario were extracted from the data. Study subjects were divided into 4 groups according to quartiles of CO concentration that were based on maternal residence. Adjusted odds ratio and 95% confidence interval were used to estimate the independent effect of CO on preeclampsia.

Results.—Rates of preeclampsia were 2.32%, 1.97%, 1.59%, and 1.26%, respectively, in the first, second, third, and fourth quartile of CO concentration. The inverse association between CO concentration and preeclampsia risk remained the same after adjustment for several important confounding factors.

Conclusion.—Maternal exposure to moderate ambient CO is associated independently with a decreased risk of preeclampsia.

▶ This study is laudable for its ambitious and exacting methods. The question as to whether ambient carbon monoxide (CO) could actually decrease preeclampsia is intriguing. It is well known that during pregnancy, the maternal increase in red blood cell mass and endogenous production by the fetus results in a slight elevation in CO hemoglobin. In addition, cigarette smokers but not smokeless tobacco users have a decreased incidence of preeclampsia. Because we know that CO functions as a vasoactive singling mechanism, the hypothesis is very reasonable. The data support the hypothesis across a wide variety of confounding variables and support a dose-response curve as well. Thus CO should be a substance that exhibits a j-shaped dose-response curve, which is too little has some untoward effects.

R. J. Hamilton, MD

Severe Poisoning After Accidental Pediatric Ingestion of Glycol Ethers
Wanga GS, Yin S, Shear B, et al (Denver Health and Hosps, CO; Children's Hosp Colorado, Denver)
Pediatrics 130:e1026-e1029, 2012

Human glycol ether poisonings are sparsely reported in the medical literature. We describe a healthy 22-month-old boy who accidentally drank up to 330 mL of brake fluid containing a 75% bleed of various glycol ethers (5%—50% polyethylene glycol monomethyl ether, 15%—40% triethylene glycol monoethyl ether, 1%—30% triethylene glycol monomethyl ether, 1%—25% triethylene glycol monobutyl ether, 1%—20% polyethylene glycol, monobutyl ether, 1%—20% triethylene glycol, and <10% of other glycol ethers). Within 4 hours, he became somnolent and developed a persistent metabolic acidosis. Thirty minutes later, he received 1 dose of fomepizole. Neither progression nor improvement in clinical or metabolic status was noted after the fomepizole. He received hemodialysis for 3 hours ~8 hours after ingestion, and his symptoms resolved resulting in an uneventfully recovery.

▶ Most of the glycol ether ingestions that I have managed have been "mouthful" or "gulp" quantities (15-30 mL) and have been asymptomatic. This ingestion is 10 times that, which explains the degree of toxicity. In defense of the potential efficacy of fomepizole, it was given after the child developed an acidosis and therefore was less likely to be effective. Therefore, I would not dismiss the use of fomepizole as a potential antidote or adjunct in similar overdoses; it just has to be given early. The dilemma is that most glycol ethers are asymptomatic.

R. J. Hamilton, MD

Accidental poisoning after ingestion of "aphrodisiac" berries: diagnosis by analytical toxicology
Nikolaou P, Papoutsis I, Stefanidou M, et al (Natl and Kapodistrian Univ of Athens, Greece)
J Emerg Med 42:662-665, 2012

Background.—A large number of plants, seeds, and berries have been used for medicinal, psychotropic, or aphrodisiac purposes for a thousand years. *Mandragora officinarum* belongs to the family of Solanaceae and is traditionally known as an aphrodisiac and is closely associated with witchcraft.

Objectives.—In this study we report a case of an accidental poisoning after ingestion of some "aphrodisiac" berries and the contribution of the toxicological analysis in the case investigation.

> *Case Report.*—A 35-year-old man was admitted to the hospital with clinical signs and symptoms of an anticholinergic syndrome. The diagnosis of the poisoning was made by the toxicological analysis of the patient's urine. The cause of the poisoning was revealed by his girlfriend's disclosure that the patient had intentionally consumed some "aphrodisiac" berries to enhance his sexual performance. Subsequently, berries similar to the ones consumed were sent to the laboratory. The analysis of the urine and the berries revealed the presence of hyoscyamine and scopolamine; the berries were identified as *Mandragora officinarum* berries. Decontamination and symptomatic treatment were proven effective for the control of this poisoning. The patient recovered completely after hospitalization for 4 days.

Conclusion.—This case report indicates the importance of analytical toxicology in diagnosis of intoxications after the consumption of unknown plants or plant products and presents the clinical aspects of *Mandragora* intoxication.

▶ The authors do a nice job of using gas chromatograph/mass spectrometry to identify the hyoscyamine and scopolamine peaks to correspond with the Mandrake ingestion. However, there was no explanation for the methaqualone peak.

R. J. Hamilton, MD

The effects of fructose-1,6-diphosphate on haemodynamic parameters and survival in a rodent model of propranolol and verapamil poisoning
Kalam Y, Graudins A (Monash Univ, Clayton, Victoria, Australia)
Clin Toxicol 50:546-554, 2012

Background.—Fructose-1,6-diphosphate (FDP) is a metabolite in the glycolytic pathway created from glucose. Exogenously administered FDP increases the yield of ATP from anaerobic glycolysis. FDP reduces ischaemic tissue area in experimentally-induced cerebral and myocardial infarction and improves haemodynamics post-cardiac bypass. We hypothesised that FDP improves haemodynamics in propranolol and verapamil poisoning.

Method.—Anesthetized Wistar rats were instrumented to record BP, heart rate (HR), cardiac output (CO) and QRS-duration. Propranolol or verapamil were infused continually. When BP dropped by 50%, propranolol-poisoned rats received one of 10% FDP125 mg/kg or 10% FDP250 mg/kg loading dose over 20 minutes followed by infusion 20 mg/kg/h. Verapamil-poisoned rats received the higher dosing regimen of FDP250.

Controls received comparable volumes of 10% glucose. Haemodynamic time-points were compared for FDP to control by unpaired t-test or Mann—Whitney test as appropriate ($p < 0.05$). Survival was assessed using Kaplan—Meier survival analysis.

Results.—FDP-treated animals survived significantly longer than glucose-treated controls at both doses in propranolol poisoning and in verapamil-poisoning. In propranolol poisoning, FDP250-treated animals showed a statistically significant increase in BP. However, there was no significant difference in cardiac output at this dose. There were also no significant differences in any haemodynamic parameters compared to control at the lower FDP dose in propranolol poisoning or in verapamil poisoning.

Conclusion.—FDP improved survival for both toxicants with an improvement in haemodynamics at the higher dose in propranolol poisoning. Future research could examine the efficacy of FDP in other beta-blocker and calcium channel-blocker poisoning as well as in concert with established inotropic therapies in drug-induced cardiovascular collapse.

▶ Fructose-1,6-diphosphate (FDP) has the potential to be a future antidote for beta-blocker and calcium channel blocker toxicity. It will be interesting to see how this research develops.

R. J. Hamilton, MD

Buprenorphine May Not Be as Safe as You Think: A Pediatric Fatality From Unintentional Exposure

Kim HK, Smiddy M, Hoffman RS, et al (New York Univ Langone Med Ctr/ Bellevue Hosp Ctr; Office of Chief Med Examiner, NY)
Pediatrics 130:e1700-e1703, 2012

Buprenorphine is a partial μ—opioid receptor agonist that is approved for the treatment of opioid dependency. It is generally believed to be safer than methadone because of its ceiling effect on respiratory depression. As more adults in US households use buprenorphine, an increasing number of children are being exposed. We report a fatal exposure to buprenorphine in a small child that occurred after ingestion of a caretaker's buprenorphine/ naloxone. Postmortem toxicology analysis showed free serum concentrations of 52 ng/mL and 39 ng/mL for buprenorphine and norbuprenorphine, respectively. No other drugs were detected. Autopsy did not find signs of injury or trauma. The theoretical safety provided by the ceiling effect in respiratory depression from buprenorphine may not apply to children, and buprenorphine may cause dose-dependent respiratory depression.

▶ Buprenorphine might be the next drug to be added to the "deadly in a large dose" list for children.

R. J. Hamilton, MD

Mistaken identity: Severe vomiting, bradycardia and hypotension after eating a wild herb

Maeda K, Idehara R, Kusaka S (Natl Hosp Organization Shiga Hosp, Higashi-oumi, Japan; Biotic and Human Interaction Res Group, Kusatsu, Shiga, Japan)
Clin Toxicol 50:532-533, 2012

A 53-year-old woman presented with severe vomiting 3.5 hours after eating a boiled wild herb thought to be *Hosta montana*. She was alert, and did not complain of diplopia or numbness of her limbs. Her vital signs were temperature of 35.9°C, blood pressure of 84/33 mmHg, and heart rate of 59 beats/minute. There was no arrhythmia or conduction block on electrocardiogram. Her blood pressure and heart rate were decreased to 75/44 mmHg and 51 beats/minute at the minimum, respectively. Complete blood count and serum chemistry were normal. The herb was correctly identified when the patient's husband brought in the herb for identification.

▶ This patient was trying to forage the edible plant *Hosta montana* and instead gathered *Veratrum album*. She developed hypotension and bradycardia, probably as a result of the toxin protoveratrine, which has been studied as an antihypertensive. Foragers are prone to this type of poisoning, and a knowledge of the look-alikes in the area can be advantageous to the patients and the physicians.

R. J. Hamilton, MD

A case of near-fatal fenpyroximate intoxication: The role of percutaneous cardiopulmonary support and therapeutic hypothermia

Lee HY, Lee BK, Jeung KW, et al (Chonnam Natl Univ Hosp, Gwangju, Republic of Korea)
Clin Toxicol 50:858-861, 2012

Introduction.—Fenpyroximate is a potent inhibitor of the mitochondrial proton-translocating NADH-quinone oxidoreductase (complex I). Although it is widely used as an acaricide, data on the acute toxicity of fenpyroximate in humans are very limited.

Case Detail.—A 44-year-old woman was brought to our hospital with a reduced level of consciousness, hypotension, and severe lactic acidosis after deliberate ingestion of 5% fenpyroximate solution. The acidosis progressively deteriorated despite maximal supportive treatment, and cardiac arrest refractory to standard cardiopulmonary resuscitation developed. The patient was successfully resuscitated with percutaneous cardiopulmonary support, therapeutic hypothermia, and intravenous acetylcysteine. Blood gases of simultaneously obtained arterial and central venous blood revealed decreased arteriovenous oxygen difference.

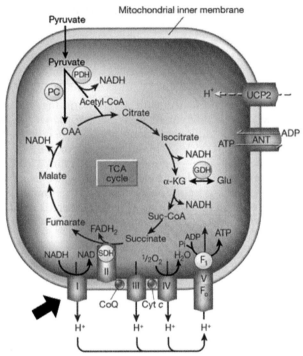

FIGURE 3.—Respiratory chain in a mitochondrion and complex I where fenpyroximate acts in the mitochondria (thick arrow). (adapted, with permission, from Maechler et al. 2001 Nature. Available at: http://www.nature.com/nature/journal/v414/n6865/images/414807a-f2.2.jpg. Accessed 6 August 2012.) ANT, adenine nucleotide translocator; GDH, glutamate dehydrogenase; Glu, glutamate; KG, keto-glutarate; OAA, oxaloacetate; PC, pyruvate carboxylase; PDH, pyruvate dehydrogenase; Suc-CoA, succinyl-CoA; SDH, succinate dehydrogenase; TCA, tricarboxylic acid; UCP2, uncoupling protein 2 (see colour version of this figure online at www.informahealthcare.com/ctx). (Reprinted from Lee HY, Lee BK, Jeung KW, et al. A case of near-fatal fenpyroximate intoxication: the role of percutaneous cardiopulmonary support and therapeutic hypothermia. *Clin Toxicol.* 2012;50:858-861, with permission of Taylor & Francis Ltd, http://www.tandf.co.uk/journals.)

Discussion.—The present case, along with previous cases of fatal complex I inhibitor poisoning, indicates that impaired oxygen utilization at the tissue level is the major mechanism underlying the fatality of this condition. Percutaneous cardiopulmonary support may help restore vital organ perfusion by increasing oxygen delivery even in the presence of decreased oxygen consumption, thereby allowing additional time for recovery and drug metabolism. Therapeutic hypothermia also may be beneficial in treating severe complex I inhibitor poisoning, since hypothermia itself attenuates oxidative processes and decreases the metabolic rate (Fig 3).

▶ An acaricide is a substance used to kill ticks and mites. This is a good example of a known-unknown material (ie, a substance with known properties but unknown human toxicity) being successfully managed by the use of intensive care as well as recently developed techniques such as therapeutic hypothermia.

I would encourage more widespread use of this technique in poisonings and overdose because the potential for recovery is great if the patient can be supported long enough to metabolize the drug.

R. J. Hamilton, MD

Pulmonary edema following scorpion envenomation: Mechanisms, clinical manifestations, diagnosis and treatment
Bahloul M, Chaari A, Dammak H, et al (Habib Bourguiba Univ Hosp, Sfax, Tunisia)
Int J Cardiol 162:86-91, 2013

Scorpion envenomation is common in tropical and subtropical regions. Cardio-respiratory manifestations, mainly cardiogenic shock and pulmonary edema, are the leading causes of death after scorpion envenomation. The mechanism of pulmonary edema remains unclear and contradictory conclusions were published. However, most publications confirm that pulmonary edema has been attributed to acute left ventricular failure. Cardiac failure can result from massive release of catecholamines, myocardial damage induced by the venom or myocardial ischemia. Factors usually associated with the diagnosis of pulmonary edema were young age, tachypnea, agitation, sweating, or the presence of high plasma protein concentrations. Treatment of scorpion envenomation has two components: antivenom

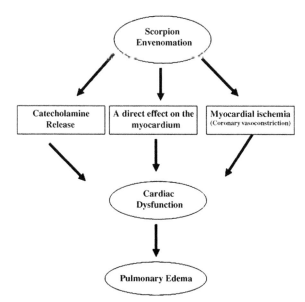

FIGURE 1.—Mechanisms of cardiac dysfunction following scorpion envenomation. (Reprinted from Bahloul M, Chaari A, Dammak H, et al. Pulmonary edema following scorpion envenomation: mechanisms, clinical manifestations, diagnosis and treatment. *Int J Cardiol*. 2013;162:86-91, Copyright 2013, with permission from International Society for Adult Congenital Heart Disease.)

TABLE 1.—Most Dangerous Scorpion Species and Type of Scorpion Antivenom in Each Country

Antivenom (reference)	Species	Country
Polyvalent scorpion antivenom [62]	*Androctonus australis garzonii, B. occitanus tunetanus, and Tityus serrulatus*	Morocco
Purified polyvalent anti-scorpion serum (equine) [66]	*Leiurus quinquestraitus Androctonus amoreuxi Androctonus crassicauda Androctonus aeneas Androctonus australis Scorpio marus palmatus Buthus occitanus*	Egypt
Scorpion antivenom (Pasteur Institute of Algeria)	*Androctonus australis*	Algeria
Polyvalent scorpion antivenom [75]	*Centruroides limpidus, C. noxius, C. suffusus*	Mexico
Soro antiescorpionico [65]	*Tityus serrulatus*	Brazil
Monovalent scorpion antivenom [65]	*Parabuthus spp.*	South Africa
Monovalent red scorpion antivenom [63,64]	Indian red scorpion (*Mesobuthus tamulus*)	India
Bivalent scorpion antivenom (Institut Pasteur, Tunis, Tunisia) [65]	*A. australis and B. occitanus*	Tunisia
Polyvalent scorpion antivenom [65]	*Leiurus quinquestriatus, Androctonus crassicauda, Buthus arenicola, Butus mimax, Buthus occitanus, Leiurus quinquestriatus hebreus and A. amoreuxi.*	Saudi Arabia
Monovalent scorpion antivenom [68]	*Leiurus quinquestriatus*	Israel
Scorpion antivenom [67]	*Tityus trivittatus*	Argentina
Scorpion antivenom [68,75]	*Tityus zulianus*	Venezuela
Polyvalent scorpion antivenom [89]	*C. limpidus limpidus, C. l. tecomanus, C. noxius noxius and C. suffusus suffusus*	North and Central America

Editor's Note: Please refer to original journal article for full references.

administration and supportive care. The latter mainly targets hemodynamic impairment and cardiogenic pulmonary edema. In Latin America, and India, the use of Prazosin is recommended for treatment of pulmonary edema because pulmonary edema is associated with arterial hypertension. However, in North Africa, scorpion leads to cardiac failure with systolic dysfunction with normal vascular resistance and dobutamine was recommended. Dobutamine infusion should be used as soon as we have enough evidence suggesting the presence of pulmonary edema, since it has been demonstrated that scorpion envenomation can result in pulmonary edema secondary to acute left ventricular failure. In severe cases, mechanical ventilation can be required (Fig 1, Table 1).

▶ Included are Fig 1 and Table 1 as a good review of scorpion envenomations by geography. Indeed, pulmonary edema from scorpion envenomation is multifactorial.

R. J. Hamilton, MD

Mechanisms of Cadmium-Induced Proximal Tubule Injury: New Insights with Implications for Biomonitoring and Therapeutic Interventions
Prozialeck WC, Edwards JR (Midwestern Univ, Downers Grove, IL)
J Pharmacol Exp Ther 343:2-12, 2012

Cadmium is an important industrial agent and environmental pollutant that is a major cause of kidney disease. With chronic exposure, cadmium accumulates in the epithelial cells of the proximal tubule, resulting in a generalized reabsorptive dysfunction characterized by polyuria and low-molecular-weight proteinuria. The traditional view has been that as cadmium accumulates in proximal tubule cells, it produces a variety of relatively nonspecific toxic effects that result in the death of renal epithelial cells through necrotic or apoptotic mechanisms. However, a growing volume of evidence suggests that rather than merely being a consequence of cell death, the early stages of cadmium-induced proximal tubule injury may involve much more specific changes in cell-cell adhesion, cellular signaling pathways, and autophagic responses that occur well before the onset of necrosis or apoptosis. In this commentary, we summarize these recent findings, and we offer our own perspectives as to how they relate to the toxic actions of cadmium in the kidney. In addition, we highlight recent findings, suggesting that it may be possible to detect the early stages of cadmium toxicity through the use of improved biomarkers. Finally, some of the therapeutic implications of these findings will be considered. Because cadmium is, in many respects, a model cumulative nephrotoxicant, these insights may have broader implications regarding the general mechanisms through which a variety of drugs and toxic chemicals damage the kidney.

▶ Cadmium toxicity crops up now and again—such as the recent recall of drinking glasses with cadmium paint and children's jewelry with high levels of cadmium. Biosurveillance for cadmium typically includes testing for increased concentrations of urinary beta-2 microglobulin. In addition, blood and urine cadmium levels can be monitored. This article describes some evolving research into cadmium toxicity and its implications for biosurveillance.

R. J. Hamilton, MD

Serum tau protein level for neurological injuries in carbon monoxide poisoning
Kilicaslan I, Bildik F, Aksel G, et al (Gazi Univ School of Medicine, Ankara, Turkey)
Clin Toxicol 50:497-502, 2012

Introduction.—Carbon monoxide (CO) poisoning causes hypoxia that results tissue injury, especially in the brain and heart. Delayed neurologic sequela is one of the most serious complications that may occur up to 40% of severe CO poisoning cases.

Objective.—The aim of the study was to determine an association between the serum tau protein and severe neurologic symptoms/signs upon presentation.

Methods.—Seventy-eight patients with CO poisoning were evaluated in this cross-sectional study. The patients were divided into two groups, Group 1: those with loss of consciousness (LOC)/syncope, seizure, coma, altered mental status (n = 19), and Group 2; without LOC (n = 59). Serum tau protein levels were studied on admission.

Results.—Mean age of the patients was 37.3 ± 15.4 and 53.6% were male. Headache was the most common presenting symptom observed among 67 patients (86%). The median serum tau protein level was 76.54 pg/mL (35.56–152.65) within group 1, 64.04 pg/mL (23.85–193.64) in patients within group 2 ($p = 0.039$), respectively. The median serum tau protein levels were 79.80 pg/mL (35.56–193.64) in patients who received HBO therapy and 65.79 pg/mL (23.85–167.29) in patients who did not receive HBO therapy ($p = 0.032$). The value of area under the curve was 0.642 for detecting CO poisoning with severe neurological symptoms.

Conclusion.—Although tau protein levels were significantly higher in patients with severe neurological symptoms; the difference did not reach a clinical significance. Further studies are needed in order to reveal the validity of tau protein for detecting neurological injuries in patients with CO toxicity.

▶ Tau protein is a soluble microtubule-associated protein in the axons of the central nervous system that is released into the extracellular space after brain trauma or injury. Once it is proteolytically cleaved and then diffuses into the cerebrospinal fluid, plasma can be measured readily. It is proposed as a central nervous system injury biomarker. Unfortunately, it is not yet ready for prime time, as it poorly differentiates from controls at this point. However, the search continues for a neurologic biomarker for injury—especially subclinical brain injury.

R. J. Hamilton, MD

Fatal gastrointestinal hemorrhage after a single dose of dabigatran
Kernan L, Ito S, Shirazi F, et al (Carl R Darnall Army Med Ctr, Fr Hood, TX; Univ of Arizona, Tucson)
Clin Toxicol 50:571-573, 2012

Introduction.—Dabigatran (Pradaxa) is a new oral anticoagulant approved by the Food and Drug Administration (FDA), available internationally and indicated as an alternative to warfarin for the prevention of stroke and systemic embolism in patients with nonvalvular atrial fibrillation. Dabigatran does not require laboratory monitoring and its kinetics allow for a more rapid onset of action with a time to peak concentration of 1.25–1.5 h. We are reporting a fatality resulting from gastrointestinal bleeding after the ingestion of a single dose of dabigatran 150 mg.

Case Details.—A 92-year-old man with a medical history of chronic obstructive pulmonary disease, hypothyroidism, and atrial flutter presented to the emergency department with complaints of weakness and rectal bleeding. He was seen by his Cardiologist the day before and was found to be in new atrial fibrillation. He was prescribed dabigatran 150 mg twice daily for anticoagulation therapy. He took one dose of dabigatran 150 mg at 2200 and woke up the following morning before 0900 with profuse rectal bleeding. The initial vital signs in the emergency department, approximately 11 h after ingestion, were heart rate 72 beats/min, blood pressure 62/30 mmHg, and lab work showed hemoglobin 9.9 g/dL, international normalization ratio (INR) 1.99, blood urea nitrogen (BUN) 66 mg/dL, and creatinine (SCr) 1.4 mg/dL (creatinine clearance (CrCl) 24.2 mL/min). He was resuscitated with intravenous fluids, two units of packed red blood cells, two units of fresh frozen plasma, platelets, and vitamin K 10 mg intravenously. He was also given an unknown dose of erythromycin early in his hospital stay. An actively bleeding gastric ulcer was discovered and treated with local epinephrine injections. Approximately 48 h after his exposure, he received an additional two units of blood to treat his decreasing blood pressure (98/41 mmHg). On day three, his hemoglobin and hematocrit were stable at 10 g/dL and 30%, INR 1.6, he was extubated and off vasoactive medications. Day six of hospitalization, he began having maroon stools, his hemoglobin decreased to 8.1 g/dL and his platelets to 81 × 1000/mcL. On day seven, the hemoglobin decreased to 6.4 mg/dL. Despite aggressive resuscitative efforts and supportive care, he died.

Discussion.—This case demonstrates the potential of a single dose of dabigatran 150 mg to result in a fatal gastrointestinal hemorrhage. This patient was started on the maximum dose with a CrCl 33.9 mL/min and on admission CrCl 24.2 mL/min, suggesting underlying renal insufficiency.

▶ Dabigatran—no antidote, no marker, no elimination, deadly in a dose. Okay, well it does not have an antidote, and you can use activated partial thromboplastin time (aPTT) to assess for nontoxic effects, and you can remove about half with hemodialysis. These overdoses can be vexing clinically. Here are my current notes on treating dabigatran overdose.

Dabigatran is a direct thrombin inhibitor that can be deadly in a dose. It is not metabolized much (few interactions) and cleared by the kidney. It will increase the international normalization ratio (INR) and partial thromboplastin time at toxic levels. Initial laboratory values should be serum creatinine, prothrombin time/INR, aPTT, thrombin clotting time, complete blood count (platelets), and thrombin time. If no renal impairment and no symptoms are seen, then 24-hour observation is sufficient because it should be cleared in that timeframe. If aPTT level is totally normal (< 1.5x), it is unlikely that significant drug effect is present.

Treatment includes fresh frozen plasma. Two to 3 hours of hemodialysis will remove roughly 60%.

Theoretical benefits include (studies equivocal for dabigatran but show that they work well for rivaroxaban-factor Xa inhibitor) (1) prothrombin complex concentrate (Profilnine®) 50 U/kg intravenous with or without fresh frozen plasma (2–4 units) and (2) recombinant factor VIIa (NovoSeven®) 90 µg/kg intravenous. Good luck!

R. J. Hamilton, MD

Detecting damaged regions of cerebral white matter in the subacute phase after carbon monoxide poisoning using voxel-based analysis with diffusion tensor imaging
Fujiwara S, Beppu T, Nishimoto H, et al (Iwate Med Univ, Morioka, Japan; et al)
Neuroradiology 54:681-689, 2012

Introduction.—The present study aimed to detect the main regions of cerebral white matter (CWM) showing damage in the subacute phase for CO-poisoned patients with chronic neurological symptoms using voxel-based analysis (VBA) with diffusion tensor imaging (DTI).

Methods.—Subjects comprised 22 adult CO-poisoned patients and 16 age-matched healthy volunteers as controls. Patients were classified into patients with transient acute symptoms only (group A) and patients with chronic neurological symptoms (group S). In all patients, DTI covering the whole brain was performed with a 3.0-T magnetic resonance imaging system at 2 weeks after CO exposure. As procedures for VBA, all fractional anisotropy (FA) maps obtained from DTI were spatially normalized, and FA values for all voxels in the whole CWM on normalized FA maps were statistically compared among the two patient groups and controls.

Results.—Voxels with significant differences in FA were detected at various regions in comparisons between groups S and A and between group S and controls. In these comparisons, more voxels were detected in deep CWM, including the centrum semiovale, than in other regions. A few voxels were detected between group A and controls. Absolute FA values in the centrum semiovale were significantly lower in group S than in group A or controls.

Conclusions.—VBA demonstrated that CO-poisoned patients with chronic neurological symptoms had already suffered damage to various CWM regions in the subacute phase. In these regions, the centrum semiovale was suggested to be the main region damaged in the subacute phase after CO inhalation.

▶ Carbon monoxide (CO)—poisoned patients with chronic neurologic sequelae are difficult to characterize, as many of the neurologic changes require psychometric testing to detect. If an objective measurement of CO injury such as the one described in this article can be established, then the value of various treatments for this condition can be addressed more precisely.

R. J. Hamilton, MD

Recipients of hyperbaric oxygen treatment for carbon monoxide poisoning and exposure circumstances

Clower JH, Hampson NB, Iqbal S, et al (Ctrs for Disease Control and Prevention, Atlanta, GA; Virginia Mason Med Ctr, Seattle, WA)
Am J Emerg Med 30:846-851, 2012

Background.—Unintentional carbon monoxide poisoning is preventable. Severe cases are often referred for hyperbaric oxygen treatment. To guide prevention efforts and treatment practices, this study provides some of the most detailed current information about patients with carbon monoxide poisoning who have been treated at hyperbaric facilities across the United States and the circumstances surrounding their exposures. This study can help improve efforts to prevent carbon monoxide poisoning and enhance treatment practices.

Methods.—From August 2008 to January 2010, nonidentifiable, patient-level data were reported by 87 hyperbaric facilities in 39 states via an online reporting system. This reporting system was developed collaboratively by the Undersea and Hyperbaric Medical Society and the Centers for Disease Control and Prevention.

Results.—Among the 864 patients reported to receive hyperbaric oxygen treatment for unintentional, non–fire-related, carbon monoxide poisoning, most of the patients were white men aged between 18 and 44 years. Only 10% of patients reported the presence of a carbon monoxide alarm at their exposure location, and 75% reported being part of a group exposure. Nineteen patients (2%) reported a prior carbon monoxide exposure. About half (55%) of the patients treated were discharged after treatment; 41% were hospitalized.

Conclusions.—The findings in this report expand the knowledge about patients with carbon monoxide poisoning. These results suggest that prevention efforts, such as educating the public about using carbon monoxide alarms and targeting the most at-risk populations, may help reduce the number of exposures, the number of persons with chronic cognitive sequelae, and the resulting burden on the health care system.

▶ This article really underscores the need for carbon monoxide (CO) alarms. Most of the other findings are reiterations of what we already know about CO epidemiology. Ask your patients if they have a CO detector! Encourage your local emergency medical service and fire rescue squads to make this part of their public awareness campaigns—it really does help save lives.

R. J. Hamilton, MD

Noninvasive pulse CO-oximetry expedites evaluation and management of patients with carbon monoxide poisoning
Hampson NB (Virginia Mason Med Ctr, Seattle, WA)
Am J Emerg Med 30:2021-2024, 2012

Purposes.—Pulse CO-oximetry (Rad-57; Masimo Corp, Irvine, CA) has been available since 2005. To date, all published clinical studies have focused on clinical reliability and whether the device enhances case finding through screening of various populations. This study examines whether use of pulse CO-oximetry shortens the time to diagnosis and treatment of patients with carbon monoxide (CO) poisoning.

Basic Procedures.—Data from the joint Undersea and Hyperbaric Medical Society/Centers for Disease Control and Prevention CO poisoning surveillance system from August 2008 to July 2011 were analyzed. Of 1711 cases of CO poisoning treated with hyperbaric oxygen in the United States and reported through the system, 1606 had their initial carboxyhemoglobin (COHb) level measured by laboratory CO-oximetry and 105 by pulse CO-oximetry. Patients were selected from the laboratory CO-oximetry group to match each of the 105 patients evaluated by pulse CO-oximetry in 5 characteristics—age, sex, race/ethnicity, intent of poisoning, and occurrence of loss of consciousness. Measures of timeliness in measurement and management were compared between the 2 groups.

Main Findings.—Patients with initial COHb measurement by pulse CO-oximetry had significantly shorter time to measurement of COHb, higher average levels of COHb, and shorter time from the end of CO exposure to the initiation of hyperbaric oxygen treatment. On average, patients evaluated by pulse CO-oximetry reached the hyperbaric chamber 1 hour faster than did patients evaluated by laboratory CO-oximetry ($P < .01$).

Principle Conclusions.—Pulse CO-oximetry is associated with more rapid diagnosis and initiation of hyperbaric oxygen therapy in CO-poisoned patients compared with laboratory CO-oximetry. The impact on clinical outcome remains to be determined.

▶ This device is something that you think you don't need until you have a mass casualty event with exposures in multiple victims—then you have to have it. The study shows that it speeds up decision making and initiation of treatment.

R. J. Hamilton, MD

Carbon Monoxide Induces Cardiac Arrhythmia Via Induction of the Late Na$^+$ Current
Dallas ML, Yang Z, Boyle JP, et al (Univ of Leeds, UK; et al)
Am J Respir Crit Care Med 186:648-656, 2012

Rationale.—Clinical reports describe life-threatening cardiac arrhythmias after environmental exposure to carbon monoxide (CO) or accidental

CO poisoning. Numerous case studies describe disruption of repolarization and prolongation of the QT interval, yet the mechanisms underlying CO-induced arrhythmias are unknown.

Objectives.—To understand the cellular basis of CO-induced arrhythmias and to indentify an effective therapeutic approach.

Methods.—Patch-clamp electrophysiology and confocal Ca^{2+} and nitric oxide (NO) imaging in isolated ventricular myocytes was performed together with protein S-nitrosylation to investigate the effects of CO at the cellular and molecular levels, whereas telemetry was used to investigate effects of CO on electrocardiogram recordings *in vivo*.

Measurements and Main Results.—CO increased the sustained (late) component of the inward Na^+ current, resulting in prolongation of the action potential and the associated intracellular Ca^{2+} transient. In more than 50% of myocytes these changes progressed to early after-depolarization—like arrhythmias. CO elevated NO levels in myocytes and caused S-nitrosylation of the Na^+ channel, $Na_v1.5$. All proarrhythmic effects of CO were abolished by the NO synthase inhibitor L-NAME, and reversed by ranolazine, an inhibitor of the late Na^+ current. Ranolazine also corrected QT variability and arrhythmias induced by CO *in vivo*, as monitored by telemetry.

Conclusions.—Our data indicate that the proarrhythmic effects of CO arise from activation of NO synthase, leading to NO-mediated nitrosylation of $Na_v1.5$ and to induction of the late Na^+ current. We also show that the antianginal drug ranolazine can abolish CO-induced early after-depolarizations, highlighting a novel approach to the treatment of CO-induced arrhythmias.

▶ This is very interesting research on arrhythmogenic effects of carbon monoxide (CO). From a clinical perspective, I can't recall the last time I had a serious arrhythmia to deal with in a CO case. However, one of the essential theories of CO poisoning is that cardiac depression leads to syncope and begins a cascade of injurious central nervous system events. I wonder if this mechanism contributes to that as well. Still, it is very helpful to understand the arrhythmia mechanism and to have a readily available drug identified that will treat it.

R. J. Hamilton, MD

Safety and Cost-Effectiveness of a Clinical Protocol Implemented to Standardize the use of Crotalidae Polyvalent Immune Fab Antivenom at an Academic Medical Center

Weant KA, Bowers RC, Reed J, et al (Univ of Kentucky HealthCare, Lexington; et al)
Pharmacotherapy 32:433-440, 2012

Study Objective.—To evaluate the safety and cost-effectiveness of a clinical protocol adopted in June 2006 that included a comprehensive, objective assessment of snake bite envenomations and standardized the use of Crotalidae polyvalent immune Fab antivenom (FabAV).

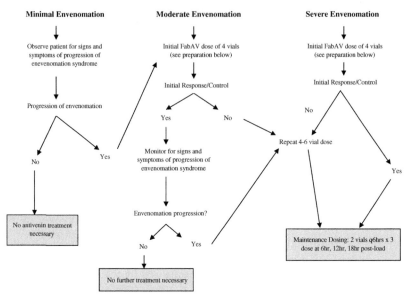

| Minimal Envenomation | Moderate Envenomation | Severe Envenomation |

FIGURE.—(Reprinted from Weant KA, Bowers RC, Reed J, et al. Safety and cost-effectiveness of a clinical protocol implemented to standardize the use of crotalidae polyvalent immune fab antivenom at an academic medical center. *Pharmacotherapy.* 2012;32:433-440, with permission from the American College of Clinical Pharmacology.)

Design.—Retrospective medical record review.

Setting.—Academic medical center that serves as the regional level I trauma center.

Patients.—Seventy-five adults treated with FabAV for snake envenomations in the emergency department between June 1, 2003, and June 1, 2009; 30 patients received treatment according to the protocol (treatment group), and 45 patients received treatment that did not adhere to the protocol (control group).

Measurements and Main Results.—Demographic and envenomation characteristics, as well as treatment details, were collected for all patients. In addition, information on quantity of FabAV vials required, length of hospital stay, and length of intensive care unit stay were compared between the treatment and control groups. In the treatment group, significantly fewer vials of FabAV were used (2.5 vs 4.727 vials, $p = 0.007$). This decreased in usage correlated to a cost savings of approximately $2000/patient. Despite no significant difference in the severity of the envenomations between the two groups ($p = 0.379$), the treatment group experienced a significantly shorter hospital length of stay (1.933 vs 2.791 days, $p = 0.030$). No significant difference in the progression to fasciotomy or the development of allergic reactions was noted between the two groups.

Conclusion.—Use of a clinical protocol related to snake envenomations resulted in approximately two fewer vials of FabAV required for each patient. In addition, the treatment group experienced a shorter hospital length of stay without a corresponding increase in adverse events or envenomation progression. Data show that use of the protocol was costeffective. The development of institution-specific multidisciplinary protocols regarding snake bite envenomations is recommended. Clinical pharmacists can play a vital role in the protocol development to ensure that optimal care is provided for this distinct patient population (Fig).

▶ I welcomed this article because as an infrequent treater of snakebites, I think I often make antivenom recommendations that lean toward overtreatment. Using the protocol in the Figure would save money and provide a solid framework for my approach.

R. J. Hamilton, MD

Acute kidney Injury in patients admitted to a liver intensive therapy unit with paracetamol-induced hepatotoxicity
O'Riordan A, Brummell Z, Sizer E, et al (King's College Hosp, London, UK)
Nephrol Dial Transplant 26:3501-3508, 2011

Background.—Paracetamol overdose can cause acute kidney injury (AKI) independent of its hepatotoxic effects. We aimed to determine the prevalence of AKI (AKI Network definition) in those with paracetamol-induced hepatotoxicity, identify factors associated with development, assess impact on the outcomes of patient survival and length of stay and determine the proportion of patients recovering renal function (estimated glomerular filtration rate > 60 mL/min) by the time of hospital discharge or transfer out.
Methods.—Between 2000 and 2007, patients admitted to a tertiary referral liver intensive therapy unit (LITU) with paracetamol-induced hepatotoxicity were identified from a prospectively maintained database and evaluated.
Results.—Those receiving a liver transplant were excluded ($n = 54$), leaving 302 patients. Renal function remained normal in 21%, the remainder developing AKI (Stages 1–8%, 2–6% and 3–65%). Vasopressor requirement, mechanical ventilation, higher admission phosphate and lower sodium levels along with a higher Day 3 lactate and lower haematocrit were associated with AKI. In survivors with AKI, 51% had recovery of renal function, while 7% remained dialysis dependant although none required it chronically. Overall, there was 25% mortality, all having Stage 3 AKI but AKI was only a univariate not multivariate predictor of reduced patient survival. AKI independently predicted longer length of stay.
Conclusions.—AKI is very common in critically ill patients with paracetamol-induced hepatotoxicity requiring LITU admission. Although outcomes are poorer with AKI than with normal renal function, they are better than those found in other intensive therapy unit populations. Gradual recovery of renal function is seen in all patients.

▶ Acute rheumatic fever was called a disease that "bites the heart and licks the joints." Rheumatoid arthritis "bites the joints and licks the heart." In the same vein, acetaminophen "bites the liver and licks the kidney." This article shows that acetaminophen-induced kidney injury and recovery follows a somewhat independent time course from what is happening with the liver.

R. J. Hamilton, MD

Octreotide for the treatment of sulfonylurea poisoning
Glatstein M, Scolnik D, Bentur Y (Tel Aviv Univ, Israel; Univ of Toronto, Ontario, Canada; Technion-Israel Inst of Technology, Haifa)
Clin Toxicol 50:795-804, 2012

Background.—Sulfonylureas are used extensively for treating type-2 diabetes mellitus. Sulfonylurea poisoning can produce sustained and profound hypoglycemia refractory to IV dextrose, particularly in children and the elderly.

Objective.—To review the use of octreotide, a long-acting somatostatin analog, in the treatment of sulfonylurea-induced hypoglycemia.

Methods.—A computerized search of U.S. National Academy of Medicine, Embase, PubMed and Toxline databases was undertaken using the keywords "octreotide", "sulfonylurea", "poisoning", "intoxication", "overdose" and "children". Textbooks of Clinical Toxicology and Pharmacology and the articles cited in their bibliographies were also searched. Twenty-four publications (19 articles and five conference abstracts) were identified; no publication was excluded.

Pharmacology of Octreotide.—Octreotide, a synthetic peptide analog of somatostatin, binds to G protein-coupled somatostatin-2 receptors in pancreatic beta-cells, resulting in decreased calcium influx and inhibition of insulin secretion. Octreotide markedly inhibited insulin secretion and decreased the number of hypoglycemic events and supplemental dextrose requirements in animal studies. In humans octreotide markedly inhibited insulin release, increased serum glucose concentration, reduced dextrose requirement, prevented recurrent hypoglycemia and was superior to IV dextrose and diazoxide after administration of sulfonylureas.

Efficacy of Octreotide in Pediatric Sulfonylurea Poisoning.—Fourteen pediatric patients were reported; 13 ingested second-generation sulfonylureas, with time to hypoglycemia of 1.5–16 hours. IV dextrose (10–25%) was administered before and after octreotide therapy. Octreotide was given after failure to correct hypoglycemia with IV dextrose in doses of 0.5–12 µg/kg IV or SC; two also required an IV octreotide infusion. Seven patients (50%) had recurrent hypoglycemia and received IV dextrose and additional octreotide.

Efficacy of Octreotide in Adult Sulfonylurea Poisoning.—Fifty-three patients were reported in prospective controlled (n = 22) and retrospective (n = 9) studies, case series (n = 6) and case reports. Fifty-one ingested second-generation sulfonylureas with time to hypoglycemia of 1–13 hours. All received IV dextrose (10–50%) before and after octreotide treatment. Octreotide 40–100 µg SC or IV was administered followed by additional doses in most patients; three patients also required an IV infusion. Octreotide significantly increased serum glucose concentrations, decreased dextrose requirement and recurrent hypoglycemic events compared with IV dextrose. Recurrent hypoglycemia was recorded in 22–50% of the patients treated with octreotide.

Therapeutic Recommendations.—Based on the published clinical and pharmacokinetic data of sulfonylureas and octreotide, we suggest the following dose regimens: in children, octreotide 1–1.5 μg/kg IV or SC, followed by 2–3 more doses 6 hours apart. In adults, octreotide 50 μg SC or IV, followed by three 50 μg doses every 6 hours. During this treatment IV dextrose infusion should be gradually tapered off.

Adverse Events.—Hypertension and apnea were recorded in one pediatric patient 30 minutes after IV octreotide; the relationship to octreotide is unclear. One adult patient with chronic renal failure treated with atenolol developed severe hyperkalemia.

Conclusions.—Although relatively limited, the available data suggest that octreotide should be considered first-line therapy in both pediatric and adult sulfonylurea poisoning with clinical and laboratory evidence of hypoglycemia. Maintenance doses of octreotide may be required to prevent recurrent hypoglycemia.

▶ This is a review article but does a nice job of coming up with concrete advice for managing sulfonylurea overdose and advancing the idea of using octreotide as first-line therapy. In fact, the cycle of hypoglycemia, dextrose bolus, insulin release, and recurrent hypoglycemia is where octreotide has its strongest role. Rather than enter into that cycle, just treat overdoses that develop hypoglycemia with octreotide.

R. J. Hamilton, MD

Unexpected late rise in plasma acetaminophen concentrations with change in risk stratification in acute acetaminophen overdoses
Dougherty PP, Klein-Schwartz W (Univ of Maryland School of Pharmacy, Baltimore)
J Emerg Med 43:58-63, 2012

Background.—The acetaminophen risk analysis nomogram is used to predict hepatotoxicity risk in acute acetaminophen overdose based on a single plasma acetaminophen concentration (PAC) measured between 4 and 24 h after ingestion. There are case reports of patients with acute overdoses of acetaminophen combination products in whom a toxic PAC occurred later after an initial non-toxic PAC at approximately 4 h.

Objectives.—The objective was to describe patients who had an initial non-toxic PAC and a subsequent toxic PAC.

Methods.—A poison center's database was searched for records in which patients were administered N-acetylcysteine. Cases were included if they involved an acute overdose of an acetaminophen-containing product with at least 2 plottable PACs, the first of which was obtained at least 4 h after ingestion and was below the treatment line on the nomogram with a subsequent toxic PAC. Data were analyzed for doses, timed PACs, specific acetaminophen preparation, coingestants, activated charcoal administration, and clinical effects.

Results.—Twenty patients were included. Thirteen patients ingested combination products. All patients experienced vomiting, neurologic, or cardiovascular effects at presentation or before obtaining the second PAC. Two patients developed hepatotoxicity, one of which died from the complications of acetaminophen-induced hepatotoxicity.

Conclusion.—The nomogram fails to predict toxicity based on a single PAC in a small subset of patients.

▶ Acetaminophen (APAP) overdose patients that "cross the nomogram line" are one of the most often discussed concerns of toxicologists. Any number of studies on kinetics of APAP preparations and APAP combination drugs show that virtually no patients should cross the nomogram line—once they have a nontoxic level at 4 hours. However, the practical matter is that determining the exact time of ingestion is not always easy. I believe that it is this error that results in a patient exhibiting prolonged clearance despite an early "nontoxic" level. Thus, if a patient arrives at midnight and says he or she took an overdose of APAP a few hours ago, when do you draw the level? I often suggest that the time range be based on the earliest possible time the patient could not have taken an overdose (seen with friends at dinner, for example) to the latest possible time the patient could have overdosed (discovered in room with pills). This creates an error bar for the start of the nomogram; in many cases, this is on the order of a half a day or so! Thus the judicious use of the nomogram and perhaps the judicious overuse of the antidote are what is indicated. This is preferable to me than deconstructing the Rumack Matthew nomogram, which has truly stood the test of time.

R. J. Hamilton, MD

Delayed Parkinsonism after CO Intoxication: Evaluation of the Substantia Nigra with Inversion-Recovery MR Imaging
Kao H-W, Cho N-Y, Hsueh C-J, et al (Natl Defense Med Ctr, Neihu, Taipei, Taiwan; et al)
Radiology 265:215-221, 2012

Purpose.—To quantitatively investigate signal alterations of the substantia nigra in patients with delayed parkinsonism following CO intoxication, as seen on gray matter (GM)-suppressed inversion-recovery (IR) magnetic resonance (MR) images.

Materials and Methods.—This prospective study was approved by the local institutional review board, and written informed consent was obtained from all subjects. Thirteen patients with delayed onset of CO-induced parkinsonism (nine men and four women; mean age, 40.3 years), 13 age-matched CO-intoxicated patients without parkinsonism, and 13

TABLE.—Summary of Clinical Variables and MR Imaging Findings of CO-intoxicated Patients

Patient No./Sex/ Age (y)	COHb (%)*	Major Clinical Symptoms	Lesion Location on MR Images	Modified H&Y Score
		CO-induced Parkinsonism		
1/F/29	0.6	Cognitive impairment, left limb weakness	Cerebral cortex, globus pallidus, white matter	2
2/M/47	16	Cognitive impairment	Globus pallidus, white matter	3
3/F/38	37.9	Bizarre behavior,	Globus pallidus	1
4/M/45	31.7	Bizarre behavior, urinary and fecal incontinence, cognitive impairment	Cerebellum, white matter	1.5
5/M/39	Not available	Bizarre behavior	Globus pallidus, white matter	4
6/M/49	Not available	Unremarkable	Globus pallidus, white matter	2.5
7/F/48	0.1	Cognitive impairment	Globus pallidus, white matter	3
8/F/22	2.8	Bizarre behavior, mutism, right limb weakness	Cerebral cortex, globus pallidus, white matter	1
9/M/31	38	Bizarre behavior, cognitive impairment	Globus pallidus, white matter	1
10/M/28	28	Unremarkable	Globus pallidus	1
11/M/43	16	Bizarre behavior	Globus pallidus, white matter	3
12/M/37	Not available	Bizarre behavior, cognitive impairment	White matter	1
13/M/68	45.5	Cognitive impairment	Globus pallidus	1
		CO Intoxication without Parkinsonism		
1/F/26	11.6	Disorientation, cognitive impairment	Globus pallidus, white matter	Not applicable
2/ M/45	16.3	Unremarkable	Globus pallidus	Not applicable
3/F/31	2.6	Bizarre behavior, cognitive impairment	Unremarkable	Not applicable
4/M/45	Not available	Bizarre behavior	Globus pallidus	Not applicable
5/M/39	21.3	Cognitive impairment	Unremarkable	Not applicable
6/M/50	10.2	Cognitive impairment	Cerebellum, globus pallidus	Not applicable
7/F/49	1.8	Unremarkable	Cerebral cortex	Not applicable
8/F/24	34.2	Cognitive impairment	White matter	Not applicable
9/M/31	13.2	Bizarre behavior	White matter	Not applicable
10/M/27	48.9	Unremarkable	Globus pallidus, white matter	Not applicable
11/F/43	24	Cognitive impairment, urinary incontinence	Globus pallidus, white matter	Not applicable
12/M/30	42.2	Unremarkable	Globus pallidus, white matter	Not applicable
13/M/59	48	Cognitive impairment	White matter	Not applicable

*COHb = carboxyhemoglobin.

age-matched healthy volunteers were examined with GM-suppressed IR MR imaging. The signal intensity of the substantia nigra was normalized to the adjacent normal-appearing white matter in the temporal lobe, followed by semiautomatic segmentation into medial, middle, and lateral parts by using a skeleton-based algorithm. Multivariate and univariate analyses and Spearman rank correlation test were performed to examine the relationships between variables. Clinical severity was assessed with the modified Hoehn and Yahr rating scale.

Results.—The normalized signal ratios in the middle and lateral segments of the substantia nigra were significantly higher in those with CO-induced parkinsonism, compared with those with CO intoxication without parkinsonism or normal volunteers ($P =.02$). For the medial segments, the ratios showed no significant differences among the groups. The normalized signal ratios of substantia nigra were correlated with the severity of parkinsonism, particularly in the lateral segments ($\rho = 0.927$, $P < .001$).

Conclusion.—CO toxicity to the substantia nigra plays a role in pathophysiologic mechanisms of CO-induced parkinsonism. GM-suppressed IR MR imaging is a useful tool in depicting substantia nigra injury following CO intoxication (Table).

▶ The enclosed Table and Fig 2 in the original article are useful data to add to the growing role of magnetic resonance (MR) imaging in diagnosing central nervous system injury from toxins, and especially from carbon monoxide. So far, I have not found any imaging techniques that can identify which toxin caused the parkinsonism and its relevant changes on MR.

R. J. Hamilton, MD

Increased Carbon Monoxide Clearance During Exercise in Humans
Zavorsky GS, Smoliga JM, Longo LD, et al (Marywood Univ, Scranton, PA; High Point Univ, NC; Loma Linda Univ, CA; et al)
Med Sci Sports Exerc 44:2118-2124, 2012

Purpose.—Hyperventilation increases the clearance of carbon monoxide (CO) from blood; thus, we hypothesized that CO elimination would be enhanced with exercise. Accordingly, this study examined the effect of exercise on the half-life of carboxyhemolobin elimination.

Methods.—Six healthy subjects (three males and three females) with mean ± SD ages of 23 ± 4 yr were exposed to CO sufficient to raise blood carboxyhemolobin concentration to 10–14% on five separate days. The half-life for CO elimination was measured breathing room air at rest and during exercise at three intensities.

Results.—Comparisons showed that the half-life decreased with exercise from that during rest in all subjects. The half-life was also measured during 100% oxygen breathing at the lowest exercise intensity of 63 ± 15 W and found to be the least of all measured (23 ± 4 min).

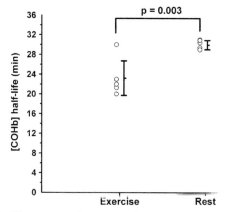

FIGURE 4.—The comparison between $t_{1/2}$ obtained in this present study using light exercise (63 W) versus the predicted $t_{1/2}$ from Takeuchi et al. (16) without exercise, matched for the same $\dot{V}_E$ and 95% to 100% O_2 supplementation. The *circles* represent the actual and matched data. The *whiskers* represent the mean and SD. $t_{1/2}$ from Takeuchi = $21 + [5059 \, (1/\dot{V}_E)]$, adjusted $r^2 = 0.87$, SEE = 9.9 min, $F(1,14) = 103$, $P < 0.001$. *Editor's Note*: Please refer to original journal article for full references. (Reprinted from Zavorsky GS, Smoliga JM, Longo LD, et al. Increased carbon monoxide clearance during exercise in humans. *Med Sci Sports Exerc.* 2012;44:2118-2124, with permission from the American College of Sports Medicine.)

Conclusions.—1) Exercise increased isocapnic ventilation, thereby decreasing the half-life of CO elimination. 2) The half-life of CO elimination represents a hyperbolic function of ventilation $[y = y0 + (a/x)]$, and so increasing ventilation by exercise reaches a point of diminishing returns. 3) Breathing 100% oxygen during mild exercise is as effective in eliminating CO as treatment with hyperbaric oxygen. 4) Moderate exercise under room air conditions is as effective in eliminating CO as breathing oxygen at rest. Thus, the combination of mild exercise, hyperventilation, and normobaric hyperoxia (100% oxygen inhalation) may be considered the "triple therapy" for CO elimination in some patients (Fig 4).

▶ The authors most definitely prove their hypothesis that exercise will hasten the elimination of carboxyhemoglobin as seen in Fig 4. The only concern I have about the applicability of this concept is that exercising in the relative hypoxia of carbon monoxide (CO) poisoning may not be safe given the combined effects of metabolic poisoning by CO and decreased oxyhemoglobin availability. Still, if I thought I had developed CO poisoning in a wilderness situation, a brisk walk in the fresh air would be a wise choice.

R. J. Hamilton, MD

The clinical toxicology of gamma-hydroxybutyrate, gamma-butyrolactone and 1,4-butanediol

Schep LJ, Knudsen K, Slaughter RJ, et al (Univ of Otago, Dunedin, New Zealand; Sahlgrenska Univ Hosp, Gothenburg, Sweden; et al)
Clin Toxicol 50:458-470, 2012

Introduction.—Gamma-hydroxybutyrate (GHB) and its precursors, gamma-butyrolactone (GBL) and 1,4-butanediol (1,4-BD), are drugs of abuse which act primarily as central nervous system (CNS) depressants. In recent years, the rising recreational use of these drugs has led to an increasing burden upon health care providers. Understanding their toxicity is therefore essential for the successful management of intoxicated patients. We review the epidemiology, mechanisms of toxicity, toxicokinetics, clinical features, diagnosis, and management of poisoning due to GHB and its analogs and discuss the features and management of GHB withdrawal.

Methods.—OVID MEDLINE and ISI Web of Science databases were searched using the terms "GHB," "gamma-hydroxybutyrate," "gamma-hydroxybutyric acid," "4-hydroxybutanoic acid," "sodium oxybate," "gamma-butyrolactone," "GBL," "1,4-butanediol," and "1,4-BD" alone

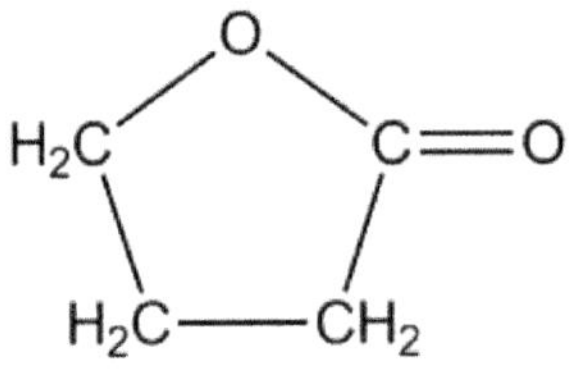

γ-Butyrolactone

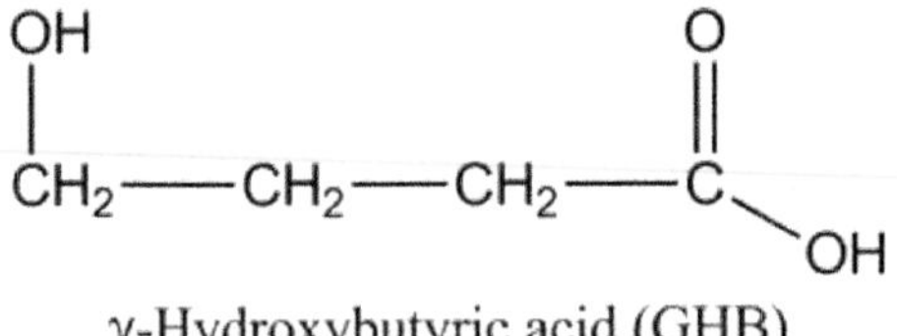

γ-Hydroxybutyric acid (GHB)

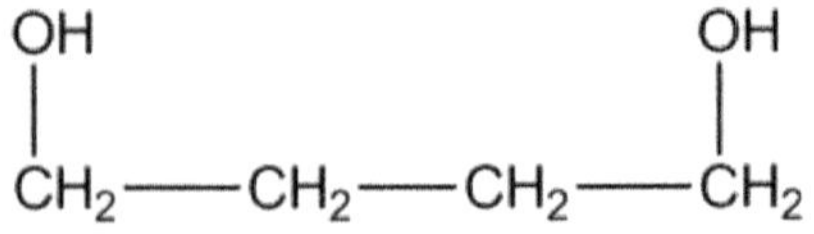

1, 4-Butanediol

FIGURE 1.—The chemical structures of gamma-butyrolactone, gammahydroxybutyric acid and 1, 4-butanediol. (Reprinted from Schep LJ, Knudsen K, Slaughter RJ, et al. The clinical toxicology of gamma-hydroxybutyrate, gamma-butyrolactone and 1,4-butanediol. *Clin Toxicol.* 2012;50:458-470, reprinted by permission of Taylor & Francis Ltd, http://www.tandf.co.uk/journals.)

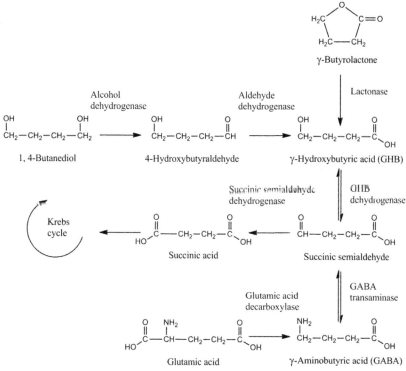

FIGURE 2.—A summary of the metabolic pathway of gamma-hydroxybutyrate. (Reprinted from Schep LJ, Knudsen K, Slaughter RJ, et al. The clinical toxicology of gamma-hydroxybutyrate, gamma-butyrolactone and 1,4-butanediol. *Clin Toxicol.* 2012;50.458-470, reprinted by permission of Taylor & Francis Ltd, http://www.tandf.co.uk/journals.)

and in combination with the keywords "pharmacokinetics," "kinetics," "poisoning," "poison," "toxicity," "ingestion," "adverse effects," "overdose," and "intoxication." In addition, bibliographies of identified articles were screened for additional relevant studies including nonindexed reports. Non-peer-reviewed sources were also included: books, relevant newspaper reports, and applicable Internet resources. These searches produced 2059 nonduplicate citations of which 219 were considered relevant.

Epidemiology.—There is limited information regarding statistical trends on world-wide use of GHB and its analogs. European data suggests that the use of GHB is generally low; however, there is some evidence of higher use among some sub-populations, settings, and geographical areas. In the United States of America, poison control center data have shown that enquiries regarding GHB have decreased between 2002 and 2010 suggesting a decline in use over this timeframe.

Mechanisms of Action.—GHB is an endogenous neurotransmitter synthesized from glutamate with a high affinity for GHB-receptors, present on both on pre-and postsynaptic neurons, thereby inhibiting GABA release.

In overdose, GHB acts both directly as a partial GABAb receptor agonist and indirectly through its metabolism to form GABA.

Toxicokinetics.—GHB is rapidly absorbed by the oral route with peak blood concentrations typically occurring within 1 hour. It has a relatively small volume of distribution and is rapidly distributed across the bloodbrain barrier. GHB is metabolized primarily in the liver and is eliminated rapidly with a reported 20–60 minute half-life. The majority of a dose is eliminated completely within 4–8 hours. The related chemicals, 1,4-butanediol and gamma butyrolactone, are metabolized endogenously to GHB.

Clinical Features of Poisoning.—GHB produces CNS and respiratory depression of relatively short duration. Other commonly reported features include gastrointestinal upset, bradycardia, myoclonus, and hypothermia. Fatalities have been reported.

Management of Poisoning.—Supportive care is the mainstay of management with primary emphasis on respiratory and cardiovascular support. Airway protection, intubation, and/or assisted ventilation may be indicated for severe respiratory depression. Gastrointestinal decontamination is unlikely to be beneficial. Pharmacological intervention is rarely required for bradycardia; however, atropine administration may occasionally be warranted.

Withdrawal Syndrome.—Abstinence after chronic use may result in a withdrawal syndrome, which may persist for days in severe cases. Features include auditory and visual hallucinations, tremors, tachycardia, hypertension, sweating, anxiety, agitation, paranoia, insomnia, disorientation, confusion, and aggression/combativeness. Benzodiazepine administration appears to be the treatment of choice, with barbiturates, baclofen, or propofol as second line management options.

Conclusions.—GHB poisoning can cause potentially life-threatening CNS and respiratory depression, requiring appropriate, symptom-directed supportive care to ensure complete recovery. Withdrawal from GHB may continue for up to 21 days and can be life-threatening, though treatment with benzodiazepines is usually effective (Figs 1 and 2).

▶ A nice review of gamma-hydroxybutyrate and its precursors. In my experience, these drugs are on the decline. Figs 1 and 2 round out the review.

R. J. Hamilton, MD

Life-treatening necrotizing fasciitis due to 'bath salts' injection
Russo R, Marks N, Morris K, et al (Louisiana State Univ Health Sciences Ctr, New Orleans)
Orthopedics 35:e124-e127, 2012

Necrotizing fasciitis is an orthopedic emergency. The ability to quickly and accurately diagnose this rapidly spreading disease can save a patient's life and limb. However, the diagnosis is complex because necrotizing fasciitis usually manifests as a less severe cellulitis or abscess while the majority of the damages rage beneath the surface of the skin. Although the diagnosis is not new, the potential causes and vectors continually change. This article reports a new source of necrotizing fasciitis in an intramuscular injection of "bath salts," a rapidly emerging street drug that is legal in some states and evades authorities with its innocuous name. The patient presented 2 days after injection of bath salts with extensive cellulitis extending to the mid portion of her upper arm. The cellulitis initially responded to broad-spectrum intravenous antibiotics, but rapidly deteriorated 48 hours later, leading to a forequarter amputation with radical mastectomy and chest wall debridement to obtain healthy tissue margins and control the disease. The patient made a full recovery after further minor debridements, negative pressure dressings, directed antibiotic therapy, and skin grafting. The recent emerging popularity of this highly obtainable, injectable substance may lead to an increase in cases of necrotizing fasciitis. Orthopedic surgeons should be vigilant in diagnosing this process early and should perform an extensive debridement.

▶ Bath salts are further evidence of the ever-evolving illicit drug epidemic. Sold as seemingly innocuous bath additives or plant food, these synthetic sympathomimetic substances have stimulant-like effects and can result in paranoia and delusions. The attached case report describes the initial presentation of a patient with complications related to intramuscular injection of bath salts and the subsequent deterioration to necrotizing fasciitis. With aggressive initial management of the cellulitis with broad-spectrum intravenous antibiotics, the patient improved over the next 2 days. Despite appropriate interventions, the patient rapidly worsened, developing skin sloughing and purulent drainage from the site. The patient rapidly received radical surgical debridement and underwent a protracted postoperative course. The case report emphasizes the sudden downward spiral in the face of appropriate interventions and apparent clinical improvement. The authors further advocate for the use of intravenous penicillin G and clindamycin as a crucial components of the treatment plan. The treating emergency physician should be vigilant in the evaluation of these challenging patients and should consider in-hospital observation. Even with detailed discharge instructions, these patients may not be reliable enough to comply with the directions.

E. C. Bruno, MD

13 Emergency Center Activities

Atraumatic headache in US emergency departments: recent trends in CT/ MRI utilisation and factors associated with severe intracranial pathology
Gilbert JW, Johnson KM, Larkin GL, et al (Yale School of Medicine, New Haven, CT)
Emerg Med J 29:576-581, 2012

Objectives.—To estimate recent trends in CT/MRI utilisation among patients seeking emergency care for atraumatic headache in the USA and to identify factors associated with a diagnosis of significant intracranial pathology (ICP) in these patients.

Design/Setting/Participants.—Data were obtained from the USA National Hospital Ambulatory Medical Care Survey of emergency department (ED) visits between 1998 and 2008. A cohort of atraumatic headache-related visits were identified using preassigned 'reason-for-visit' codes. Sample visits were weighted to provide national estimates.

Results.—Between 1998 and 2008 the percentage of patients presenting to the ED with atraumatic headache who underwent imaging increased from 12.5% to 31.0% ($p < 0.01$) while the prevalence of ICP among those visits decreased from 10.1% to 3.5% ($p < 0.05$). The length of stay in the ED was 4.6 h (95% CI 4.4 to 4.8) for patients with headache who received imaging compared with 2.7 (95% CI 2.6 to 2.9) for those who did not. Of 18 factors evaluated in patients with headache, 10 were associated with a significantly increased odds of an ICP diagnosis: age $\geq$ 50 years, arrival by ambulance, triage immediacy < 15 min, systolic blood pressure $\geq$ 160 mm Hg or diastolic blood pressure $\geq$ 100 mm Hg and disturbance in sensation, vision, speech or motor function including neurological weakness

Conclusions.—The use of CT/MRI for evaluation of atraumatic headache increased dramatically in EDs in the USA between 1998 and 2008. The prevalence of ICP among patients who received CT/MRI declined concurrently, suggesting a role for clinical decision support to guide more judicious use of imaging.

▶ The authors of this database review conclude that emergency physicians are increasingly ordering diagnostic imaging for the evaluation of patients with atraumatic headaches. Encompassing the decade of patients, they found that computed tomography of the head (CT head) and magnetic resonance imaging of the brain

(MRI brain) have increased from 12.5% to 31.0%, although intracranial pathology has decreased from 10.1% to 3.5%. The increased utilization is, in part, explained by resource availability and quality. More facilities have the capability to perform the tests, and 24-hour reporting makes ordering the imaging study a less arduous decision. The unrelenting malpractice climate and its defensive medical practice repercussions also undoubtedly contribute to the number of diagnostic procedures performed. Patients do not escape blame, occasionally demanding the imaging and describing their symptoms as "the worst headache of my life" to maximize pharmaceutical response by the treating physician. National organizations may benefit and defend their memberships, providing reasonable practice guidelines regarding the ordering of diagnostic imaging in patients with atraumatic headaches.

E. C. Bruno, MD

Fetal loss in symptomatic first-trimester pregnancy with documented yolk sac intrauterine pregnancy
Hessert MJ, Juliano M (Naval Med Ctr Portsmouth, VA)
Am J Emerg Med 30:399-404, 2012

Background.—The possibility of spontaneous miscarriage is a common concern among pregnant women in the emergency department (ED).

Objective.—This study sought to determine fetal outcomes for women following ED evaluation for firsttrimester abdominopelvic pain or vaginal bleeding who had an intrauterine pregnancy (IUP) on ultrasound before a visible fetal pole ("yolk sac IUP").

Methods.—A retrospective chart review of consecutive ED charts from December 2005 to September 2006 identified patients with a yolk sac IUP. Demographic data, obstetric/gynecologic history, and presenting symptoms were obtained. Outcomes were determined via computerized records. Fetal loss was diagnosed by falling β-human chorionic gonadotropin or pathology specimen. Live birth was diagnosed by viable fetus at 20-week ultrasound or delivery.

Results.—A total of 131 patients were enrolled in this study. Of these, 14 were lost to follow-up (12%), leaving 117 patient encounters. Of the 117 women, 82 carried their pregnancies to at least 20-week gestation. Thirty-five patients miscarried. Fetal loss rate by chief complaint were as follows: 8 of 46 patients presenting with pain only, 14 of 34 presenting with vaginal bleeding only, and 13 of 37 with both vaginal bleeding and pain.

Conclusion.—Seventy percent of women diagnosed with a yolk sac IUP in the ED carried their pregnancy to at least 20 weeks. The remaining women (30%) experienced fetal loss. Vaginal bleeding (with or without pain) increased the rate of fetal loss compared with women with pain only. These data will assist the emergency physician in counseling women with symptomatic first-trimester pregnancies.

▶ Female patients commonly present with concerns surrounding their early pregnancy. While the patients focus on pregnancy conception date, duration, viability, and sometimes sex, emergency physicians center in on the location, ectopic or not. Once an intrauterine pregnancy (IUP) has been identified, in the presence of pain and/or vaginal bleeding, patients will routinely return to queries about viability. Using obstetrical and gynecology baselines that cite a 20% to 25% spontaneous abortion rate in all pregnancies and a 3% to 6% rate once the IUP is determined, the authors of this retrospective review looked to determine how often women would carry the pregnancy to term (beyond 20 weeks) if an IUP was established during the emergency department visit. Pregnant patients with a documented IUP had to be symptomatic, excluding those who ventured to the emergency department just to get the urine human chorionic gonadotropin test. Thirty percent of the included patients encountered spontaneous miscarriage, which is higher than previously reported. Vaginal bleeding also increased the frequency of abortion (41% vs 17%). These results do not impact clinical practice in terms of an intervention but emergency physicians can give realistic information to uneasy patients.

E. C. Bruno, MD

Impact of physician-assisted triage on timing of antibiotic delivery in patients admitted to the hospital with community-acquired pneumonia (CAP)
Capp R, Soremekun OA, Biddinger PD, et al (Brigham & Women's Hosp and Massachusetts General Hosp, Boston; Harvard Med School, Boston, MA)
J Emerg Med 43:502-508, 2012

Background.—Time to antibiotic delivery in patients with diagnosis of pneumonia is a publicly reported quality measure.

Objective.—We aim to describe the impact of emergency department (ED) physician-assisted triage (PAT) on The Joint Commission (TJC) and Centers for Medicare and Medicaid Services (CMS) pneumonia core quality measures of timing to antibiotic delivery.

Methods.—Retrospective case series studies of patients admitted to the hospital through the ED with diagnosis of community-acquired pneumonia were identified over a period of 48 months. Patients were included in the study if they met TJC/CMS PN-5 (antibiotic timing) criteria. We compared antibiotic delivery timing before and after implementation of PAT in moderate-acuity patients using Wilcoxon rank sum tests. A linear regression analysis was done to account for age, sex, ED volume, and acuity level.

Results.—A total of 659 patients were identified: 497 patients and 162 patients enrolled pre- and post-implementation of a PAT, respectively. The median antibiotic delivery times for moderate-acuity patients during open hours of operation of PAT were 180 min (pre) and 195 min (post), $p = 0.027$; this was unchanged when ED volume, age, sex, and acuity level were accounted for. A total of 43 patients (9%) and 13 patients (8%) failed to receive antibiotics within 6 h of ED presentation before and after implementation of PAT, respectively.

Conclusion.—In this study, implementation of PAT did not result in overall decrease in antibiotic delivery time in patients admitted to the hospital with CAP. We postulate several explanations for this delay in antibiotic delivery time.

▶ Since at least 2004 when The Joint Commission (TJC) and Centers for Medicare and Medicaid Services (CMS) began to require that emergency department (ED) patients admitted with a diagnosis of community-acquired pneumonia (CAP) receive antibiotics within 4 hours, hospitals have implemented various systems of care to achieve this goal. In 2007, TJC/CMS lengthened the requirement to 6 hours and included a question of diagnostic uncertainty to account for limitations in diagnosis of pneumonia in the ED. Nevertheless, many EDs are still unable to meet the antibiotic time limit, and it has been postulated that the delay in antibiotic administration is caused by a delay in physician evaluation. Previous investigations have found that having a physician in triage who can provide a rapid evaluation and begin an appropriate workup will improve ED performance metrics such as ED length of stay, time spent on ambulance diversion, and patients who leave without being seen; however, the effect on quality measures has not been researched.

This study from the Division of Emergency Medicine at Harvard Medical School shows that after the implementation of physician-assisted triage, the median antibiotic delivery times actually increased by 15 minutes. Further analysis with linear regression discovered that an increased ED volume was the main predictor in the delay of antibiotic delivery in patients with CAP. The major limitation of a study like this is the before and after design. Confounding variables, in this case increased ED volume, may obscure any effect from the intervention.

The result from this analysis seems to suggest that physician-assisted triage will not have a beneficial effect on quality measures. However, we do not know what would have happened without this change in the ED operational flow; perhaps the time to antibiotics would have increased even more. Further study into the effect of physician-assisted triage on quality measures appears warranted.

E. A. Ramoska, MD, MPHE

Characteristics of frequent geriatric users of an urban emergency department
Wajnberg A, Hwang U, Torres L, et al (Mount Sinai School of Medicine, NY)
J Emerg Med 43:376-381, 2012

Background.—As the population ages, it is projected that older adults will increase emergency department (ED) utilization and contribute to ED crowding. Older patients are at risk of decreased health-related quality of life after an ED visit. Characteristics of older adults that frequently use the ED have not been well studied, and prior studies have shown that lack of access to primary care may influence ED utilization.

Objective.—Determine factors associated with frequent Emergency Department (ED) utilization by older adults.

Methods.—Retrospective chart review of all patients ≥ 65 years of age seen in an urban ED between December 2007 and September 2008. A prospective telephone survey was done of "frequent" (≥4 ED visits over a 6-month period) geriatric users. "Frequent" and "infrequent" geriatric ED users were compared using chi-squared and *t*-test. Survey results are univariate descriptive statistics.

Results.—There were 8520 ED visits of adults ≥ 65 years of age analyzed, of which 5718 were unique patients. Of these, 268 (5%) were frequent ED users. Frequent geriatric ED users were more likely to be Black or Hispanic and were considered less urgent at triage. Of the 59 surveyed frequent users of the ED, 95% reported having a usual source of care, though only 36% contacted their outpatient provider before a visit to the ED.

Conclusion.—Frequent geriatric users of the ED were considered less urgent at triage, and although most identified themselves as having a primary care provider in the community, many did not contact them before going to the ED.

▶ This study, like others of its kind, is useful for understanding why certain patients use the emergency department (ED) more frequently than others. The results suggest that frequent geriatric users are not all that different from nonfrequent geriatric users. The authors did find that black and Hispanic patients were more likely to be frequent users when compared with white patients; however, the authors admit that this may be the result of the location of their particular ED. In addition, the authors' analysis revealed that frequent ED users had a higher emergency severity index (ESI) triage score (higher scores are considered less urgent) than infrequent users; however, the difference was only 0.11 on the 5-point ESI scale. Although this may be a statistically different result, whether it is clinically significant is uncertain. Frequent ED users also were more likely to have problems related to cardiac or pulmonary conditions when compared to infrequent ED users, which certainly makes intuitive sense since cardiopulmonary disease is quite prevalent in this population. There were no significant differences in age, gender, or the rates of hospital admission or mortality in the ED between frequent and nonfrequent ED users.

Contrary to the common assumption that frequent ED users may lack health insurance or access to primary care, this admittedly small prospective survey (only 59 of the 148 patients eligible for telephone survey) revealed that the vast majority of patients did indeed have health insurance (92%) and a usual source of primary care (95%). Reasons that may have contributed to frequent ED use by these geriatric patients were related to perceptions about the ED providing better care, the ease of access to a vast array of diagnostic tests and other resources (one-stop shopping), and a lack of knowledge about or difficulty navigating the primary care telephone system. For many of these patients, the use of the ED may be an affirmative choice rather than a provider of last resort.

E. A. Ramoska, MD, MPHE

A National Depiction of Children With Return Visits to the Emergency Department Within 72 Hours, 2001–2007

Cho CS, Shapiro DJ, Cabana MD, et al (Univ of California, San Francisco; et al)
Pediatr Emerg Care 28:606-610, 2012

Objectives.—The objectives of this study were to estimate the frequency of pediatric 72-hour return visits (RVs) to the emergency department (ED) between 2001 and 2007 and to determine demographic and clinical characteristics associated with these RVs.

Methods.—Data from the National Hospital Ambulatory Medical Care Survey between 2001 and 2007 were analyzed to estimate the frequency of RVs to EDs by children. Patient demographics and clinical variables were compared for RVs and non-RVs using the χ^2 test; RVs were further characterized using multivariable logistic regression.

Results.—Between 2001 and 2007, there was an annual average of 698,000 RVs by children (2.7% of all ED visits). The RV rate significantly increased from 2001 to 2007. Factors associated with an RV included age younger than 1 year or 13 to 18 years, arrival to the ED between 7 A.M. and 3 P.M., recent discharge from the hospital, and western region of the United States. During ED RVs, a complete blood count was more likely to be obtained, and the patient was more likely to be admitted. Insurance was not associated with an RV to the ED. On RV, patients were less likely to have a diagnosis related to trauma or injury.

Conclusions.—Analysis of the National Hospital Ambulatory Medical Care Survey database offers a national perspective into ED RVs in children. In this era of increasing utilization, these results can help physicians and policy makers address the unique needs of this population and create interventions that will optimize patient service while attempting to control potentially unnecessary RVs.

▶ This report does not propose firm recommendations about how to address pediatric 72-hour return visits (RVs), but offers an assessment of the current national state of affairs with regard to this issue. RVs within 72 hours accounted for 3.0% of all visits to emergency departments nationally in 2001 and 3.8% of visits in 2007 according to the National Hospital Ambulatory Medical Care Survey (NHAMCS). Pediatric (younger than 19 years old) 72-hour RVs were at 2.6% in 2001 and increased to 3.6% in 2007, according to this study. So RVs appear to be increasing both generally and in the pediatric population.

This analysis reveals that both infants (younger than 1 year of age) and teenagers (13–18 years old) were associated with an increased RV rate. The diagnosis category for symptoms/signs/ill-defined conditions was more common in the 72-hour RVs than in non-RVs, whereas the diagnosis categories for injury/poisoning and asthma were less common. The diagnosis category for infection did not differ significantly between the 2 types of visits. Interestingly, 72-hour RVs were more likely to have a complete blood count and be admitted to the hospital than non-RVs, but they were less likely to use diagnostic imaging. The complete blood count was used as a proxy for blood work as it is one of the most common blood tests and is included in the NHAMCS data collection form.

E. A. Ramoska, MD, MPHE

Answering the myth: use of emergency services on Friday the 13th
Lo BM, Visintainer CM, Best HA, et al (Eastern Virginia Med School, Norfolk)
Am J Emerg Med 30:886-889, 2012

Objective.—The aim of the study was to evaluate the risk of Friday the 13th on hospital admission rates and emergency department (ED) visits.

Methods.—This was a retrospective chart review of all ED visits on Friday the 13th from November 13, 2002, to December 13, 2009, from 6 hospital-based EDs. Thirteen unlikely conditions were evaluated as well as total ED volumes. As a control, the Friday before and after and the month before and after were used. χ^2 Analysis and Wilcoxon rank sum tests were used for each variable, as appropriate.

Results.—A total of 49 094 patient encounters were evaluated. Average ED visits for Friday the 13th were not increased compared with the Friday before and after and the month before. However, compared with the month after, there were fewer ED visits on Friday the 13th (150.1 vs 134.7, $P = .011$). Of the 13 categories evaluated, only penetrating trauma was noted to have an increase risk associated with Friday the 13th (odds ratio, 1.65; 95% confidence interval, 1.04-2.61). No other category was noted to have an increase risk on Friday the 13th compared with the control dates.

Conclusions.—Although the fear of Friday the 13th may exist, there is no worry that an increase in volume occurs on Friday the 13th compared with the other days studies. Of 13 different conditions evaluated, only penetrating traumas were seen more often on Friday the 13th. For those providers who work in the ED, working on Friday the 13th should not be any different than any other day.

▶ When I saw the title of this article, I knew I wanted to read it. We all know someone who is a "black cloud" and it seems whenever he or she is working, all sorts of badness ensues. Likewise, you should never bring a book to read or some paperwork to complete, because that is just going to make the shift busy. And finally, there is the "Q" word—never, ever say it is quiet in the emergency department. Everyone from the medical director to the nurses, techs, secretary, housekeeping to security know that will cause all sorts of maladies to present in short order. It seems that highly educated and otherwise rational medical care professionals are superstitious.

This study from Eastern Virginia Medical School looked at 13 categories of medical conditions that presented on 13 consecutive Fridays that fall on the 13th. They discovered that Friday the 13th was no busier than the week before or the week after; in fact it was slower than the Friday 1 month after. There were no more acute coronary syndromes, strokes, seizures, motor vehicle crashes, animal bites, or psychiatric evaluations on Friday the 13th when compared with other Fridays. There were slightly more penetrating traumas, however. So it seems that if you are lucky enough to be scheduled to work on a Friday the 13th, you have nothing to fear. Then again, there is still that full moon to contend with.

E. A. Ramoska, MD, MPHE

Diagnostic and Prognostic Stratification in the Emergency Department Using Urinary Biomarkers of Nephron Damage: A Multicenter Prospective Cohort Study

Nickolas TL, Schmidt-Ott KM, Canetta P, et al (Columbia Univ College of Physicians and Surgeons, NY; et al)
J Am Coll Cardiol 59:246-255, 2012

Objectives.—This study aimed to determine the diagnostic and prognostic value of urinary biomarkers of intrinsic acute kidney injury (AKI) when patients were triaged in the emergency department.

Background.—Intrinsic AKI is associated with nephron injury and results in poor clinical outcomes. Several urinary biomarkers have been proposed to detect and measure intrinsic AKI.

Methods.—In a multicenter prospective cohort study, 5 urinary biomarkers (urinary neutrophil gelatinase—associated lipocalin, kidney injury molecule-1, urinary liver-type fatty acid binding protein, urinary interleukin-18, and cystatin C) were measured in 1,635 unselected emergency department patients at the time of hospital admission. We determined whether the biomarkers diagnosed intrinsic AKI and predicted adverse outcomes during hospitalization.

Results.—All biomarkers were elevated in intrinsic AKI, but urinary neutrophil gelatinase—associated lipocalin was most useful (81% specificity, 68% sensitivity at a 104-ng/ml cutoff) and predictive of the severity and duration of AKI. Intrinsic AKI was strongly associated with adverse in-hospital outcomes. Urinary neutrophil gelatinase—associated lipocalin and urinary kidney injury molecule 1 predicted a composite outcome of dialysis initiation or death during hospitalization, and both improved the net risk classification compared with conventional assessments. These biomarkers also identified a substantial subpopulation with low serum creatinine at hospital admission, but who were at risk of adverse events.

Conclusions.—Urinary biomarkers of nephron damage enable prospective diagnostic and prognostic stratification in the emergency department.

▶ This study was supported by Abbott Laboratories and evaluated the utility of various urinary biomarkers to diagnose intrinsic acute kidney injury (AKI) and to predict hospital course. AKI is a common clinical event occurring in up to 1 million hospitalized patients each year in the United States. It is associated with severe consequences including chronic kidney disease, dialysis, and death. About one-third of the patients in this study who were diagnosed with intrinsic AKI experienced the composite outcome of in-hospital mortality or the requirement to initiate in-hospital hemodialysis, whereas less than 4% of patients with normal kidney function, stable chronic kidney disease, or prerenal AKI experienced this outcome. Having a urinary biomarker that could help to identify patients who would be at risk for intrinsic AKI would be helpful. These biomarkers are certainly not ready for prime time yet; however, once one is found to be clinically useful and an easy to use assay is developed, then expect a company representative to tout them as the next miracle test that you have to have.

E. A. Ramoska, MD, MPHE

Emergency Medical Services for Children: The New Jersey Model
Sacchetti A, Kelly-Goodstein N, Sweeney R, et al (Our Lady of Lourdes Med Ctr, Camden; Dept of Health and Senior Services Trenton, NJ; Jersey Shore Univ Med Ctr, Neptune, NJ; et al)
Pediatr Emerg Care 28:310-312, 2012

Identification of specific facilities within a community for the emergency department (ED) treatment of children is a traditional component of Emergency Medical Services for Children systems. In such models, these Emergency Departments Approved for Pediatrics are the preferred EDs to receive patients from Emergency Medical Services providers. This article examines an alternative model developed in New Jersey in which every ED in the state is required by regulation to meet the standards of a traditional Emergency Departments Approved for Pediatrics. The New Jersey model leads to more accessible care and more rapid stabilization of children regardless of their mode of delivery to the ED.

▶ The New Jersey model (NJM) requires that any physician practicing in an emergency department (ED) must be either board certified or board eligible in emergency medicine or pediatric emergency medicine. If the physician is trained in another specialty, he or she must meet the following additional educational criteria: maintain a current course completion card in Advanced Cardiac Life Support, Advanced Trauma Life Support, and either Pediatric Advanced Life Support (PALS) or Advanced Pediatric Life Support (APLS). In addition, nursing regulations mandate that, at all times within the hospital, there must be a nurse present with pediatric capabilities as defined by certification in PALS, APLS, or the Emergency Nurse Pediatric Course. All EDs in the state are also required to maintain specialized equipment and supplies as defined by the document "Emergency Preparedness for the Care of Children." This is a policy statement that defines the optimal parameters for an ED prepared to treat any potential pediatric emergency and is jointly sponsored by the American Academy of Pediatrics, the American College of Emergency Physicians, and the Emergency Nurses Association.

As opposed to the standard Emergency Medical Services for Children model, in which dedicated emergency departments approved for pediatrics are identified within a given geographic area, in the NJM, every hospital ED in the state becomes a hospital capable of accepting pediatric patients. This unique model

(New Jersey is the only state that has adopted this archetype) leads to a number of interesting implications and unanswered questions. First, it means that the state of New Jersey, rather than the hospital medical staff, regulates the credentials of physicians practicing in a hospital. Whether this is a good precedent to set remains unclear. Second, there are costs involved in requiring every hospital to maintain a pediatric-capable nurse on duty and to have the appropriate equipment and supplies available. In a densely populated urban area where there are hospitals in close proximity, this may not be a good way to spend limited health care dollars. Finally, the authors state, "this model permits a baseline pediatric exposure for all EDs that maintain the skills necessary to care for a critically ill or injured child." Whether this is true is a matter of conjecture. It is not apparent that routinely treating colds, falls from bicycles, asthma, and insect bites prepares an emergency physician for the cyanotic infant with congenital heart disease or the child who is in shock from multiple trauma. In any case, New Jersey has a distinctive system for handling pediatric emergency care that works well in this densely populated sprawling suburban state. How this system compares with the standard model is unknown.

E. A. Ramoska, MD, MPHE

Early Pediatric Emergency Department Return Visits: A Prospective Patient-Centric Assessment
Ali AB, Place R, Howell J, et al (Inova Fairfax Hosp, Falls Church, VA)
Clin Pediatr 51:651-658, 2012

Background.—A substantial percentage of emergency department (ED) patients return within 72 hours of their initial evaluation. Quality reviews typically demonstrate that most revisits do not seem to be directly related to problematic care provided on the first evaluation. We examined the possibility that return visits are related to nonmedical issues on the first visit, most notably patient discharge education.

Objective.—We prospectively surveyed a convenience sample of caregivers in a pediatric ED to determine why they returned with their children within 72 hours of their initial ED visit.

Design/Methods.—All patients who returned within 72 hours of a previous visit were identified and prospectively interviewed using a survey instrument with nominal (multiple choice) and brief descriptive responses.

Results.—Caregivers of 124 children were prospectively surveyed; 93 children (75%) returned because their symptoms had not improved or worsened. Only 50 (53%) had contacted their primary medical doctor (PMD) prior to the second visit; of these, 14 (28%) could not get an appointment, and 32 (64%) were told to return to the ED. Discharge instructions were felt to be informative by 94% (n = 86) of caregivers with the same number (94%) reported being satisfied with the first ED physician. Twenty-nine children (30%) were admitted on the second visit.

Conclusions.—Among children who are discharged from the emergency department and return within 72 hours, most caregivers are satisfied with the care and instructions provided on their first visits. Though most patients have a PMD, many do not call them prior to their return ED visit, and those who do either cannot schedule an appointment or are told to return to the ED. The majority of patients return for clinical progression of illness.

▶ Emergency department (ED) 72-hour return visits (RVs) are an almost universal measure of ED quality of care. This thought-provoking study from the pediatric ED of Inova Fairfax Hospital in Virginia suggests that RVs may not be what we think they are. Most studies of 72-hour returns look at the problem retrospectively from the physician side and in doing so find errors in diagnosis or treatment, poor patient education and inadequate discharge instructions, or ineffective doctor-patient rapport and patient dissatisfaction. This analysis found that most patients (94%) were satisfied with their physician and thought that their discharge instructions were clear and informative.

Of the 124 patients with RVs, 14% had scheduled revisits and 11% returned for a completely different reason; this left 93 patients (75%) in the study. Slightly over one-half of these patients (53%) contacted their primary medical doctor (PMD) prior to the RV, and the overwhelming majority of these (98%) either could not get an appointment, were told by the office staff (nurse or physician) on the telephone to return to the ED, or were seen by their PMD that same day and sent back to the ED for reevaluation. Only 4 of the 93 children (4.3%) with unscheduled RVs for the same complaint did not have a PMD.

These data suggest that most 72-hour RVs are due to progression of disease or inadequacies within the primary care system, and that the ED, at least in the patients' eyes, is not at fault for their unscheduled return nor is it a cause of patient dissatisfaction. Of course, this study has a major limitation in that less than 5% of the patients in this population did not have a PMD. This is certainly in contrast to most EDs where I have ever practiced and most EDs in the country. Nonetheless, it is intriguing to note the authors' conclusions: "Retrospective chart review of RVs cannot reliably be used as a quality indicator for patient satisfaction with the initial medical encounter or quality of discharge."

E. A. Ramoska, MD, MPHE

Cancer diagnosis and outcomes in Michigan EDs vs other settings
Sikka V, Ornato JP (Virginia Commonwealth Univ, Richmond)
Am J Emerg Med 30:283-292, 2012

Objective.—This study determined the proportion of incident colorectal and lung cancers with a diagnosis associated with an emergency department (ED) visit. The characteristics of these patients and the correlation between diagnosis near an ED visit and stage at diagnosis were also examined.

Methods.—A population-based sample of all Michigan cancer cases diagnosed in all EDs and other health care settings was used to extract a sample of patients >65 years old, diagnosed with colorectal and lung cancers between January 1, 1996, and June 30, 2000 (n = 20 311). Logistic regressions were used for the statistical analysis.

Results.—Patients with a colorectal cancer diagnosis associated with an ED visit were more likely insured by Medicaid before diagnosis (odds ratio [OR], 1.37; 95% confidence interval [CI], 1.17-1.60), had an inpatient admission before diagnosis (OR, 1.29; 95% CI, 1.06-1.56), had 3 or more comorbidities (OR, 4.11; 95% CI, 3.53-4.79), were more likely to be female (OR, 1.18; 95% CI, 1.07-1.31), and were more likely to be aged 85 years and older (OR, 1.89; 95% CI, 1.57-2.27). Patients who had at least one primary care physician (PCP) visit before diagnosis were less likely to have a diagnosis associated with an ED visit (OR, 0.68; 95% CI, 0.61-0.76). Patients diagnosed with lung cancer in association with an ED visit were also more likely to have an inpatient admission before diagnosis (OR, 1.21; 95% CI, 1.02-1.43), a higher comorbidity burden (OR, 12.44; 95% CI, 10.18-15.20), be female (OR, 1.13; 95% CI, 1.02-1.25), African-American (OR, 1.42; 95% CI, 1.21-1.66), and older (80 years and older) (ages 80-84 years: OR, 1.33; 95% CI, 1.13-1.57; age 85 years and older: OR, 1.52; 95% CI, 1.25-1.85). Patients with an ED visit near a colorectal cancer (OR, 1.28; 95% CI, 1.15-1.42) or lung cancer diagnosis (OR, 1.65; 95% CI, 1.44-1.88) were more likely to be diagnosed at a later stage compared with patients diagnosed in other settings.

Conclusions.—An examination of patients' patterns of care leading to a cancer diagnosis in association with an ED visit lends insight to conditions precipitating a more immediate diagnosis and their associated outcomes.

▶ This study revealed that almost one-quarter (23%) of elderly patients (65 years or older) with colorectal cancer and nearly one-fifth (19%) of elderly patients with lung cancer in the state of Michigan had an emergency department (ED) visit associated with their initial diagnoses. Patients who were diagnosed in the ED had a statistically significant higher average number of ED visits in the 12 months before the diagnosis was made when compared with patients who were diagnosed in other settings. Moreover, the patients diagnosed in the ED tended to be older, African-American, on Medicaid, and had more comorbidities and more advanced stages of their cancers. This suggests that patients with a usual source of care are more likely to have appropriate cancer screening and detection of their cancer at earlier stages.

The authors then suggest that these findings have policy and practice implications for raising patients' cancer screening awareness in the ED, since a large number of the 2 most prevalent cancers in the United States are associated with an ED visit. However, their data imply that these patients do not have patient care providers (PCPs), or if they do have PCPs, they do not visit them, which is why they are in the ED in the first place. So sending them to a PCP, who they either do not have or do not visit, is not helpful. Furthermore, just because the ED has the opportunity to identify health problems in a population should not lead to the conclusion that those problems should be addressed in the ED. Emergency physicians face increasing pressures from growing numbers of patients, ED crowding, and expanded regulations from the Joint Commission and Centers for Medicare and Medicaid Services. Perhaps a better solution is to augment the linkage between the ED and the primary care setting. Getting these patients to a PCP or a clinic may be a better alternative than attempting to have the ED solve the problem.

E. A. Ramoska, MD, MPHE

Can Asymptomatic Patients With a Supratherapeutic International Normalized Ratio Be Safely Treated as Outpatients?

Levine M, Ruha A-M, Goldstein JN (Banner Good Samaritan Med Ctr, Phoenix, AZ; Massachusetts General Hosp, Boston, MA)
Ann Emerg Med 59:318-320, 2012

To determine whether asymptomatic patients with a supratherapeutic international normalized ratio (INR) warrant admission, a MEDLINE and EMBASE search was performed with the terms "warfarin AND anticoagulation," "warfarin AND bleeding," "warfarin and plications," and "warfarin and INR." The references in relevant articles were also searched. A secondary objective was to determine the risk of hemorrhage within 1 week. No randomized trials comparing inpatient versus outpatient management of asymptomatic patients with an increased INR were identified. Several studies examining outcomes after outpatient management, however, were identified. According to this review, it is certainly within the standard of care to manage patients with an asymptomatic, supratherapeutic INR as outpatients.

▶ Some other doctor may be sending home patients that you would not. Is there a method to the madness?

What is your practice for disposition of asymptomatic patients with elevated INR (international normalized ratio)? Unfortunately, it is apparent that the literature is lacking any great study (prospective, randomized, or controlled) to answer what the best course of action is.

Most likely, we practice according to the way our mentors taught us, with the exception of a few anecdotal horror stories of our own. Perhaps because of these latter situations, a memorable malpractice case comes to mind each time we consider what to do with our patients. We just do not have the evidence that will support sending these patients home with or without vitamin K.

There is no doubt that a major problem of warfarin use is bleeding and a supratherapeutic INR level marks an increased risk of bleeding. The problem we face is how to better define that risk well enough to decide what kind of monitoring is appropriate.

N. B. Handly, MD, MSc, MS

IV access difficulty: incidence and delays in an urban emergency department

Witting MD (Univ of Maryland School of Medicine, Baltimore)
J Emerg Med 42:483-487, 2012

Background.—Intravenous access difficulty (IVAD) has long been recognized as a problem for emergency departments (ED), but epidemiologic data are lacking.

Objective.—To estimate the incidence of IVAD and its associated delays in an urban ED.

Methods.—We conducted this prospective cohort study in an urban ED at an academic medical center, enrolling adult patients who were likely to require an IV line. We recorded patients' history of IVAD and the time from the initial skin puncture to IV line establishment, noting the need for a second provider and the type of provider who was successful. We defined IVAD as follows: none, requiring a single skin puncture; mild, requiring multiple skin punctures; moderate, requiring a second non-physician provider; and severe, requiring a physician. We used descriptive statistics and calculated the relative risk (and 95% confidence interval [CI]) for the association between prior IVAD and observed moderate or severe IVAD.

Results.—We enrolled 125 patients, 107 of whom had an IV line placed in the ED. Their median age was 48 (interquartile range 38−60) years. The incidence and median delays associated with IVAD categories were as follows: none, 61%/1 min; mild, 11%/5 min; moderate, 23%/15 min; and severe, 5%/120 min. Prior IVAD was associated with a 2.5-fold greater risk of observed IVAD (95% CI 1.3−4.7).

Conclusion.—In an urban, tertiary care ED, mild and moderate IVAD was common and led to mild delays, but severe IVAD, requiring a physician, caused substantial delays.

▶ Just the other day, 1 of our patients had to wait several hours for a disposition. A second intravenous (IV) line had to be placed. The first cannulation was already delayed because the nurses were unable to place a line and the resident had to use ultrasound-guided technique. But the first line failed (fluid extravasated, which was noted about 45 minutes after placement); meanwhile, the laboratory reported that several tubes of blood were hemolyzed 25 minutes after that. So the resident would need to place another IV under ultrasound guidance. At the same time, we as a team were busy in a trauma so no further work-up was possible for approximately 30 minutes. The patient was eventually admitted, although the rationale for an IV was just for admission. This was a clear case that delayed IV access would affect patient throughput.

Witting reports a study of factors that may influence success of IV placement, what manpower was required, and the amount of time spent in accessing the vessel. Additionally, the research assistants recorded the purpose for which the IV would be used, whether for blood tests, fluid administration, or even just for satisfying an admissions criterion.

If a patient does not need an IV, then it would be possible to bypass the problem of the delays identified in this study. Rigorous review of the kinds of clinical presentations that do not require an IV (whether low acuity, or eventual discharge, or blood sampling only) would be useful to help reduce the effect of delayed IV access.

This study was performed at a single clinical site and should be repeated to further characterize patterns of IV delays. It may be that each site has different practice cultures as far as IV use is concerned; nevertheless having an expectation of difficult IV access, the clinical team can prepare for the task ahead.

N. B. Handly, MD, MSc, MS

International evidence-based recommendations on ultrasound-guided vascular access
Lamperti M, Bodenham AR, Pittiruti M, et al (Neurological Inst Besta, Milan, Italy; Leeds General Infirmary, UK; Catholic Univ, Rome, Italy; et al)
Intensive Care Med 38:1105-1117, 2012

Purpose.—To provide clinicians with an evidence-based overview of all topics related to ultrasound vascular access.

Methods.—An international evidence-based consensus provided definitions and recommendations. Medical literature on ultrasound vascular access was reviewed from January 1985 to October 2010. The GRADE and the GRADE-RAND methods were utilised to develop recommendations.

Results.—The recommendations following the conference suggest the advantage of 2D vascular screening prior to cannulation and that real-time ultrasound needle guidance with an in-plane/long-axis technique optimises the probability of needle placement. Ultrasound guidance can be used not only for central venous cannulation but also in peripheral and arterial cannulation. Ultrasound can be used in order to check for immediate and life-threatening complications as well as the catheter's tip position. Educational courses and training are required to achieve competence and minimal skills when cannulation is performed with ultrasound guidance. A recommendation to create an ultrasound curriculum on vascular access is proposed. This technique allows the reduction of infectious and mechanical complications.

Conclusions.—These definitions and recommendations based on a critical evidence review and expert consensus are proposed to assist clinicians in ultrasound-guided vascular access and as a reference for future clinical research.

▶ When I first encountered this title, I thought, "Wait, do we need consensus this far into the practice of ultrasound for vascular access?" But then it dawned on me that of course any effort to use evidence means that there needs to be agreement on what we call things and how we measure the effects of using ultrasound-based techniques.

One study may present ultrasound as a tool to identify whether adequate veins are available but not use it to guide a catheter; another study may present the use of ultrasound to determine whether the catheter is adequately positioned in the vessel. Similar to the consensus process that occurred at Utstein for describing data collected for resuscitation, definitions for what names apply to various possible ultrasound-related processes are needed. Then we need to agree on outcomes both process-oriented (did we succeed at the defined task?) and patient-oriented (did the patient get an infection because of the process? did the patient have pain due to the process?).

The use of ultrasound has been well incorporated in emergency medicine for many years, so we are likely to shrug our shoulders. But emergency physicians who trained before ultrasound was part of residency or those practicing in environments in which ultrasound is not available are not likely to think of ultrasound in the same way. When it comes time for these doctors to make a case for or against the use of ultrasound, judgment depends on good evidence and the information identified in this article is going to be useful.

N. B. Handly, MD, MSc, MS

Seasonality of Testicular Torsion: A 10-Year Nationwide Population Based Study

Chiu B, Chen C-S, Keller JJ, et al (Far Eastern Memorial Hosp, Ban Ciao, New Taipei; Natl Taipei Univ, Taiwan; Taipei Med Univ, Taiwan)
J Urol 187:1781-1785, 2012

Purpose.—Using a 10-year nationwide data set, we examined seasonal variability in the monthly incidence of testicular torsion in Taiwan. We also investigated the association between meteorological factors (ambient temperature, relative humidity, atmospheric pressure, rainfall and total hours of sunshine) and testicular torsion, stratified by age group.

Materials and Methods.—This study retrieved data from the National Health Insurance Research Database. We identified 1,782 hospitalizations for testicular torsion between 2000 and 2009. Spearman's rank correlation was used to explore possible associations between climatic parameters and the monthly incidence of testicular torsion. In addition, we used the ARIMA method (Auto-Regressive Integrated Moving Average) to test for seasonality in the incidence of testicular torsion.

Results.—The results demonstrated a fairly similar seasonal pattern in monthly incidence rates for testicular torsion across both age groups and the combined groups. January (midwinter) had the highest rates, which decreased in April to a trough in June (early summer). After adjusting for the time trend effect and climatic parameters, the ARIMA regression revealed that January had a significantly higher monthly incidence of testicular torsion compared to February. In addition, our results indicated that the monthly incidence of testicular torsion was negatively associated with ambient temperature.

Conclusions.—Our results suggest that the monthly incidence of testicular torsion was significantly associated with seasonality and ambient temperature.

▶ When I first looked at the title of this article, I thought, "Oh, boy—a data-dredging effort." But as I thought more about it, it made some sense that temperature might be associated with risk of torsion. After all, in colder temperatures, more numerous and perhaps more confining clothing would be worn and these temperatures can also cause ascent of the testes.

Okay, there is a logical connection between temperature and torsion. The authors find a negative correlation (lower temperatures and higher incidence of torsion), but clearly there must be something else that is involved because torsion is not happening to every male when the weather turns cold. What about the comparison of those patients coming from outdoor versus indoor controlled temperatures—how long is the effect of exposure to cold temperature on the incidence of torsion? Just how cold does it need to be?

Still, one of the problems with retrospective studies like this is that it could be possible that the seasonal pattern may occur because of something other than temperature. Perhaps it is a change in activity or a change in some circadian pattern?

N. B. Handly, MD, MSc, MS

Effectiveness of Tai Chi as a Community-Based Falls Prevention Intervention: A Randomized Controlled Trial
Taylor D, Hale L, Schluter P, et al (AUT Univ, New Zealand; Univ of Otago, Dunedin, New Zealand; et al)
J Am Geriatr Soc 60.841-848, 2012

Objectives.—To compare the effectiveness of tai chi and low-level exercise in reducing falls in older adults; to determine whether mobility, balance, and lower limb strength improved and whether higher doses of tai chi resulted in greater effect.

Design.—Randomized controlled trial.

Setting.—Eleven sites throughout New Zealand.

Participants.—Six hundred eighty-four community-residing older adults (mean age 74.5; 73% female) with at least one falls risk factor.

Intervention.—Tai chi once a week (TC1) (n = 233); tai chi twice a week (TC2) (n = 220), or a low-level exercise program control group (LLE) (n = 231) for 20 wks.

Measurements.—Number of falls was ascertained according to monthly falls calendars. Mobility (Timed-Up-and-Go Test), balance (step test), and lower limb strength (chair stand test) were assessed.

Results.—The adjusted incident rate ratio (IRR) for falls was not significantly different between the TC1 and LLE groups (IRR = 1.05, 95% confidence interval (CI) = 0.83–1.33, $P = .70$) or between the TC2 and

LLE groups (IRR = 0.88, 95% CI = 0.68–1.16, P =.37). Adjusted multi-level mixed-effects Poisson regression showed a significant reduction in logarithmic mean fall rate of −0.050 (95% CI = −0.064 to −0.037, P < .001) per month for all groups. Multilevel fixed-effects analyses indicated improvements in balance (P < .001 right and left leg) and lower limb strength (P < .001) but not mobility (P =.54) in all groups over time, with no differences between the groups (P =.37 (right leg), P =.66 (left leg), P =.21, and P =.44, respectively).

Conclusion.—There was no difference in falls rates between the groups, with falls reducing similarly (mean falls rate reduction of 58%) over the 17-month follow-up period. Strength and balance improved similarly in all groups over time.

▶ The authors evaluated a scheme for primary prevention of falls in an older population by randomly assigning the subjects into 1 of 3 different exercise regimens. Two were based on Tai Chi activity and 1 was a standardized limited exercise activity. (There was no "sham" activity—no trip to the exercise center without activity—for comparison.)

Subjects in all groups showed similar decreases in fall rates. It was also noted that a fair number of subjects continued exercise activities after the 5-month acute intervention was completed (subjects were followed for up to an additional 12 months).

How much of the risk of falling in this sample could be attributed to baseline problems with balance or weakness is not clear; however, subjects in each exercise activity did improve function over the course of the study.

Keeping patients from falls via exercise activities like this is directly valuable but community activities like these also have the advantage of getting people out of the house, helping maintain relationships, and providing opportunities to provide support and health monitoring.

N. B. Handly, MD, MSc, MS

An Over-the-Counter Simulation Study of a Single-Tablet Emergency Contraceptive in Young Females

Raine TR, Ricciotti N, Sokoloff A, et al (Kaiser Permanente Northern California, Oakland, CA; Teva Women's Health Res, North Wales, PA; Univ of California, San Francisco)
Obstet Gynecol 119:772-779, 2012

Objectives.—To evaluate use of a single-tablet (levonorgestrel 1.5 mg) emergency contraceptive administered to young females under simulated over-the-counter conditions. Secondary objectives were to assess repeat use, pregnancy, and adverse events.

Methods.—Females aged 11–17 years requesting emergency contraception at teen reproductive health clinics in five cities were eligible to participate. Participants read the study product label and determined whether and how to use the product without interacting with providers. Study product was dispensed to participants who appropriately selected to use it; participants were contacted 1, 4, and 8 weeks later to assess use, pregnancy, and adverse events. The incidences of outcomes were calculated and regression analysis was used to assess the effect of age and use status (ever used or no previous use) on primary outcomes.

Results.—Of the 345 females enrolled, 279 were younger than age 17 years. Among the 340 participants included in the selection analysis, 311 (91.5%) (97.5% confidence interval 87.5−94.5%) participants appropriately selected to use or not use product. Among the 298 participants who used product, 274 (92.9%) (97.5% confidence interval 88.8−95.8%) correctly used it as labeled. Selection and correct use were not associated with age. Fifty-seven participants (18.8%) used additional emergency contraception over the study period and seven (2.3%) participants who used product became pregnant; there were no unusual adverse events.

Conclusion.—Restricting young females' use of a single-tablet emergency contraceptive by prescription only is not warranted, because females younger than 17 years can use it in a manner consistent with over-the-counter access.

Level of Evidence.—II.

▶ A significant challenge to making a pharmaceutical available for over-the-counter sale is testing to show that the drug will be properly selected and safely used by the consumer. If the drug has a narrow therapeutic index and is dangerous at the high end of its window, then it should not be legal to buy alongside gum and bread.

Once safety is no longer an issue, then it is time to determine if the general population can read a package label and make an appropriate decision to both buy and use. This study did not test the buying part of the consumerization step but did examine the decision-making process by young women ages 13 to 17 to use the drug levonorgestrel.

A read of the limitations of the study is enlightening about how complicated it is to devise a way to test decision-making among younger women. Consider the consent process: some states do not allow unemancipated minors to give consent independently of their parents. Additionally, the venue for recruiting subjects is tricky, too. I cannot imagine walking through the mall stopping every young female and asking if she would like to participate in a study about emergency contraception—it seems like it would be a creepy request.

The authors found that 13- to 17-year-old females could make decisions to take levonorgestrel and generally use it appropriately. In a few cases in which the pill was taken after the 72-hour window after intercourse, all of the surveyed subjects reported that they had taken the pill by 120 hours, which is currently considered as a possible extension to the current practice. It was not possible to determine if the young women had some exposure to knowledge about the 120-hour window or if there is enough of a sense of urgency that all of these women would try to take the pill in this enlarged timeframe.

N. B. Handly, MD, MSc, MS

Consultation in the emergency department: a qualitative analysis and review
Kessler C, Kutka BM, Badillo C (Univ of Illinois of Illinois-Chicago; Advocate Christ Med Ctr, Oak Lawn, IL)
J Emerg Med 42:704-711, 2012

Background.—No studies have evaluated the consultation process or attempted to define a standardized approach that could improve communication and patient outcomes.

Objective.—To perform a qualitative analysis of emergency medicine (EM) consultation to reveal its complexity and elucidate strategies and frameworks for physician-to-physician communication.

Methods.—Data were collected in three phases: informal interviews conducted in an emergency department (ED), 10-question surveys given to a subset of EM and specialty physicians, and semi-structured 1-h group interviews using open-ended questions to further explore issues and trends elicited from the survey responses. In addition, we conducted an extensive literature search focused on health care and business consultation and communication.

Results.—Seventy-six percent (29 of 38) of emergency and specialty physicians completed the 10-question survey in its entirety. Three themes were identified from the survey responses: organizational skills, interpersonal and communication skills, and medical knowledge. Of 95 total comments, 41 (43%) focused on organizational skills, 26 (27%) on interpersonal and communication skills, and 28 (30%) on medical knowledge. There were 29 comments regarding poor consultations: 15 issues with organization, 6 with interpersonal and communication skills, and 8 with medical knowledge. The literature search revealed several models and types of consultation, but no standard algorithm currently exists.

Conclusions.—We recommend focusing on organizational skills, interpersonal and communication skills, and medical knowledge when teaching ED consultation and present a conceptual framework of the Five Cs Consultation Model: contact, communication, core question, collaboration, and closing the loop.

▶ There is an art (and a developing science as suggested by this article) for effective consultation.

Culture clearly will play a role (perhaps the major role) in the interactions between the requester of a consultation and potential consultant. Unfortunately, much of culture in the clinical world is obscure, unmentioned, or nebulous, as would be found in other organizations.

Graduates of a residency program may find that the cultural practices of consultation at their hospitals may not be present in another. Subcultural aspects may exist depending on who is the supervising physician for either the requester or provider of the consultation. These variations can be confusing to the learner. So it is helpful that the authors provide structure to debrief participants in the consultation experience and guidance for effective communication.

A specific problem of consultations is to know enough about your consultants' specialty skills and practices to know what advice or skill to expect from them. Good knowledge about the consultants would also affect the choice of information to be provided during the consultation request. This would seem to be something that would not be learned during a medical student clinical rotation. Instead, this is likely to be learned in the practice of requesting consults as a resident. If this knowledge could be structured, it would go a long way toward improving the consultation experience.

I have been listening to a lot of the Freakonomics podcasts lately. So when I read the report of this study, I thought about incentives. Are there rational drivers of behavior? What are the incentives for the consultant to be an effective partner in the consultation process? Both rational and irrational incentives should be called into play for effective consultation to occur.

N. B. Handly, MD, MSc, MS

Effect on Injuries of Assigning Shoes Based on Foot Shape in Air Force Basic Training
Knapik JJ, Brosch LC, Venuto M, et al (U.S. Army Ctr for Health Promotion and Preventive Medicine, Aberdeen Proving Ground, MD; U.S. Air Force, San Antonio, TX; Dept of Health and Human Services Food and Drug Administration, College Park, MD; et al)
Am J Prev Med 38:S197-S211, 2010

Background.—This study examined whether assigning running shoes based on the shape of the bottom of the foot (plantar surface) influenced injury risk in Air Force Basic Military Training (BMT) and examined risk factors for injury in BMT.

Methods.—Data were collected from BMT recruits during 2007; analysis took place during 2008. After foot examinations, recruits were randomly consigned to either an experimental group (E, $n = 1042$ men, 375 women) or a control group (C, $n = 913$ men, 346 women). Experimental group recruits were assigned motion control, stability, or cushioned shoes for plantar shapes indicative of low, medium, or high arches, respectively. Control group recruits received a stability shoe regardless of plantar shape. Injuries during BMT were determined from outpatient visits provided from the Defense Medical Surveillance System. Other injury risk factors (fitness, smoking, physical activity, prior injury, menstrual history, and demographics) were obtained from a questionnaire, existing databases, or BMT units.

Results.—Multivariate Cox regression controlling for other risk factors showed little difference in injury risk between the groups among men (hazard ratio [E/C] = 1.11, 95% CI = 0.89−1.38) or women (hazard ratio [E/C] = 1.20, 95% CI = 0.90−1.60). Independent injury risk factors among both men and women included low aerobic fitness and cigarette smoking.

Conclusions.—This prospective study demonstrated that assigning running shoes based on the shape of the plantar surface had little influence on injury risk in BMT even after controlling for other injury risk factors.

▶ Running a military basic training operation is tough enough with trying to bring a varied group of recruits up to a standard of ability. It might not be surprising that those in charge of basic training may not have the expertise to make judgments about which type of shoe is best for candidates to avoid injuries.

So where would someone in charge learn about the value of different types of shoes for different types of feet? It would probably be described in an advertisement or a fluff piece in a health magazine (doesn't this sound familiar—where do many physicians learn about new drugs and devices?).

This is a report from a well-constructed, prospective study of recruits who, as members of the control group, were assigned to wear standard running shoes or, in the experimental group, were assigned to wear shoes to specifically match their arch size. The subjects were then followed through basic training to assess if wearing shoes matched to arch size made any difference in the types and numbers of injuries suffered when compared with control subjects.

The authors found no statistically significant association of shoe wearing to the injury patterns surveyed. It may be possible that there would be very specific injuries associated with shoe fit; however, the authors did not look for patterns of this type.

The Army is already using custom shoe assignments. This study would suggest that the Army should properly test the value of custom shoe wearing among the recruits. It is possible that there are differences in the types of activities in each service's basic training, so for some experiences, the type of shoe may be important. Otherwise, the results of this study would suggest that there is no benefit to buying custom shoes for recruits.

N. B. Handly, MD, MSc, MS

From Hot Hands to Declining Effects: The Risks of Small Numbers
Lauer MS (Natl Heart, Lung, and Blood Inst (NHLBI) of the Natl Insts of Health (NIH), Bethesda, MD)
J Am Coll Cardiol 60:72-74, 2012

About 25 years ago, a group of researchers demonstrated that there is no such thing as the "hot hand" in professional basketball. When a player hits 5 or 7 shots in a row (or misses 10 in a row), what's at work is random variation, nothing more. However, random causes do not stop players, coaches, fans, and media from talking about and acting on "hot hands," telling stories and making choices that ultimately are based on randomness. The same phenomenon is true in medicine. Some clinical trials with small numbers of events yielded positive findings, which in turn led clinicians, academics, and government officials to talk, telling stories and sometimes making choices that were later shown to be based on randomness. I provide some cardiovascular examples, such as the use of angiotensin receptor blockers for chronic heart failure, nesiritide for acute heart failure, and cytochrome P-450 (CYP) 2C19 genotyping for the acute coronary syndromes. I also review the more general "decline effect," by which drugs appear to yield a lower effect size over time. The decline effect is due at least in part to over interpretation of small studies, which are more likely to be noticed because of publication bias. As funders of research, we at the National Heart, Lung, and Blood Institute seek to support projects that will yield robust, credible evidence that will affect practice and policy in the right way. We must be alert to the risks of small numbers.

▶ Let's play a game of statistics. No, wait, it will not be that bad. We are going to try to discover how likely it is to find a result that seems significant but is actually a result of a random outcome.

Consider a standard (control) treatment that is associated with an outcome of 4% survival (found over such a very large number of subjects tested that it may be accepted as a real value). A new therapy is considered (perhaps identified after performance of some cell or animal study) that seems worthy of testing on humans. The control treatment is not great (only 4% survival) so your Institutional Review Board (IRB) considers your study worthy but it needs to be performed with caution. You are approved to recruit 25 subjects since it is a complicated protocol. If your new therapy appears to put your patients at greater risk of death than the standard therapy, then study will be canceled.

Let us look at the case that the new treatment is no better than the standard treatment.

I will simulate this experiment with resampling using Statistics101, version 2.6 (www.statistics101.net), and spare you the hard work. First I create a pool of 100 subjects, of which 96 are dead after standard treatment and 4 survive after standard treatment. The null hypothesis that there is no difference between the standard and new treatments would mean that 4 of 100 or 1 of 25 would survive treatment. Then I sample 25 subjects randomly from the pool of 100 subjects as a possible outcome of one experiment using the new treatment. In fact, what I will do is draw samples of a group of 25 subjects many thousands of times and find the greatest number of subjects that would survive with at least 5% probability. The simulation reveals that 3 survivors of 25 subjects (an amazing 12% survival after the new treatment!) could be found after 1 experiment that would still be consistent with the null hypothesis. Note that no assumptions about normality or variance are needed to simulate this result.

If you did report back to the IRB that your new treatment was better when you found 3 survivors when you expected 1 survivor for equivalence of the 2 treatments, you would be making a mistake. You present an abstract of your work, and after your report you and others begin to study the new treatment further. The results of these studies are less dramatic than originally thought—essentially, now enough sampling has occurred to find the real values for new treatment success.

Sure, your new treatment might actually be better, but without enough testing, it just might be an incorrect assumption of the "hot hand."

N. B. Handly, MD, MSc, MS

Cost-effectiveness and budget impact analyses of a long-term hypertension detection and control program for stroke prevention

Yamagishi K, Sato S, Kitamura A, et al (Univ of Tsukuba, Japan; Osaka Ctr for Cancer and Cardiovascular Disease Prevention, Japan; et al)
J Hypertens 30:1874-1879, 2012

Objectives.—The nation-wide, community-based intensive hypertension detection and control program, as well as universal health insurance coverage, may well be contributing factors for helping Japan rank near the top among countries with the longest life expectancy. We sought to examine the cost-effectiveness of such a community-based intervention program, as no evidence has been available for this issue.

Methods.—The hypertension detection and control program was initiated in 1963 in full intervention and minimal intervention communities in Akita, Japan. We performed comparative cost-effectiveness and budget-impact analyses for the period 1964—1987 of the costs of public health services and treatment of patients with hypertension and stroke on the one hand, and incidence of stroke on the other in the full intervention and minimal intervention communities.

Results.—The program provided in the full intervention community was found to be cost saving 13 years after the beginning of program in addition to the fact of effectiveness that; the prevalence and incidence of stroke were consistently lower in the full intervention community than in the minimal intervention community throughout the same period. The incremental cost was *minus* 28 358 yen per capita over 24 years.

Conclusion.—The community-based intensive hypertension detection and control program was found to be both effective and cost saving. The national government's policy to support this program may have contributed in part to the substantial decline in stroke incidence and mortality, which was largely responsible for the increase in Japanese life expectancy.

▶ A lot of energy has been added to discussions about use of prevention to deal with the problems of high numbers of persons suffering from chronic disease and the costs associated with the management of these diseases.

In Japan, insurance and public health plans were established to deal with the problems of hypertension and stroke. The authors were able to take advantage of a natural experiment (based on 2 communities that provided different levels of intervention for these 2 medical problems) to compare the cost of a minimal and a high-intensity intervention system. In doing so, the authors found costs associated with screenings, education, and treatment for both hypertension and stroke.

Based on these costs, the authors were able to estimate that after 13 years from the start of the programs, the high-intensity interventions had an overall cost that was lower than found in community subject to the minimal-intensity intervention. It was also noted that there was a lower incidence and prevalence of hypertension and stroke in the community subject to the high-intensity intervention. This is an important finding if one wanted to take away lessons for other demonstrations of cost effectiveness of care—any trial of intervention needs to have the commitment of perhaps 15 years to demonstrate its value. It is likely in our current political and economic situation, there is no stomach to wait this long for results.

The authors raised the issue of quality of life (QoL) for both the sufferers of stroke and their family members; however, no measurement of QoL was available to compare between the 2 communities.

Another not surprising finding was that when blood pressure screenings were no longer free, the number of participants dropped by about 30%. We do not know if these dropouts were more or less likely to suffer from the burden of hypertension and stroke; nevertheless, the overall community suffered from higher incidence and prevalence of hypertension and stroke.

It would be hard to directly apply these results to the United States. We do not have a structured antihypertension and antistroke system in place starting at age 30 years. We also know little about how to provide the community-oriented education and motivation to get our citizens to participate in hypertension and stroke reduction.

N. B. Handly, MD, MSc, MS

Carotid intima-media thickness progression to predict cardiovascular events in the general population (the PROG-IMT collaborative project): a meta-analysis of individual participant data
Lorenz MW, on behalf of the PROG-IMT Study Group (J W Goethe-Univ, Frankfurt am Main, Germany; et al)
Lancet 379:2053-2062, 2012

Background.—Carotid intima-media thickness (cIMT) is related to the risk of cardiovascular events in the general population. An association between changes in cIMT and cardiovascular risk is frequently assumed but has rarely been reported. Our aim was to test this association.

Methods.—We identified general population studies that assessed cIMT at least twice and followed up participants for myocardial infarction, stroke, or death. The study teams collaborated in an individual participant data meta-analysis. Excluding individuals with previous myocardial infarction or stroke, we assessed the association between cIMT progression and the risk of cardiovascular events (myocardial infarction, stroke, vascular death, or a combination of these) for each study with Cox regression. The log hazard ratios (HRs) per SD difference were pooled by random effects meta-analysis.

Findings.—Of 21 eligible studies, 16 with 36 984 participants were included. During a mean follow-up of 7·0 years, 1519 myocardial infarctions, 1339 strokes, and 2028 combined endpoints (myocardial infarction, stroke, vascular death) occurred. Yearly cIMT progression was derived from two ultrasound visits 2—7 years (median 4 years) apart. For mean common carotid artery intima-media thickness progression, the overall

HR of the combined endpoint was 0.97 (95% CI $0.94-1.00$) when adjusted for age, sex, and mean common carotid artery intima-media thickness, and 0.98 ($0.95-1.01$) when also adjusted for vascular risk factors. Although we detected no associations with cIMT progression in sensitivity analyses, the mean cIMT of the two ultrasound scans was positively and robustly associated with cardiovascular risk (HR for the combined endpoint 1.16, 95% CI $1.10-1.22$, adjusted for age, sex, mean common carotid artery intima-media thickness progression, and vascular risk factors). In three studies including 3439 participants who had four ultrasound scans, cIMT progression did not correlate between occasions (reproducibility correlations between $r = -0.06$ and $r = -0.02$).

Interpretation.—The association between cIMT progression assessed from two ultrasound scans and cardiovascular risk in the general population remains unproven. No conclusion can be derived for the use of cIMT progression as a surrogate in clinical trials.

Funding.—Deutsche Forschungsgemeinschaft.

▶ It has been suggested that the intima-media thickness in the carotid (cIMT) measured by ultrasound can provide a meaningful risk measure for vascular diseases. One particular measurement is progression, the rate of increase of cIMT over time, which has been assumed to be useful for prediction but never has been studied specifically.

The authors were able to find a number of prior studies of cIMT in which multiple measures of cIMT were performed and the individual patient data could be accessed (in some cases, the authors contacted the prior study authors to obtain these data). Several models were constructed to consider several covariates including age, gender, and mean cIMT value. In each model, no significant association between cIMT progression and vascular events was found. What the authors did confirm was that the mean cIMT value was related to likelihood of vascular events including myocardial infarctions and strokes.

One of the problems with assembling data is that of missing values. A simple approach is to drop the records that do not have all values present. However, to do so could change the actual picture of what is going on. If all records that had missing values were truly representative of the entire data set, then dropping these values would have little bearing on the analysis. But if the records with missing values were not representative of the entire set then a biased impression of the sample would be generated.

The authors used techniques of imputation to essentially "fill in the blanks" of the missing values. There are a number of techniques that can be used to do imputation. For example, one might calculate a missing value based on relationships to other known values of that variable such as the mean; eg, the missing systolic blood pressure could be imputed as the average of all the known systolic blood pressures. This does assume that we really do know something about the distribution of these values and those that are missing. Likely more reliable values could be generated by a function of a collection of different variables. In this case, a missing systolic blood pressure could be imputed as a more complicated function of age, gender, and cIMT value. What this function is seems complicated to derive; however, modern statistical software can do this work for us. Several different imputation results can be assembled and provide some sense of variance and confidence limits to the resulting model's prediction.

There are right times and wrong times to do imputation. Certainly, if you know a lot about the distribution of the values for a particular variable/factor, in that they do not vary much at all, then imputation would be more work than it would be worth.

Pay attention when reading about methods of assembling retrospective studies or meta-analyses about how the authors deal with missing data.

N. B. Handly, MD, MSc, MS

Contomporory Evidence About Hospital Strategies for Reducing 30-Day Readmissions: A National Study

Bradley EH, Curry L, Horwitz LI, et al (Yale School of Public Health, New Haven, CT; Yale Univ School of Medicine, New Haven, CT; et al)
J Am Coll Cardiol 60:607-614, 2012

Objectives.—This study sought to determine the range and prevalence of practices being implemented by hospitals to reduce 30-day readmissions of patients with heart failure or acute myocardial infarction (AMI).

Background.—Readmissions of patients with heart failure or AMI are both common and costly; however, evidence on strategies adopted by hospitals to reduce readmission rates is limited.

Methods.—We used a Web-based survey to conduct a cross-sectional study of hospitals' reported use of specific practices to reduce readmissions for patients with heart failure or AMI. We contacted all hospitals enrolled in the Hospital to Home (H2H) quality improvement initiative as of July 2010. Of 594 hospitals, 537 completed the survey (response rate of 90.4%). We used standard frequency analysis to describe the prevalence of key hospital practices in the areas of: 1) quality improvement resources and performance monitoring; 2) medication management efforts; and 3) discharge and follow-up processes.

Results.—Nearly 90% of hospitals agreed or strongly agreed that they had a written objective of reducing preventable readmission for patients with heart failure or AMI. More hospitals reported having quality improvement teams to reduce preventable readmissions for patients with heart failure (87%) than for patients with AMI (54%). Less than one-half (49.3%) of hospitals had partnered with community physicians and only 23.5% had partnered with local hospitals to manage patients at high risk for readmissions. Inpatient and outpatient prescription records were electronically linked usually or always in 28.9% of hospitals, and the discharge summary was always sent directly to the patient's primary medical doctor in only 25.5% of hospitals. On average, hospitals used 4.8 of 10 key practices; < 3% of hospitals utilized all 10 practices.

Conclusions.—Although most hospitals have a written objective of reducing preventable readmissions of patients with heart failure or AMI, the implementation of recommended practices varied widely. More evidence establishing the effectiveness of various practices is needed.

▶ The Center for Medicare and Medicaid Services (CMS) has established a policy that will reduce payments for patient care when the patient has an unscheduled readmission within 30 days after discharge for events of acute myocardial infarct or congestive heart failure. How much incentive does a hospital need to figure out how to reduce these readmissions?

A number of hospitals have joined together to share strategies for and evidence about reducing these readmission (the Hospital to Home [H2H] consortium). These authors surveyed those hospitals that joined the H2H consortium at the time of its formation in 2009 to identify what systems were in place to monitor three aspects of a quality effort: Is there a quality team to manage readmission? What steps have been taken for medication reconciliation? What steps have been taken to coordinate the handoff from hospital inpatient to outpatient care?

The last of these three, the handoff, seems to be the hardest to do. Perhaps this is because this is something that has not been well incorporated in these hospitals' cultures. Meanwhile, most of the hospitals have quality improvement teams whose focus is readmission and medication reconciliation systems are present in an intermediate extent between team operation and handoff systems.

It would not surprise me that hospitals have to rely on nonphysician team members, such as pharmacists, nurse educators, and case managers, for reducing readmissions. Hospitals will need to do a better job of passing discharge summaries and medications lists to primary care practitioners, where the obstacles are largely dependent of information systems and hospitals' risk management policies as to what can be sent out from a patient's medical record. Hospital physicians will need to complete documentation more rapidly to get information to outpatient practices.

It should not be thought that there are no other ways to reduce readmission rates. Besides these approaches, your ideas are certainly welcome, especially if they can be more easily integrated into your own hospital culture.

N. B. Handly, MD, MSc, MS

Are Patients With Longer Emergency Department Wait Times Less Likely to Consent to Research?
Limkakeng AT Jr, Glickman SW, Shofer F, et al (Duke Univ Med Ctr, Durham, NC; Univ of North Carolina at Chapel Hill)
Acad Emerg Med 19:396-401, 2012

Objectives.—There are unique challenges to enrolling patients in emergency department (ED) clinical research studies, including the time-sensitive nature of emergency conditions, the acute care environment, and the lack of an established relationship with patients. Prolonged ED wait times have been associated with a variety of adverse effects on patient care. The objective of this study was to assess the effect of ED wait times on patient participation in ED clinical research. The hypothesis was that increased ED wait times would be associated with reduced ED clinical research consent rates.

Methods.—This was a retrospective cohort study of all patients eligible for two diagnostic clinical research studies from January 1, 2008, through December 31, 2008, in an urban academic ED. Sex, age, race, study eligibility, and research consent decisions were recorded by trained study personnel. The wait times to registration and to be seen by a physician were obtained from administrative databases and compared between consenters and nonconsenters. An analysis of association between patient wait times for the outcome of consent to participate was performed using a multivariate logistic regression model.

Results—A total of 903 patients were eligible for enrollment and were asked for consent. Overall, 589 eligible patients (65%) gave consent to research participation. The consent rates did not change when patients were stratified by the highest and lowest quartile wait times for both time from arrival to registration (68% vs. 65%, $p = 0.35$) and time to be seen by a physician (65% vs. 66%, $p = 0.58$). After adjusting for patient demographics (age, race, and sex) and study, there was still no relationship between wait times and consent ($p > 0.4$ for both wait times). Furthermore, median time from arrival to registration did not differ between those who consented to participate (15 minutes; interquartile range [IQR] = 9 to 36 minutes) versus those who did not (15.5 minutes; IQR = 10 to 39 minutes; $p = 0.80$; odds ratio [OR] = 1.00, 95% confidence interval [CI] = 0.99 to 1.01). Similarly, there was no difference in the median time to be seen by a physician between those who consented (25 minutes; IQR = 15 to 55 minutes) versus those who did not (25 minutes; IQR = 15 to 56 minutes; $p = 0.70$; OR = 1.00, 95% CI = 0.99 to 1.01).

Conclusions.—Regardless of wait times, nearly two-thirds of eligible patients were willing to consent to diagnostic research studies in the ED. These findings suggest that effective enrollment in clinical research is possible in the ED, despite challenges with prolonged wait times.

▶ This is an interesting investigation of the type of relationship we are building with our patients and how it may be influenced by the waiting experience.

To have patients agree to participate in research studies implies that there is some trust between the possible subject and the consenter. But there must also be some confidence in those performing the study because subjects likely decide to participate in a study because they can identify a value to them. It may be that the value is offered to the subject personally or to society in general (our consent documents have to include whether the subject can expect to personally benefit).

Another possible motive for patients to agree to participate in a study is that they feel that they may owe something to the investigators (possibly, in return for the care they have been or will be given), which at least might be some goodwill. Does waiting pay down some of this debt and reduce the likelihood that a patient will choose to join a study?

The authors did not find that the length of time that patients have been waiting influences whether patients will agree to participate in a study. However, it could be that once a patient has been seen by the doctor and evaluation and care has started, a new debt has been created. To see if this is the case, consider a study in which patients consented while they were still in the waiting room to see what effect waiting has on the consent process.

N. B. Handly, MD, MSc, MS

Impact of nasogastric lavage on outcomes in acute GI bleeding
Huang ES, Karsan S, Kanwal F, et al (Massachusetts General Hosp, Boston; Cedars Sinai Med Ctr, Los Angeles, CA; Saint Louis Univ, MO; et al)
Gastrointest Endosc 74:971-980, 2011

Background.—Nasogastric lavage (NGL) is often performed early in the management of GI bleeding. This practice assumes that NGL results can assist with timely risk stratification and management.

Objective.—We performed a retrospective analysis to test whether NGL is associated with improved process measures and outcomes in GI bleeding.

Design.—Propensity-matched retrospective analysis.

Setting.—University-based Veterans Affairs medical center.

Patients.—A total of 632 patients admitted with GI bleeding.

Main Outcome Measurements.—Thirty-day mortality rate, length of hospital stay, transfusion requirements, surgery, and time to endoscopy.

Results.—Patients receiving NGL were more likely to take nonsteroidal anti-inflammatory drugs and be admitted to intensive care, but less likely to have metastatic disease or tachycardia, be taking warfarin, or present on weekdays. After propensity matching, NGL did not affect mortality (odds ratio [OR] 0.84; 95% confidence interval [CI], 0.37-1.92), length of hospital stay (7.3 vs 8.1 days, $P = .57$), surgery (OR 1.51; 95% CI, 0.42-5.43), or transfusions (3.2 vs 3.0 units, $P = .94$). However, NGL was associated with earlier time to endoscopy (hazard ratio 1.49; 95% CI, 1.09-2.04), and bloody aspirates were associated high-risk lesions (OR 2.69; 95% CI, 1.08-6.73).

Limitations.—Retrospective design.

Conclusions.—Performing NGL is associated with the earlier performance of endoscopy, but does not affect clinical outcomes. Performing NGL at initial triage may promote more timely process of care, but further studies will be needed to confirm these findings.

▶ Every now and again a well-structured study comes along. Even better, this study attempts to provide information about an important topic: does the use of nasogastric (NG) lavage have practical value in patients with acute gastrointestinal (GI) bleeding? We in the emergency department want to know the answer to this question since we are often dealing with more than just a GI bleeder. You make the phone call to your GI specialist and as part of the conversation you are asked whether you placed an NG tube and what you saw in the lavage aspirate. Did you even place an NG tube? What is the value to the patient (and you) of placing the NG tube and lavaging the stomach?

So what in this study was well done? The authors sought to examine the outcomes of patients who had NG lavage performed early in their care. The authors are off to a good start when they recognize the difference between disease and patient-oriented outcomes. It is a retrospective study and thus has expected weaknesses. Grouping patients based on whether they were treated with NG lavage alone might ignore the fact that physicians may decide to use NG lavage based on how the patients look, and appearance is not available among the data.

One approach to dealing with the absent appearance data is to use propensity. Essentially, you first investigate (among the data available) which variables separate those patients who received NG lavage and those who did not. Once there is a good model to distinguish between these 2 situations, it may be expected that there will be some patients who did not get NG lavage who by the model would have been expected to have received NG lavage. It is possible then to pair patients for comparison, including all the likely variables that might play a role in outcomes as well as the propensity to receive NG lavage, where one patient did get NG lavage and the other patient did not.

The results are not entirely unexpected: the patient-oriented outcomes studied do not appear to be affected by treatment with early NG lavage; however, it was noted that process outcomes, such as having endoscopy before discharge, were affected by the patient who had early NG lavage.

N. B. Handly, MD, MSc, MS

A community intervention trial to evaluate emergency care practitioners in the management of children
O'Keeffe C, Mason S, Bradburn M, et al (Univ of Sheffield, UK)
Arch Dis Child 96:658-663, 2011

Objective.—To evaluate the impact of emergency care practitioners (ECPs) on the patient care pathway for children presenting with minor conditions in unscheduled care settings.

Design.—A pragmatic quasi-experimental multi-site community intervention trial comparing ECPs with usual care providers.

Setting.—Three pairs of emergency and urgent care services in the UK: minor injury unit (MIU), urgent care centre (UCC) and general practitioner out of hours.

Patients.—Paediatric acute episodes (n=415 intervention and n=748 control) in participating services presenting with minor conditions.

Main Outcome Measures.—Percentage of patients discharged following care episode and percentage of patients referred to hospital and primary care services.

Interventions.—ECPs operational in emergency and unscheduled care settings.

Results.—ECPs discharged significantly fewer patients than usual care providers (percentage difference 7.3%, 95% CI 13.6% to 0.9%). ECPs discharged fewer patients within all three pairs of services (out of hours percentage difference 6.33%, 95% CI 15.17% to 2.51%; UCC percentage difference 8.73%, 95% CI 19.22% to 1.76%; MIU percentage difference 6.80%, 95% CI 24.36% to 10.75%). ECPs also referred more patients to hospital (percentage difference 4.6%, 95% CI −2.9% to 12.0%) and primary care providers (percentage difference 3.0%, 95% CI 3.7% to 9.7%).

Conclusions.—ECPs are not as effective as usual health providers in discharging children after assessment of urgent healthcare problems. This has implications for the workload of other paediatric providers such as the emergency department. ECPs may be better targeted to settings and patients groups in which there is more evidence of their effectiveness in patient care pathways.

▶ It is unlikely that the numbers of patients heading for emergency departments (ED) will decrease any time soon. To help deal with this, it is worth considering a role for care extenders in some outside hospital settings to help reduce the number of patients needing ED care.

Some of the patients arriving at EDs are referred by primary care physicians after their offices have closed. If there were a way to treat these patients using the facilities of these primary care practices, this could help mitigate some of the flow of patients. Another possibility of diverting patients from the ED is to take advantage of free-standing clinics.

Important to the operation of these alternatives to ED care is the performance of the staff at these sites. In the United Kingdom there is what is called an emergency care practitioner (ECP) physician extender. Although this was a study in the United Kingdom, physician extenders are practicing in the United States as well; thus it is worth looking at this study for its application.

If ECPs are able to divert care from EDs, they would be a valuable resource. In this study, the authors examined the ability of ECPs to divert pediatric patients from the ED and primary care physicians.

The authors suggested that ECPs are not effective in reducing pediatric burden on the health care system in the United Kingdom. (ECPs, when compared with physicians or nurse practitioners, were more likely to refer their pediatric patients to EDs.) However, I think a more cautious interpretation is in order.

The performance of ECPs practicing when neither a physician nor nurse practitioner is available might be better compared to a setting of parents alone making the decisions. Can ECPs divert more children from EDs than parents? This comparison was not done.

Another issue is the cost of systems using ECPs as is currently done, replacing ECPs with physicians or nurse practitioners or not having any extender available. ECPs tended to do less testing and they may add to cost savings, but to truly assess any savings based on testing, it would be useful to compare the amount of testing that the children referred to EDs or physician offices ultimately received. These were not done.

It may not be sufficient to only compare the amount of children diverted. Perhaps one should compare the performance of ECPs to determine how many patients seen by each provider type ended up in the ED or physician's office within 1 week (a measure of ultimate success of diversion from the ED or physician's office).

The decisions to use extenders need to be made carefully. This study is instructive of how better analysis is needed yet.

N. B. Handly, MD, MSc, MS

Management of an Apparent Life-Threatening Event: A Survey of Emergency Physicians Practice

Kundra M, Duffy E, Thomas R, et al (Children's Hosp of Michigan, Detroit)
Clin Pediatr 51:130-133, 2012

Objective.—The etiology of an apparent life-threatening event (ALTE) has been attributed to a wide range of causes. Physicians rely on caregiver narratives, which are often unreliable given the distressing nature of the event, which in turn leads to variation in the evaluation and management. The objective of this study was to study this variation in the management of ALTE among emergency physicians in Michigan.

Design and Methods.—The authors developed and conducted a survey that contained questions on the evaluation and management of 2 common ALTE scenarios. These surveys were then mailed to 1000 randomly selected emergency physicians from a comprehensive physician database.

Results.—A total of 25.5% responded. Majority of the respondents were trained in emergency medicine residency. Fourth-seven percent of the respondents work in suburban areas. Most respondents said that they would perform diagnostic laboratory workup on children presenting with ALTE although there is wide variation in the extent of the workup. Ninety-two percent of ALTE patients are likely to get pediatric subspecialist consultation from the emergency department.

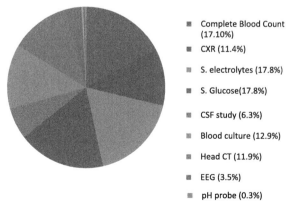

- Complete Blood Count (17.10%)
- CXR (11.4%)
- S. electrolytes (17.8%)
- S. Glucose(17.8%)
- CSF study (6.3%)
- Blood culture (12.9%)
- Head CT (11.9%)
- EEG (3.5%)
- pH probe (0.3%)

FIGURE 3.—Diagnostic workups for clinical vignettes. (Reprinted from Kundra M, Duffy E, Thomas R, et al. Management of an apparent life-threatening event: a survey of emergency physicians practice. *Clin Pediatr.* 2012;51:130-133, with permission from The Author(s).)

Conclusions.—There is a wide variation in the evaluation and management of ALTE among emergency medicine physicians in Michigan. These children with ALTE are very likely to be seen by pediatric subspecialists subsequently (Fig 3).

▶ An apparent life-threatening event (ALTE) causes distress for the patient, the caregiver(s), and the physician charged with evaluating the patient. The authors of this study surveyed emergency physicians to establish practice patterns when faced with an ALTE. Although based solely in Michigan, the results can likely be generalized to a North American population.

The authors address significant variations in the etiologies, presenting symptoms, histories provided, diagnostic workups, consultations, and ultimate dispositions. With so many variables, practice disparity may be unavoidable. Based on the presented vignettes, the surveyed physicians proceeded with a theoretical management plan. Workups most commonly included diagnostic tests readily available in the emergency department, such as complete blood count, serum electrolytes, serum glucose, and chest radiograph (Fig 3). Bronchiolitis and idiopathic etiologies were the most common reasons for admission, but the researchers do not present what percentage of physicians admitted the patients.

The most appropriate management may be to perform pertinent diagnostic tests followed by in-hospital observation.

E. C. Bruno, MD

The importance of a proper against-medical-advice (AMA) discharge: how signing out AMA may create significant liability protection for providers
Levy F, Mareiniss DP, Iacovelli C (Johns Hopkins Univ School of Medicine, Baltimore, MD)
J Emerg Med 43:516-520, 2012

Background.—Every year, patients leave the Emergency Department against medical advice (AMA) and before an adequate evaluation can be performed. It is well known that many of these patients are at risk of subsequent complications.

Objective.—The goal of this article is to explain the potential legal protections that may be created from a proper AMA discharge.

Discussion.—In this article, the authors review the steps that need to be taken when performing an AMA discharge, including an assessment of capacity, proper documentation, and adequate disclosure. The authors then review the potential legal protections that can result from a properly documented and performed discharge. Among these protections are: proof that the provider's duty to the patient ended with discharge and that the patient assumed the risk of a subsequent complication.

Conclusion.—The authors conclude that a properly executed discharge can provide significant legal protection from liability risks.

▶ Emergency physicians (EP) are routinely faced with patients who leave without being seen by a qualified medical provider, leave without complete treatment, or leave against medical advice (AMA). The reasons for leaving can be as varied as the chief complaints. Occasionally, a patient's decision to leave AMA is not necessarily a negative situation, especially when the patient is malingering. However, AMA patients carry significant risk for adverse events and subsequent medical malpractice claims. The authors of the attached informational article describe the critical components of a proper AMA process and provide additional information regarding potential malpractice defense strategies. The authors repeatedly portray how to properly complete an AMA operation, including the assessment of capacity, the disclosure of risks, and the requisite documentation. The emphasis is on a bona fide AMA process specific to the individual patient, not simply going through the motions in order to expedite the patient's removal from the emergency department. Although the EP is not always given the opportunity to properly dismiss these patients, every attempt should be made to provide the risks, benefits, and alternatives of AMA decision and to afford the EP malpractice protection later.

E. C. Bruno, MD

Emergency Department Triage: Do Experienced Nurses Agree on Triage Scores?

Dallaire C, Poitras J, Aubin K, et al (Université Laval, Québec, Canada; Axe de recherche en médecine d'urgence du Centre de recherche du Centre hospitalier affilié universitaire Hôtel-Dieu de Lévis, Québec, Canada; et al)
J Emerg Med 42:736-740, 2012

Background.—The reproducibility of the Canadian Triage & Acuity Scale (CTAS), designed and introduced in the late 1990s in all Canadian emergency departments (EDs), has been studied mostly using measures of interrater agreement. However, each of these studies shares a common limitation: the nurses had received fresh CTAS training, which is likely to have led to an overestimation of the reproducibility of CTAS.

Objectives.—This study aims to assess the interrater reliability of the CTAS in current clinical practice, that is, as used by experienced ED nurses without recent certification or recertification.

Methods.—A prospective sample of 100 patients arriving by ambulance was identified and yielded a set of 100 written scenarios. Five experienced ED nurses reviewed and blindly assigned a CTAS score to each scenario. The agreement among nurses was measured using the Kappa statistic calculated with quadratic weights. Kappa values were generated for each pair of nurses and a global Kappa coefficient was calculated to measure overall agreement.

TABLE 2.—Interrater Agreement between Paired Nurses

Nurses	1	2	3	4	5
1	-	0.30 (0.20–0.40)	0.39 (0.27–0.52)	0.31 (0.18–0.43)	0.53 (0.40–0.66)
2	-	-	0.48 (0.35–0.62)	0.61 (0.51–0.71)	0.44 (0.33–0.56)
3	-	-	-	0.49 (0.35–0.64)	0.44 (0.26–0.60)
4	-	-	-	-	0.42 (0.28–0.56)

Results.—Overall interrater agreement was moderate, with a global Kappa of 0.44 (95% confidence interval 0.40–0.48). However, pairwise, Kappa values were heterogeneous (0.30 to 0.61, $p = 0.0013$).

Conclusions.—The moderate interrater agreement observed in this study is disappointingly low and suggests that CTAS reliability may be lower than expected, and this warrants further research. Intra-observer reliability of CTAS should be ascertained more extensively among experienced nurses, and a future evaluation should involve several institutions (Table 2).

▶ Most emergency departments (EDs) use a 5-level triage scale. The 3 in most common use are the Canadian Triage and Acuity Scale (CTAS), the National Triage Scale, and the Emergency Severity Index (ESI). This study involves the CTAS, and it was conducted in an academic urban hospital ED located within the Chaudière-Appalaches region of Québec, Canada. The authors found that, in contrast with various other studies, the global interrater reliability of this scale was only moderate, and that variation in pairwise interrater agreement ranged from fair to good (see Table 2). This study is unique in that the 5 nurses involved in the study were not retrained in the use of the triage scale. They were all senior ED nurses with between 2 and 6 years of experience. Assuming that these results have external validity and are therefore generalizable (after all, this was a single-institution study and it involved written case scenarios as opposed to live patients), this gives us a real-world look at what happens when patients are triaged. Nurses will disagree with one another about who should be evaluated next and who can wait.

I am more familiar with the ESI, as are probably most US-based emergency physicians. The ESI is novel because it incorporates both patient acuity and a prediction of resource utilization to assign a triage level. It would be interesting to see if the ESI has as disappointing an interrater reliability as the CTAS. Perhaps we need to rethink these expanded triage scales. They may not be as dependable as originally suggested.

E. A. Ramoska, MD, MPHE

Article Index

Chapter 1: Trauma

Do we glow? Evaluation of trauma team work habits and radiation exposure 1

Are All Level I Trauma Centers Created Equal? A Comparison of American College of Surgeons and State-Verified Centers 2

Epidemiology of out-of hospital pediatric cardiac arrest due to trauma 3

In a Mature Trauma System, There Is No Difference in Outcome (Survival) Between Level I and Level II Trauma Centers 5

Effect of comorbid illness on the long-term outcome of adults suffering major traumatic injury: a population-based cohort study 6

Are general surgeons behind the curve when it comes to disaster preparedness training? A survey of general surgery and emergency medicine trainees in the United States by the Eastern Association for the Surgery for Trauma Committee on Disaster Preparedness 7

Chronic consequences of acute injuries: Worse survival after discharge 8

A decade of experience with a selective policy for direct to operating room trauma resuscitations 9

Screening for traumatic stress among survivors of urban trauma 11

Neighborhood Social Inequalities in Road Traffic Injuries: The Influence of Traffic Volume and Road Design 12

Association Between Helicopter vs Ground Emergency Medical Services and Survival for Adults With Major Trauma 13

A web-based model to support patient-to-hospital allocation in mass casualty incidents 15

Factors Associated With the Interfacility Transfer of the Pediatric Trauma Patient: Implications for Prehospital Triage 17

Analysis of radiation exposure in trauma patients at a level I trauma center 18

A Multisite Assessment of the American College of Surgeons Committee on Trauma Field Triage Decision Scheme for Identifying Seriously Injured Children and Adults 19

Diagnostic Accuracy of Focused Assessment with Sonography for Trauma (FAST) Examinations Performed by Emergency Medical Technicians 20

Repeat imaging in trauma transfers: A retrospective analysis of computed tomography scans repeated upon arrival to a Level I trauma center 22

A prehospital shock index for trauma correlates with measures of hospital resource use and mortality 24

A prehospital shock index for trauma correlates with measures of hospital resource use and mortality 25

Changing Characteristics of Facial Fractures Treated at a Regional, Level 1 Trauma Center, From 2005 to 2010: An Assessment of Patient Demographics, Referral Patterns, Etiology of Injury, Anatomic Location, and Clinical Outcomes 26

Immediate and Delayed Traumatic Intracranial Hemorrhage in Patients With Head Trauma and Preinjury Warfarin or Clopidogrel Use 27

Evaluating Age in the Field Triage of Injured Persons 29

Management of Minor Head Injury in Patients Receiving Oral Anticoagulant
Therapy: A Prospective Study of a 24-Hour Observation Protocol 30

Immediate and Delayed Traumatic Intracranial Hemorrhage in Patients With Head
Trauma and Preinjury Warfarin or Clopidogrel Use 31

Subdural Hematomas and Emergency Management in Infancy and Childhood:
A Single Institution's Experience 33

Risk factors that predict mortality in patients with blunt chest wall trauma:
A systematic review and meta-analysis 34

Patients With Rib Fractures Do Not Develop Delayed Pneumonia: A Prospective,
Multicenter Cohort Study of Minor Thoracic Injury 35

Chapter 2: Resuscitation

Implication of cardiac marker elevation in patients who resuscitated from out-of-
hospital cardiac arrest 37

Time to first compression using Medical Priority Dispatch System compression-first
dispatcher-assisted cardiopulmonary resuscitation protocols 38

Mild hypothermia treatment in patients resuscitated from non-shockable cardiac
arrest 40

Lightweight noninvasive trauma monitor for early indication of central
hypovolemia and tissue acidosis: A review 41

Damage Control Immunoregulation: Is There a Role for Low-Volume Hypertonic
Saline Resuscitation in Patients Managed with Damage Control Surgery? 42

Chapter 3: Cardiovascular

A new site for venous access: superficial veins of portal collateral circulation 45

Gender Differences in Calls to 9-1-1 During an Acute Coronary Syndrome 46

Intraosseous Versus Intravenous Vascular Access During Out-of-Hospital Cardiac
Arrest: A Randomized Controlled Trial 47

Prehospital care of left ventricular assist device patients by emergency medical
services 49

Potential utility of near-infrared spectroscopy in out-of-hospital cardiac arrest: an
illustrative case series 50

Impact of delayed and infrequent administration of vasopressors on return of
spontaneous circulation during out-of-hospital cardiac arrest 52

Prehospital Point-of-Care Testing for Troponin: Are the Results Reliable? 54

Cardiac arrest survival is rare without prehospital return of spontaneous circulation 56

Genetics of myocardial infarction: a progress report 58

Effect of Long-Term Thoracic Epidural Analgesia on Refractory Angina Pectoris:
A 10-Year Experience 59

Community-based gender perspectives of triage and treatment in suspected
myocardial infarction 60

A new electrocardiographic criteria for emergent reperfusion therapy   62

Body Mass Index and Mortality in Acute Myocardial Infarction Patients   63

Posterior myocardial infarction: are we failing to diagnose this?   64

Electrocardiographic Differentiation of Early Repolarization From Subtle Anterior
ST-Segment Elevation Myocardial Infarction   65

Chapter 4: Respiratory Distress

Feasibility of continuous positive airway pressure by primary care paramedics   67

Ordering CT pulmonary angiography to exclude pulmonary embolism: defense
versus evidence in the emergency room   68

Evaluation of pulmonary embolism in the emergency department and consistency
with a national quality measure: quantifying the opportunity for improvement   70

Normalization of Vital Signs Does Not Reduce the Probability of Acute Pulmonary
Embolism in Symptomatic Emergency Department Patients   71

Risk factors associated with delayed diagnosis of acute pulmonary embolism   72

Chapter 5: Infections and Immunologic Disorders

Lower mortality in sepsis patients admitted through the ED vs direct admission   75

Advanced endotracheal tube biofilm stage, not duration of intubation, is related to
pneumonia   76

Viral Meningitis: Which Patients Can Be Discharged from the Emergency
Department?   77

The degree of bandemia in septic ED patients does not predict inpatient mortality   79

Acute meningitis prognosis using cerebrospinal fluid interleukin-6 levels   80

Ambulatory Intravenous Antibiotic Therapy for Children With Preseptal Cellulitis   81

U.S. Emergency Department Visits for Meningitis, 1993–2008   82

Chapter 6: Neurology

Cheerio, Laddie! Bidding Farewell to the Glasgow Coma Scale   85

Does primary stroke center certification change ED diagnosis, utilization, and
disposition of patients with acute stroke?   86

Effect of Functional Status on Survival in Patients With Stroke: Is Independent
Ambulation a Key Determinant?   88

Effects of microbubbles on transcranial Doppler ultrasound-assisted intracranial
urokinase thrombolysis   89

Neuroprotective Effect of Curcumin in an Experimental Rat Model of
Subarachnoid Hemorrhage   90

Variables Associated With Discordance Between Emergency Physician and
Neurologist Diagnoses of Transient Ischemic Attacks in the Emergency
Department   91

Stroke Mimics and Intravenous Thrombolysis   92

Chapter 7: Psychiatry

Can Activation of Coagulation and Impairment of Fibrinolysis in Patients With
Anxiety and Depression Be Reversed After Improvement of Psychiatric Symptoms?
Results of a Pilot Study 95

Chapter 8: Gastrointestinal

Eliminating routine oral contrast use for CT in the emergency department: impact
on patient throughput and diagnosis 97

Clinical triage decision vs risk scores in predicting the need for endotherapy in
upper gastrointestinal bleeding 98

Adult intussusception: presentation, management, and outcomes of 148 patients 100

Ondansetron Use in the Pediatric Emergency Room for Diagnoses Other Than
Acute Gastroenteritis 101

Chapter 9: Endocrinology

Prevalence of hypokalemia in ED patients with diabetic ketoacidosis 103

Emergency Department Patients With Diabetes Have Better Glycemic Control
When They Have Identifiable Primary Care Providers 104

Chapter 10: Pediatric Emergency Medicine

Reasons for Nonurgent Pediatric Emergency Department Visits: Perceptions of
Health Care Providers and Caregivers 107

Pediatric clavicular fractures: assessment of fracture patterns and predictors of
complicated outcome 108

Epidemiology of pediatric hand injuries presenting to United States emergency
departments, 1990 to 2009 109

Cardiac Troponin T as a Screening Test for Myocarditis in Children 110

Accuracy of plain radiographs to exclude the diagnosis of intussusception 112

A Clinical Decision Rule to Identify Infants With Apparent Life-Threatening Event
Who Can Be Safely Discharged From the Emergency Department 114

Age variability in pediatric injuries from falls 116

Emergency Department Transport Rates of Children From the Scene of Motor
Vehicle Collisions: Do Booster Seats Make a Difference? 117

Utilization of a Pediatric Observation Unit for Toxicologic Ingestions 119

Conducted Electrical Weapon (TASER) Use Against Minors: A Shocking Analysis 121

Petechaiae/Purpura in Well-Appearing Infants 123

Adherence of families to a group a streptococcal pharyngitis protocol used in a
pediatric emergency department 124

Delayed Versus Immediate Antimicrobial Treatment for Acute Otitis Media 126

The management of bite wounds in children—A retrospective analysis at a level I trauma centre — 127

Accuracy of Ultrasonography Versus Computed Tomography Scan in Detecting Parapharengeal Abscess in Children — 128

Procalcitonin as a Marker of Bacteremia in Children With Fever and a Central Venous Catheter Presenting to the Emergency Department — 129

Comparison of Amoxicillin/Clavulanic Acid High Dose with Cefdinir in the Treatment of Acute Otitis Media — 130

The frequency of cerebral ischemia/hypoxia in pediatric severe traumatic brain injury — 132

Sports-Related Concussions — 133

Implementation of Adapted PECARN Decision Rule for Children With Minor Head Injury In the Pediatric Emergency Department — 135

Implementation of Adapted PECARN Decision Rule for Children With Minor Head Injury in the Pediatric Emergency Department — 136

Utility of Plain Radiographs in Detecting Traumatic Injuries of the Cervical Spine in Children — 138

Contact Lens Removal: The "Chopstick" Approach — 140

Etomidate for Short Pediatric Procedures in the Emergency Department — 141

Diagnosis of Intussusception by Physician Novice Sonographers in the Emergency Department — 143

Children With and Without Developmental Disabilities: Sedation Medication Requirements and Adverse Events Related to Sedation — 145

Adherence to PALS Sepsis Guidelines and Hospital Length of Stay — 147

ED point-of-care ultrasound in the diagnosis of ankle fractures in children — 149

Sonographic Diagnosis of Metaphyseal Forearm Fractures in Children: A Safe and Applicable Alternative to Standard X-Rays — 151

Randomized Trial Comparing Wound Packing to No Wound Packing Following Incision and Drainage of Superficial Skin Abscesses in the Pediatric Emergency Department — 153

Topical anesthetic cream is associated with spontaneous cutaneous abscess drainage in children — 155

Dehydration Treatment Practices Among Pediatrics-Trained and Non—Pediatrics Trained Emergency Physicians — 156

Induction Dose of Propofol for Pediatric Patients Undergoing Procedural Sedation in the Emergency Department — 157

Intranasal Fentanyl and High-concentration Inhaled Nitrous Oxide for Procedural Sedation: A Prospective Observational Pilot Study of Adverse Events and Depth of Sedation — 158

Triage Nurse Initiation of Corticosteroids in Pediatric Asthma is Associated With Improved Emergency Department Efficiency — 159

Capnometry as a Predictor of Admission in Bronchiolitis — 160

Complicated and Dislodged Airway Foreign Body in an Intubated Child: Case Report — 161

Fatal and Near-Fatal Asthma in Children: The Critical Care Perspective — 164

Effect of Honey on Nocturnal Cough and Sleep Quality: A Double-blind, Randomized, Placebo-Controlled Study — 165

Trampoline Safety in Childhood and Adolescence — 166

Are routine pelvic radiographs in major pediatric blunt trauma necessary? — 167

Spinal cord trauma in children under 10 years of age: clinical characteristics and prevention — 168

Race disparities in firearm injuries and outcomes among Tennessee children — 170

The acute compartment syndrome following fractures of the lower leg in children — 171

Support for blood alcohol screening in pediatric trauma — 172

Theoretical increase of thyroid cancer induction from cervical spine multidetector computed tomography in pediatric trauma patients — 175

Serum troponin-I as an indicator of clinically significant myocardial injury in paediatric trauma patients — 177

The Predictive Value of a Normal Radiographic Anterior Fat Pad Sign Following Elbow Trauma in Children — 179

Hidden attraction: a menacing meal of magnets and batteries — 180

Diagnosis and treatment of tracheobronchial foreign bodies in 1024 children — 182

C-Reactive Protein and Procalcitonin Are Predictors of the Severity of Acute Appendicitis in Children — 185

Chapter 11: Emergency Medical Service Systems

Global rating scale for the assessment of paramedic clinical competence — 187

Comparison of emergency medical services systems across Pan-Asian countries: a Web-based survey — 188

HEMS in Slovenia: One Country, Four Models, Different Quality Outcomes — 189

The core content of emergency medical services medicine — 191

Disparities in Trauma Center Access of Older Injured Motor Vehicular Crash Occupants — 193

A pilot study of emergency medical technicians' field assessment of intoxicated patients' need for ED care — 194

Can nebulized naloxone be used safely and effectively by emergency medical services for suspected opioid overdose? — 195

Intravenous Access During Out-of-Hospital Emergency Care of Noninjured Patients: A Population-Based Outcome Study — 197

Life Flight Network — 198

Effects of physician-based emergency medical service dispatch in severe traumatic brain injury on prehospital run time — 199

Medical preparation for the 2008 Republican National Convention: A practical guide — 200

The methodology of the Australian Prehospital Outcomes Study of Longitudinal Epidemiology (APOStLE) Project — 203

Three insulation methods to minimize intravenous fluid administration set heat loss 205

The 60-Day Temperature-Dependent Degradation of Midazolam and Lorazepam in the Prehospital Environment 206

Successful Administration of Intranasal Glucagon in the Out-of-Hospital Environment 207

Lithium Battery Fires: Implications for Air Medical Transport 208

Major incident preparation for acute hospitals: Current state-of-the-art, training needs analysis, and the role of novel virtual worlds simulation technologies 210

Factors associated with ambulance use among patients with low-acuity conditions 211

Ten-year trends in intoxications and requests for emergency ambulance service 213

Helicopter Emergency Medical Service in Tehran, Iran: A Descriptive Study 215

Effects of an emergency medical services–based resource access program on frequent users of health services 216

Inappropriate helicopter emergency medical services transports: results of a national cohort utilization review 217

Accuracy of prehospital diagnosis and triage of a Swiss helicopter emergency medical service 219

The impact of distance on triage to trauma center care in an urban trauma system 221

Effect of gender on prehospital refusal of medical aid 223

Termination of resuscitation for adult traumatic cardiopulmonary arrest 225

Non-Urgent Commercial Air Travel After Acute Myocardial Infarction: A Review of the Literature and Commentary on the Recommendations 226

EMS Medical Direction and Prehospital Practices for Acute Cardiovascular Events 228

Occult traumatic loculated tension pneumothorax—a sonographic diagnostic dilemma 229

Chapter 12: Toxicology

A Case of Histamine Fish Poisoning in a Young Atopic Woman 231

Long-term neurotoxic effects of dimethylamine borane intoxication 232

Use of haloperidol in PCP-intoxicated individuals 232

Severe Colchicine Intoxication in a Renal Transplant Recipient on Cyclosporine 233

A rare cause of poisoning in childhood: yellow phosphorus 234

A Review of Disaster-Related Carbon Monoxide Poisoning: Surveillance, Epidemiology, and Opportunities for Prevention 235

A rare cause of atrial fibrillation: mad honey intoxication 235

Aminorex poisoning in cocaine abusers 236

Anaphylaxis at image-guided epidural pain block secondary to corticosteroid compound 237

Rapid and Complete Bioavailability of Antidotes for Organophosphorus Nerve Agent and Cyanide Poisoning in Minipigs After Intraosseous Administration 237

Gastro-intestinal poisoning due to consumption of daffodils mistaken for vegetables at commercial markets, Bristol, United Kingdom — 238

Maternal exposure to moderate ambient carbon monoxide is associated with decreased risk of preeclampsia — 239

Severe Poisoning After Accidental Pediatric Ingestion of Glycol Ethers — 240

Accidental poisoning after ingestion of "aphrodisiac" berries: diagnosis by analytical toxicology — 240

The effects of fructose-1,6-diphosphate on haemodynamic parameters and survival in a rodent model of propranolol and verapamil poisoning — 241

Buprenorphine May Not Be as Safe as You Think: A Pediatric Fatality From Unintentional Exposure — 242

Mistaken identity: Severe vomiting, bradycardia and hypotension after eating a wild herb — 243

A case of near-fatal fenpyroximate intoxication: The role of percutaneous cardiopulmonary support and therapeutic hypothermia — 243

Pulmonary edema following scorpion envenomation: Mechanisms, clinical manifestations, diagnosis and treatment — 245

Mechanisms of Cadmium-Induced Proximal Tubule Injury: New Insights with Implications for Biomonitoring and Therapeutic Interventions — 247

Serum tau protein level for neurological injuries in carbon monoxide poisoning — 247

Fatal gastrointestinal hemorrhage after a single dose of dabigatran — 248

Detecting damaged regions of cerebral white matter in the subacute phase after carbon monoxide poisoning using voxel-based analysis with diffusion tensor imaging — 250

Recipients of hyperbaric oxygen treatment for carbon monoxide poisoning and exposure circumstances — 251

Noninvasive pulse CO-oximetry expedites evaluation and management of patients with carbon monoxide poisoning — 252

Carbon Monoxide Induces Cardiac Arrhythmia Via Induction of the Late Na^+ Current — 252

Safety and Cost-Effectiveness of a Clinical Protocol Implemented to Standardize the use of Crotalidae Polyvalent Immune Fab Antivenom at an Academic Medical Center — 253

Acute kidney injury in patients admitted to a liver intensive therapy unit with paracetamol-induced hepatotoxicity — 255

Octreotide for the treatment of sulfonylurea poisoning — 256

Unexpected late rise in plasma acetaminophen concentrations with change in risk stratification in acute acetaminophen overdoses — 257

Delayed Parkinsonism after CO Intoxication: Evaluation of the Substantia Nigra with Inversion-Recovery MR Imaging — 258

Increased Carbon Monoxide Clearance During Exercise in Humans — 260

The clinical toxicology of gamma-hydroxybutyrate, gamma-butyrolactone and 1,4-butanediol — 262

Life-treating necrotizing fasciitis due to 'bath salts' injection — 264

Chapter 13: Emergency Center Activities

Atraumatic headache in US emergency departments: recent trends in CT/MRI utilisation and factors associated with severe intracranial pathology 267

Fetal loss in symptomatic first-trimester pregnancy with documented yolk sac intrauterine pregnancy 268

Impact of physician-assisted triage on timing of antibiotic delivery in patients admitted to the hospital with community-acquired pneumonia (CAP) 269

Characteristics of frequent geriatric users of an urban emergency department 270

A National Depiction of Children With Return Visits to the Emergency Department Within 72 Hours, 2001–2007 272

Answering the myth: use of emergency services on Friday the 13th 273

Diagnostic and Prognostic Stratification in the Emergency Department Using Urinary Biomarkers of Nephron Damage: A Multicenter Prospective Cohort Study 274

Emergency Medical Services for Children: The New Jersey Model 275

Early Pediatric Emergency Department Return Visits: A Prospective Patient-Centric Assessment 276

Cancer diagnosis and outcomes in Michigan EDs vs other settings 277

Can Asymptomatic Patients With a Supratherapeutic International Normalized Ratio Be Safely Treated as Outpatients? 279

IV access difficulty: incidence and delays in an urban emergency department 280

International evidence-based recommendations on ultrasound-guided vascular access 281

Seasonality of Testicular Torsion: A 10-Year Nationwide Population Based Study 282

Effectiveness of Tai Chi as a Community-Based Falls Prevention Intervention: A Randomized Controlled Trial 283

An Over-the-Counter Simulation Study of a Single-Tablet Emergency Contraceptive in Young Females 284

Consultation in the emergency department: a qualitative analysis and review 286

Effect on Injuries of Assigning Shoes Based on Foot Shape in Air Force Basic Training 287

From Hot Hands to Declining Effects: The Risks of Small Numbers 288

Cost-effectiveness and budget impact analyses of a long-term hypertension detection and control program for stroke prevention 290

Carotid intima-media thickness progression to predict cardiovascular events in the general population (the PROG-IMT collaborative project): a meta-analysis of individual participant data 291

Contemporary Evidence About Hospital Strategies for Reducing 30-Day Readmissions: A National Study 293

Are Patients With Longer Emergency Department Wait Times Less Likely to Consent to Research? 294

Impact of nasogastric lavage on outcomes in acute GI bleeding 296

A community intervention trial to evaluate emergency care practitioners in the management of children   297

Management of an Apparent Life-Threatening Event: A Survey of Emergency Physicians Practice   299

The importance of a proper against-medical-advice (AMA) discharge: how signing out AMA may create significant liability protection for providers   300

Emergency Department Triage: Do Experienced Nurses Agree on Triage Scores?   301

Author Index

A

Abrahamson E, 81
Ackermann O, 151
Adducci MdC, 80
Adguzel S, 234
Aguirrebarrena G, 229
Aksel G, 247
Alexander ME, 110
Ali AB, 276
Alzanki M, 237
Amram O, 15
Arora S, 103
Artto V, 92
Attof R, 15
Aubin K, 301
Avila S, 11

B

Babl FE, 158
Badillo C, 286
Bahloul M, 245
Bajaj L, 141
Ball CG, 6
Ballard DW, 86
Baren JM, 114
Barnes S, 8
Barnett PLJ, 123
Bartolini V, 236
Battle CE, 34
Bayram NA, 235
Bellolio MF, 100
Bentur Y, 256
Beppu T, 250
Best HA, 273
Bhullar I, 24-25
Biddinger PD, 269
Bildik F, 247
Block SL, 130
Blumberg SM, 179
Bodenham AR, 281
Boet S, 187
Bonomo JB, 79
Borland E, 198
Bowers RC, 253
Boyle JP, 252
Bozeman WP, 121
Bradburn M, 297
Bradley EH, 293
Brady WJ, 226
Brandt M-M, 7
Brens-Heldens V, 199
Bressan S, 135-136

Brosch LC, 287
Brown JC, 180
Brugha RE, 81
Brummell Z, 255
Buatsi J, 68
Bucholz EM, 63
Buffo-Sequeira I, 177
Bulloch B, 129
Burns B, 24-25
Burns BJ, 229

C

Cabana MD, 272
Cabeza B, 185
Caidahl K, 60
Camacho MA, 97
Camargo CA Jr, 82
Canetta P, 274
Cantrell CL Jr, 52
Capp R, 269
Carey TP, 108
Carey TS, 22
Casey JR, 130
Cassidy-Smith T, 155
Castillo EM, 216
Cederholm I, 59
Chaari A, 245
Chan TC, 216
Channel J, 1
Charles AG, 22
Chauhan A, 64
Chauny JM, 35
Chen C-S, 282
Cheng D, 103
Cheskes S, 67
Chiu B, 282
Chiu H-T, 88
Cho CS, 272
Cho N-Y, 258
Christich AC, 157
Cichon ME, 54
Clower JH, 235, 251
Cohen DC, 210
Cohen HA, 165
Cole F, 9
Coll C, 80
Collett L, 56
Cone DC, 203, 232
Conrad R, 95
Cooke CR, 197
Cornwall AH, 194
Corredor DM, 71
Courtney DM, 70, 75

Cox K, 217
Crain EF, 179
Curry L, 293

D

Dallaire C, 301
Dallas ML, 252
Dammak H, 245
Das A, 98
Davidson KW, 46
de Amoreira Gepp R, 168
De Maio VJ, 3
Dennis AJ, 7
Dischinger PC, 193
Dougherty PP, 257
Doumouras AG, 221
Downs M, 217
Dries DJ, 200
Duchesne JC, 42
Dudley NC, 119
Duffy E, 299
Durant E, 211
Durmaz T, 235

E

Eckert K, 151
Eddleston M, 237
Edwards JR, 247
Egan KR, 175
Eisenberg MA, 110
El-Shammaa E, 140
Emick DM, 22
Émond M, 35
Erdmann J, 58
Evans M, 238
Evans PA, 34
Eviatar E, 128
Exadaktylos AK, 219

F

Fahimi J, 211
Farooq FT, 98
Ferlic PW, 171
Fertel BS, 79
Fesmire FM, 62
Finalle C, 223
Frank R, 50
Franschman G, 199

Frascone RJ, 200
Fredrikson M, 59
Frisch A, 50
Fujiwara S, 250

G

Galvagno SM Jr, 13
Gang W, 182
Gardner AR, 121
Garrouste C, 233
Gauvin L, 12
Gavela T, 185
Gavriel H, 128
Geiser F, 95
Gergelé L, 45
Geske JB, 72
Gessler K, 95
Ghali WA, 231
Gilbert JW, 267
Glasenapp M, 91
Glatstein M, 256
Glickman SW, 294
Gobin M, 238
Goldstein JN, 279
Gomez D, 221
Gosserand JK, 133
Graudins A, 241
Graw-Panzer KD, 161
Gray D, 76
Green SM, 85
Green-Hopkins I, 110
Greer S, 228
Grünauer J, 127
Guidry C, 42
Guo Y, 239

H

Haas B, 221
Hafner JW, 217
Hale L, 283
Hampson NB, 251, 252
Hartford M, 60
Hasler RM, 219
Hassan M, 1
Hassani SA, 215
Hauda WE II, 121
Haut ER, 13
Hebert PL, 197
Hedley N, 15
Hedrick J, 130
Hennings JR, 62
Henry M, 129
Henry TD, 65

Herman BE, 119
Hernandez SA, 235
Hessert MJ, 268
Hick JL, 200
Hock Ong ME, 188
Hoffman JD, 195
Hoffman RS, 242
Hogg MM, 71
Holzer BM, 213
Homan MB, 17
Hongbo L, 182
Horn E, 97
Horwitz DA, 104
Horwitz LI, 293
House DR, 117
Howe R, 208
Howell J, 276
Howell JM, 160
Hsiao AL, 143
Hsueh C-J, 258
Huang ES, 296
Huang J, 86
Huang Z-Z, 89
Hubble MW, 38, 52
Huffman G, 117
Hutchings H, 34
Hwang U, 270

I

Iacovelli C, 300
Idehara R, 243
Inaba K, 2
Iqbal S, 235, 251
Irvine KA, 203
Ito S, 248
Izenberg S, 9

J

Jacobsen R, 207
Jaindl M, 127
Jasiak KD, 157
Javid PJ, 180
Jeng J-S, 88
Jeung KW, 243
Johnson KM, 267
Juliano M, 268

K

Kalam Y, 241
Kalmovich LM, 128
Kamdar G, 112

Kannikeswaran N, 145
Kanwal F, 296
Kao H-W, 258
Karakiozis J, 76
Karch SB, 236
Karsan S, 296
Kasem AJ, 129
Kaysi S, 233
Kazanci B, 33
Kehl C, 219
Keles T, 235
Keller JJ, 282
Kelly-Goodstein N, 275
Kernan L, 248
Kersnik J, 189
Kessler C, 286
Kessler DO, 153
Khalil A, 65
Khan JN, 64
Khare RK, 75
Kilicaslan I, 247
Kim CH, 20
Kim HJ, 37
Kim HK, 242
Kim YM, 37
Kirkpatrick AW, 6
Kitamura A, 290
Klein-Schwartz W, 257
Klemenc-Ketis Z, 189
Kline JA, 70, 71
Knapik JJ, 287
Knudsen K, 262
Krantz A, 153
Kraus T, 171
Kristal H, 165
Kundra M, 299
Kunkov S, 179
Kuo C-P, 90
Kusaka S, 243
Kutka BM, 286

L

Lagisetty J, 167
Laine MK, 126
Lamperti M, 281
Landman MP, 170
Langhan ML, 143
Larkin GL, 267
Lashkeri T, 160
Lauer MS, 288
Lee BK, 243
Lee H, 161
Lee HY, 243
Lee JC, 5

Lee MH, 98, 123
Levenson RB, 97
Levine M, 279
Levy F, 300
Ley EJ, 172
Limkakeng AT Jr, 294
Lin K-J, 232
Lindor RA, 100
Liu C-H, 232
Liu DR, 156
Liu W-S, 89
Lo BM, 273
Locklair MR, 116
Longo LD, 260
Lorenz MW, 291
Lu C H, 90
Lucci M, 30

M

Macneal JJ, 232
Maeda K, 243
Mandt MJ, 141
Manifold CA, 56
Mareiniss DP, 300
Mari F, 236
Marks N, 264
Martin CA, 170
Martin M, 9
Mason S, 297
Matulkova P, 238
McMullan JT, 206
McNab A, 24-25
Menditto VG, 30
Middleton PM, 203
Mills G, 208
Minder CE, 213
Mion T, 135-136
Mistry RD, 155
Mittal MK, 114
Moharari RS, 215
Mohseni MM, 77
Mojica M, 153
Monuteaux MC, 147
Moran DE, 237
Morency P, 12
Morgenthaler TI, 72
Morris K, 264
Morrow SE, 116
Moynagh MR, 237
Mozdiak E, 64
Muchow RD, 175
Murray DB, 237
Murray KF, 180
Musto RJ, 231

N

Nadal LG, 168
Nager AL, 156
Nakamura Y, 29
Nee J, 40
Neuman MI, 147
Newgard CD, 19
Newman JD, 46
Newth CJL, 164
Nickolas TL, 274
Nigrovic LE, 138
Nikolaou P, 240
Nishijima DK, 27, 31
Nishimoto H, 250
Niven DJ, 6
Nunez J, 156

O

O'Connor RE, 226
Oh SH, 37
O'Keeffe C, 297
O'Riordan A, 255
Ornato JP, 277
Osler T, 5
Osmond MH, 159
Oswanski MF, 18

P

Padayachy LC, 132
Papoutsis I, 240
Patel V, 210
Patil A, 1
Paul R, 147
Pederson T, 11
Pepelassis D, 177
Peppler WW, 175
Phan H, 157
Philipponnet C, 233
Piek R, 205
Pierzchala A, 101
Pittiruti M, 281
Place R, 160, 276
Plante C, 12
Platzer P, 127
Plint A, 159
Plourde M, 35
Plumb J, 119
Plurad D, 2
Pockett CR, 124
Poitras J, 301
Polonara S, 30

Powell ES, 75
Prozialeck WC, 247
Putaala J, 92

R

Raine TR, 284
Rathore SS, 63
Ravn-Fischer A, 60
Reades R, 47
Reed J, 253
Reed ME, 86
Reese C, 11
Reid KJ, 63
Renfro LA, 8
Rewers A, 17
Ricciotti N, 284
Richards ME, 52
Richter A, 59
Riera A, 143
Roback MG, 141
Rochette LM, 109
Roden KS, 26
Rogers FB, 5
Rohacek M, 68
Rohlwink U, 132
Romanato S, 135-136
Roser M, 40
Roskind CG, 112
Ross DW, 17
Rozen J, 165
Ruha A-M, 279
Russo CJ, 155
Russo R, 264
Ruuskanen O, 126
Ruzal-Shapiro CB, 112
Ryan KL, 41
Ryb GE, 193

S

Sacchetti A, 275
Sadosty AT, 100
Salami O, 107
Salomone J, 207
Salvador J, 107
Samani NJ, 58
Sangha GS, 177
Sarvar M, 215
Sato S, 290
Schätti G, 213
Schep LJ, 262
Schluter P, 283
Schmidt-Ott KM, 274
Schrock JW, 91

Schunkert H, 58
Schuurman N, 15
Schwarz ES, 104
Schweiger B, 151
Schweiger M, 49
Scolnik D, 256
Scott MG, 104
Seabrook JA, 108
Seith RW, 158
Serrano A, 185
Sethuraman U, 145
Sevdalis N, 210
Seymour CW, 197
Shafi S, 8
Shah S, 149
Shah SS, 109
Shapiro DJ, 272
Sharma OP, 18
Shear B, 240
Shin SD, 20, 188
Shirazi F, 248
Shofer F, 294
Short SS, 172
Sibley T, 207
Sidhu R, 18
Sikka V, 277
Simms E, 42
Simon HK, 101
Singer G, 171
Singer MB, 172
Sinha V, 232
Sivaswamy L, 145
Sizer E, 255
Slaughter RJ, 262
Slovis T, 167
Smiddy M, 242
Smith G, 239
Smith GA, 109
Smith J, 2
Smith SB, 72
Smith SW, 65
Smoliga JM, 260
Sokoloff A, 284
Soller BR, 41
Song KJ, 20
Soremekun OA, 269
Stake CE, 54
Stefanidou M, 240
Stein C, 205
Steinberg J, 7
Stiegler P, 49
Stockdale J, 140
Storm C, 40
Strauss BJ, 108
Strbian D, 92

Studnek JR, 47
Sturm JJ, 101
Suffoletto BP, 50
Sun G, 114
Surrusco M, 26
Sweeney R, 275
Szucs-Farkas Z, 68

T

Tadros AS, 216
Taggart I, 149
Tähtinen PA, 126
Takhar SS, 82
Tanaka H, 188
Taskesen M, 234
Tataris KL, 195
Tavares W, 187
Taylor D, 283
Tehli O, 33
Theophilos T, 158
Theriault R, 187
Thomas F, 208
Thomas R, 167, 299
Thomas S, 237
Thompson GC, 124
Thomson S, 67
Ting SA, 82
Tomazin I, 189
Tong W, 26
Torres L, 270
Tsang J, 223
Turc J, 45
Türkoğlu E, 33
Turner L, 67

U

Unni P, 116, 170
Upshaw JE, 133

V

Valderrama AL, 228
Van Vleet LM, 38
Vandeventer S, 47
Vázquez JA, 80
Vega R, 107
Venkatesh AK, 70
Venturini JM, 54

Venuto M, 287
Verburg N, 199
Victor A, 91
Vierecke J, 49
Visintainer CM, 273
Voskoboynik N, 149

W

Wadowski SJ, 161
Wajnberg A, 270
Waldron R, 223
Walthall JDH, 117
Wampler DA, 56
Wang H-M, 232
Wang W, 226
Wang X-W, 89
Wang Y-H, 88
Wanga GS, 240
Ward MJ, 79
Warren O, 194
Weant KA, 253
Weber JM, 195
Wen L-L, 90
Wilde JA, 77
Williams I, 228
Williams N, 133
Wilson A, 76
Wilson BJ, 231
Witting MD, 280
Wyler B, 103

Y

Yamagishi K, 290
Yang Z, 252
Ye S, 46
Yin S, 240

Z

Zafar SN, 13
Zaller N, 194
Zavorsky GS, 260
Zemek R, 159
Zhai D, 239
Zhengxia P, 182
Zou F, 41
Zwane E, 132

Printed and bound by CPI Group (UK) Ltd, Croydon, CR0 4YY

08/05/2025

01864755-0009